Treating Addictive Behaviors

Second Edition

APPLIED CLINICAL PSYCHOLOGY

Series Editors:
Alan S. Bellack
University of Maryland at Baltimore, Baltimore, Maryland
Michel Hersen
Pacific University, Forest Grove, Oregon

A Continuation Order Plan is available for this series. A continuation order will bring delivery of each new volume immediately upon publication. Volumes are billed only upon actual shipment. For further information please contact the publisher.

Treating Addictive Behaviors

Second Edition

Edited by

William R. Miller

University of New Mexico
Albuquerque, New Mexico

and

Nick Heather

Centre for Alcohol and Drug Studies
Newcastle upon Tyne, United Kingdom

Plenum Press • New York and London

Library of Congress Cataloging-in-Publication Data

Treating addictive behaviors / edited by William R. Miller and Nick
  Heather. -- 2nd ed.
        p.   cm. -- (Applied clinical psychology)
    Includes bibliographical references and index.
    ISBN 0-306-45852-7
    1. Compulsive behavior--Treatment. 2. Substance abuse--Treatment.
  3. Attitude change. 4. Motivation (Psychology)   I. Miller, William
  R. II. Heather, Nick. III. Series.
    [DNLM: 1. Behavior, Addictive--therapy. 2. Substance-Related
  Disorders--therapy.   WM 176T784 1998]
  RC533.T73 1998
  616.86'06--dc21
  DNLM/DLC
  for Library of Congress   98-27475
                                                                  CIP

ISBN 0-306-45852-7

©1998, 1986 Plenum Press, New York
A Division of Plenum Publishing Corporation
233 Spring Street, New York, N.Y. 10013

http://www.plenum.com

10 9 8 7 6 5 4 3 2 1

Printed in the United States of America

To the remarkable team of people known as CASAA

—W. R. M.

To Jean, with love and thanks for everything

—N. H.

Contributors

Nichole R. Andrews, Department of Psychology, University of New Mexico, Albuquerque, New Mexico 87131

Melanie E. Bennett, Department of Psychology, University of New Mexico, Albuquerque, New Mexico 87131

Janice M. Brown, Department of Psychology, University of Arkansas, Fayetteville, Arkansas 72701

Kelly D. Brownell, Department of Psychology, Yale University, New Haven, Connecticut 06520

Kathleen M. Carroll, Division of Substance Abuse, Yale University, New Haven, Connecticut 06519

Robin Davidson, Department of Psychology, Belvoir Park Hospital, Belfast BT8 8JR, Northern Ireland

Carlo C. DiClemente, Department of Psychology, University of Maryland Baltimore County, Baltimore, Maryland 21250

Dennis M. Donovan, Alcohol and Drug Abuse Institute and Department of Psychiatry and Behavioral Sciences, University of Washington, Seattle, Washington 98105

David A. F. Haaga, Department of Psychology, American University, Washington, D.C. 20016

Nick Heather, Centre for Alcohol and Drug Studies, Newcastle City Health NHS Trust, Newcastle upon Tyne NE1 6UR, England

Katherine Battle Horgen, Department of Psychology, Yale University, New Haven, Connecticut 06520

Barry T. Jones, Department of Psychology, University of Glasgow, Glasgow G12 8QQ, Scotland

Lindsey Kirk, Department of Psychology, American University, Washington, D.C. 20016

Katharine L. Loeb, Eating Disorders Clinic, Rutgers University, Piscataway, New Jersey 08854

G. Alan Marlatt, Department of Psychology, University of Washington, Seattle, Washington 98195

Margaret E. Mattson, Treatment Research Branch, National Institute on Alcohol Abuse and Alcoholism, Bethesda, Maryland 20892

James R. McKay, Department of Psychiatry, University of Pennsylvania, Philadelphia, Pennsylvania 19104

A. Thomas McLellan, Department of Psychiatry, University of Pennsylvania, and Philadelphia Department of Veterans Affairs Medical Center, Philadelphia, Pennsylvania 19104

John McMahon, Centre for Alcohol and Drug Studies, University of Paisley, Paisley PA2 6BY, Scotland

Robert J. Meyers, Center on Alcoholism, Substance Abuse, and Addictions, University of New Mexico, Albuquerque, New Mexico 87106

Erica J. Miller, Center on Alcoholism, Substance Abuse, and Addictions, University of New Mexico, Albuquerque, New Mexico 87106

William R. Miller, Department of Psychology, University of New Mexico, Albuquerque, New Mexico 87131

James O. Prochaska, Department of Psychology, University of Rhode Island, Kingston, Rhode Island 02881

Stephen Rollnick, Department of General Practice, University of Wales College of Medicine, Llanedeyrn, Cardiff CF3 7PN, Wales

Natasha Slesnick, Department of Psychology, University of New Mexico, Albuquerque, New Mexico 87131

Jane Ellen Smith, Center on Alcoholism, Substance Abuse, and Addictions, University of New Mexico, Albuquerque, New Mexico 87106

Linda C. Sobell, Center for Psychological Studies, Nova Southeastern University, Fort Lauderdale, Florida 33314

Mark B. Sobell, Center for Psychological Studies, Nova Southeastern University, Fort Lauderdale, Florida 33314

J. Scott Tonigan, Center on Alcoholism, Substance Abuse, and Addictions, Family and Child Guidance Center, University of New Mexico, Albuquerque, New Mexico 87106

Radka T. Toscova, Albuquerque Family and Child Guidance Center, Albuquerque, New Mexico 87108

Jalie A. Tucker, Department of Psychology, Auburn University, Auburn, Alabama 36849

Vanessa C. López Viets, Department of Psychology, University of New Mexico, Albuquerque, New Mexico 87131

Rudy E. Vuchinich, Department of Psychology, Auburn University, Auburn, Alabama 36849

Holly Barrett Waldron, Department of Psychology, University of New Mexico, Albuquerque, New Mexico 87131

Kenneth R. Weingardt, Department of Psychology, University of Washington, Seattle, Washington 98195

Verner S. Westerberg, Center on Alcoholism, Substance Abuse, and Addictions, University of New Mexico, Albuquerque, New Mexico 87106

Paula Wilbourne, Department of Psychology, University of New Mexico, Albuquerque, New Mexico 87131

G. Terence Wilson, Graduate School of Applied and Professional Psychology, Rutgers University, Piscataway, New Jersey 08855

Preface

In the early 1980s the transtheoretical model of change was still in its infancy. Seminal publications were just appearing, but the model already seemed to hold such promise that we made it the organizing theme for the Third International Conference on Treatment of Addictive Behaviors (ICTAB-3), which convened in Scotland in 1984. That meeting gave rise to the first edition of this volume (Miller & Heather, 1986), which focused on processes involved in moving people from one stage to the next.

With the volume still in print more than a decade later, we were approached by Plenum Press with the idea of preparing this second edition. We were, obviously, persuaded that there was merit to the idea. Since 1986 the work of Prochaska and DiClemente has grown exponentially in popularity and influence. In Britain and the Americas, it is now unusual to find an addiction professional who has not at least heard about the stages of change, and more sophisticated applications of the transtheoretical model are spreading through health care systems and well beyond. The model has influenced professional training, health care delivery, and the design of many studies including a number of large clinical trials.

Another measure of a model's influence is the degree to which it attracts commentary and critique. This, too, has expanded since our first edition appeared. It seemed appropriate, therefore, to reflect not only advances but also criticisms that have arisen. Part I thus contains an update of the model by its authors, a review of critiques, and a rejoinder.

Because the transtheoretical model has been largely descriptive of *how* change unfolds and, in a sense, atheoretical with regard to the *why* of change, we sought in Part II to provide a broader conceptual context through five chapters on the process of change. From here on, we adhered to the original organization of the book, paralleling the transtheoretical stages of change. Part III contains chapters on approaches for increasing readiness to change. These address the motivational challenges of working with people characterized as being in the precontemplation, contemplation, and preparation stages. Motivation for change has also been a rapidly growing area of interest and study during the 1990s, and it is a natural companion topic whenever stages of change are considered.

What about clients in the action stage? Here the challenge is in facilitating strategies for change, although it can be a serious mistake to assume that motivational issues have been resolved at this point. A popular aspect of the first edition was a set of reviews of the state of knowledge with regard to treatment outcomes. These are updated and expanded in Part IV of this book. Since 1986 there has been steady and substantial progress in research on the treatment of addictive behaviors. Hundreds of new outcome studies have been reported, and major collaborative trials have been undertaken and completed. The rise of metanalysis has been evident in the addiction field, as has recognition of the limits of this method. Pharmacotherapies have gained in prominence in clinical research and, to a lesser extent, in practice. Gambling problems seem to be on the rise and are receiving increased attention. In a number of areas of addictive behavior, a public health perspective is increasing in popularity. All of this prompted us to retain and expand the clinical reviews of the first edition, summarizing state-of-the-art scientific knowledge.

This left a final section focusing on the ever present problem of maintaining change once it has been achieved, clearly an enduring challenge in the addiction field. When our first edition appeared, the focus was on "aftercare" and the prevention of relapse. Part V in this volume offers three chapters focusing respectively on predictors of maintenance, on strategies for maintaining change through continuing care, and on ways of helping clients whose substance use persists. These chapters reflect substantial evolution in thinking about maintenance during the past decade.

The resulting volume is, we hope, much more than a second edition, in the usual sense of a revised and updated version of an existing book. Rather it is a completely new book, not only updated but reconceptualized in light of developments in the field. The first edition was assembled from the invited addresses of ICTAB-3, and some of the same authors have been invited to contribute again. However, three-fourths of the chapters in this second edition are written by new authors. We trust that we have retained the spirit of an active collaboration between basic and applied research, between science and practice. We are certainly grateful to the outstanding contributors to this new edition, who bring their varied and provocative insights about one of humankind's most enduring problems. It is our wish that this volume will prove at least as useful to the field as was its predecessor, offering fresh ideas to inform theory, research, and practice in the twenty-first century.

Contents

Treating Addictive Behaviors

Second Edition

I

The Transtheoretical
Model of Change

The transtheoretical model that again serves as an organizing structure for this book is best thought of as a work in progress. When our first edition appeared in 1986, it was a fresh approach of mostly heuristic value. The didactic appeal of the model, and particularly of the stages of change, is evident in its widespread adoption and adaptation. It has also generated a large body of empirical research, and as would be expected with a maturing model, no small amount of controversy. Debate has emerged as to whether the descriptive aspects of the model oversimplify or even misrepresent the more complex reality of human change.

This volume opens, therefore, with its progenitors' statement of developments in the model (Chapter 1) since the first edition appeared. This is followed by Robin Davidson's thoughtful summary, in Chapter 2, of criticisms of the model that have been raised. Some of these are characteristic critiques of stage models more generally: that the stages are arbitrarily imposed on what is really a continuum, are artifacts of language or measurement, or do not behave in an orderly, progressive fashion. Difficulties are also noted in the clear classification of individuals and in theoretically grounded prediction of movement through the stages. Chapter 3 provides Prochaska and DiClemente's rejoinder on these issues. As acknowledged in the concluding words of the chapter, readers can judge for themselves the extent to which the accumulated criticisms of the model detract from its usefulness in theory and practice.

1

Toward a Comprehensive, Transtheoretical Model of Change

Stages of Change and Addictive Behaviors

CARLO C. DICLEMENTE AND JAMES O. PROCHASKA

OVERVIEW OF THE TRANSTHEORETICAL MODEL

The transtheoretical model (TTM) offers an integrative framework for understanding and intervening with human intentional behavior change. Although the model has been used with a variety of health risk and health protective behaviors, much of the original and continuing research on the model has focused on initiation and cessation of addictive behaviors (Prochaska, DiClemente, & Norcross, 1992). The model emerged from the research efforts of the authors as they attempted to apply a set of common processes of change, identified from existing theories of therapy (Prochaska, 1979), to successful smoking cessation (DiClemente, 1978; Prochaska & DiClemente, 1982, 1984). There are three organizing constructs of the model: the stages of change, the processes of change, and the levels of change.

CARLO C. DICLEMENTE • Department of Psychology, University of Maryland Baltimore County, Baltimore, Maryland 21250.   JAMES O. PROCHASKA • Department of Psychology, University of Rhode Island, Kingston, Rhode Island 02881.

Treating Addictive Behaviors, 2nd ed., edited by Miller and Heather. Plenum Press, New York, 1998.

Stages of Change

The stages represent the dynamic and motivational aspects of the process of change over time. They are a way of segmenting the process into meaningful steps consisting of specific tasks required to achieve successful, sustained behavior change. Five sequential stages have been identified. In the precontemplation stage, individuals are either ignorant of the nature and extent of a problem needing to be changed or are unwilling to change the problematic behavior. The contemplation stage involves thinking seriously about change and includes a decision-making evaluation of the pros and cons of both the problem behavior and the change. The preparation stage* represents resolution of the decision-making task and a commitment to a change plan to be implemented in the near term. During the action stage the change plan is implemented, active coping is initiated, and the actual behavior change is made. If successful action is sustained for a period of three to six months, the individual moves into the maintenance stage, in which behavior change must become integrated into lifestyle. Once this change becomes completely integrated into the lifestyle, the individual can exit from or terminate this process of change.

Processes of Change

The processes of change are the engines that facilitate movement through the stages of change. These principles of change have been derived from many diverse theories of behavior change and are at the heart of the transtheoretical model (Prochaska & DiClemente, 1986, 1992; Prochaska et al., 1992; Prochaska, Norcross, & DiClemente, 1994). Ten processes have been reliably identified: consciousness raising, self-reevaluation, environmental reevaluation, dramatic relief, social liberation, self-liberation, counterconditioning, stimulus control, reinforcement management, and helping relationship. These processes represent change principles identified by the various cognitive, experiential, behavioral, and humanistic existential theories of psychotherapy. According to the model, these processes employed at particular stages are responsible for movement through the stages of change.

Levels of Change

Clinicians working with addictive behaviors recognize that individuals often have multiple problems that complicate and interact with the process of changing any single addictive behavior. In addition to the stages and processes of change, the model recognizes that changing any one problem behavior is usually complicated by other problems that interfere with or facilitate the process of change. The concept of levels of change incorporates the realization that individuals are in different stages of change with respect to problem areas (see Figure 1).

---

*Originally labeled as a determination or decision-making stage, this stage was not included in some earlier versions of the model because of difficulties in measuring and making an operational definition of this stage. Currently the preparation stage is defined by a near-term intention to take action (in the next 30 days) and a marker of a behavioral commitment to take action (e.g., an attempt to quit smoking in the past year).

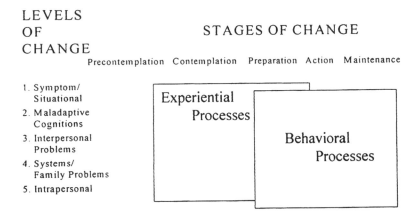

FIGURE 1. Substance Abuse Intervention Template viewed through the stages, levels, and processes of change of the TTM.

The five levels of change identified in the transtheoretical model are symptom/situational, maladaptive cognitions, interpersonal conflicts, family/systems problems, and intrapersonal conflicts (Prochaska & DiClemente, 1984). The levels of change concept has been the least studied of the three basic constructs of the TTM. However, the reality of multiple complicating problems dominates current discussions about addictions, particularly in the areas of drug abuse and alcohol dependence (see Chapter 13, this volume). Polydrug abuse has become the norm among drug abusers. There is a growing recognition of how clinical depression, marital problems, spousal violence, and personality disorders complicate treatment of drug addiction and alcohol dependence. Addiction treatment must have a multidimensional problem perspective, as the current focus on dual diagnosis treatment combining interventions for both psychiatric and substance abuse problems emphasizes (DiClemente, 1994; DiClemente, Carbonari, & Velasquez, 1992). The levels of change concept can guide interventions with the problems at these levels of change. When substance abusers are given services to address the multiple problems that they are facing, the treatment outcomes are often better (DiClemente & Scott, 1997; McLellan, Arndt, Metzger, Wooky, & O'Brien, 1993).

CURRENT STATUS OF RESEARCH ON THE TTM

A comprehensive model of change for addictive behaviors must be able to provide a framework for change that establishes reliable and replicable relationships among constructs. In addition, such a model must be applicable across different addictive behaviors, able to document change that occurs by various methods including self-change, consistent with the experience of the addicted individual, and useful for planning interventions. These qualities are similar to those required to support any theoretical framework: utility, parsimony, explanatory value, heuristic value, and empirical support (Rychlak, 1968). Over the past 15 years empirical and clinical support for the scope and utility of the TTM with addictive behaviors has been accumulating. Although much of the initial research on the model used smoking cessation as the prototypic addictive behavior, the model has been applied to most behaviors typically considered addictive: abuse of and dependence on alcohol, nicotine, cocaine, heroin, and other illegal drugs (Belding, Iguchi, & Lamb, 1996; DiClemente & Hughes, 1990; Donovan & Marlatt, 1988; Rossi et al., 1996; Tsoh, 1995); obesity and eating disorders (Norcross, Prochaska, & DiClemente, 1995); and gambling (DiClemente, in preparation). In addition, the TTM constructs have been used to examine health behaviors that interact with addictive behaviors, such as regular physical exercise (Marcus, Rossi, Selby, Niaura, & Abrams, 1992), condom use (Bowen & Trotter, 1995; Grimley, Riley, Bellis, & Prochaska, 1993), and other health behaviors (Emmons, Marcus, Linnan, Rossi, & Abrams, 1994; Prochaska et al., 1992). The application of the model in research studies and intervention projects has been extensive. The extent of its use has been surprising even to those of us who believe that the TTM constructs reflect important dimensions of the process of human intentional behavior change. Such widespread use brings with it more critical appraisals and some misinterpretations and misapplications as well as supportive evaluations and dissemination.

The stages and the processes of change remain the basic constructs at the heart of the TTM. Addictive behavior change occurs in a segmentable sequence (stages) and as a function of certain specific coping activities (processes of change) (DiClemente, 1993; Prochaska et al., 1992). Over the past few years researchers using the transtheoretical model have been able to gain a better understanding of the movement through the stages as cyclical. Extensive relapse and recycling occurs across the population of addicted individuals who are attempting to take action to stop the behavior (DiClemente, 1994; Fava, Velicer, & Prochaska, 1995; Martin, Velicer, & Fava, 1996; Prochaska et al., 1992; Sewell, Carbonari, & DiClemente, 1994). Recycling through the stages multiple times until reaching sustained maintenance and termination from the cycle of change appears to be the norm. In addition to this better understanding of the natural process of cycling through the stages, the relationships among stage status, participation in treatment, and successful outcomes are being examined and clarified (DiClemente et al., 1991; Piotrowski, Delucchi, Presti, Tunis, & Young, 1995; Prochaska, DiClemente, Velicer, & Rossi, 1993; Prochaska, Velicer, Fava, Rossi, & Tsoh, 1997; Smith, Subich, & Kalodner, 1995).

Conceptually the most interesting and useful research advances for the TTM are the continued documentation of the reliable relationship between the stages and processes of change. The ten processes of change identified in our original research with smokers (Prochaska & DiClemente, 1986, 1992) have been replicated with various populations with varied addictive behavior problems (DiClemente, Carbonari, Addy, & Rothfleisch, 1996; Martin et al., 1996; Norcross et al., 1995). The ten individual processes represent two second-order factors with a set of five labeled cognitive/experiential processes and another set of five labeled behavioral processes (Prochaska & DiClemente, 1992). Both cross-sectional and longitudinal research indicate that experiential processes are most helpful and more often used in the earlier stages of change (contemplation and preparation), while the behavioral processes are most important and more often utilized in the later stages (action and maintenance) (Perz, DiClemente, & Carbonari, 1996; Prochaska, Velicer, Guadagnoli, Rossi, & DiClemente, 1991) (see Figure 1).

Finally, over the past 15 years there have been numerous efforts to develop and evaluate different approaches to intervening with addictive behaviors based on the constructs of the model. Strategies have been developed to address the needs of individuals in specific stages of change, for example, motivational interviewing (Miller & Rollnick, 1991) for early-stage individuals (precontemplation and contemplation), manuals and materials designed to address stage status and movement (American Lung Association, 1987; Glynn, Boyd, & Gruman, 1990; Prochaska et al., 1993), and computer-based efforts to tailor interventions to stage and provide stage and process specific feedback (Prochaska, Velicer, Fava, Ruggiero, et al., 1997; Velicer et al., 1993; Velicer, Prochaska, Fava, LaForge, & Rossi, 1997). In addition, numerous programs and clinicians have been actively engaged in using the constructs of the TTM to construct better intervention strategies in their clinics, treatments, and public health practices (Abrams et al., 1996; Miller, Zweben, DiClemente, & Rychtarik, 1992; Shaffer, 1992; Sorenson et al., 1996). Another important discovery is that proactive approaches involving persons with addictive behaviors, in contrast to the more traditional reactive approaches of waiting until motivation for treatment is fully developed, can be helpful in reaching individuals who are not currently interested in changing the addictive behavior (Prochaska, Velicer, Fava, Rossi, & Tsoh, 1997).

UNDERSTANDING THE STAGES OF CHANGE

STAGE-SPECIFIC TASKS

The concept of stages segments the process of change into various steps with specific tasks required to achieve successful, sustained behavior change. There are several preaction stages, an action stage, during which the targeted behavior change initially takes place, and a maintenance stage, in which the change is sustained and consolidated into a new lifestyle. Each of the stages has unique problems and tasks. Individuals moving through a particular stage must successfully resolve the key task(s) of that stage. Acknowledgment of the problem is needed to move from the precontemplation stage; making the decision to change, to move from contemplation to preparation; generalization and consolidation of the change, to reach maintenance. However, there can be important differences among individuals who are classified in the same stage of change (DiClemente, 1991; Dijkstra, DeVries, & Bakker, 1996).

It is unusual for an individual to go through these stages in a linear fashion, for example, realizing there is a problem, recognizing the need for change, making the decision, and then taking action that would be successfully sustained for a lifetime. For the addictive behaviors, but also with most health behavior change, movement through the stages is not best represented by a single, successful series of transitions from one stage to the next. In fact, such a change would represent what has been identified in the learning literature as "one-trial learning," which is actually rather rare for most animals and humans and most closely associated with traumatic learning. Most individuals move through these stages of change in a cyclical rather than a linear fashion. Most successful behavior change requires several cycles through the stages of change before the individual is able to achieve sustained change. Cycling and recycling through the stages is the norm for human intentional behavior change.

Staging addictive behaviors has been accomplished rather successfully not only with cigarette smokers who have quit on their own, with minimal interventions, or through treatment programs, but also with alcoholics in treatment (DiClemente & Hughes, 1990; Isenhart, 1994), cocaine dependent individuals (Martin *et al.,* 1996; Rothfleisch, 1997; Tsoh, 1995), individuals in treatment for obesity (Norcross *et al.,* 1995), methadone maintained individuals (Belding *et al.,* 1996); polysubstance abusers (Carney & Kivlahan, 1995), dually diagnosed individuals (Velasquez, 1997), and other individuals with various multiple risk behaviors (Emmons *et al.,* 1994). Moreover, meaningfully segmenting change into stages has been accomplished with very different types of assessment instruments and by a varied pool of investigators, indicating the robustness of the construct of stages of change.

The debate continues over whether these stages represent distinct, separate steps that require successful completion of the unique tasks of that stage or are simply arbitrary points on a continuum. Theoretically, we have posited distinct stages with specific, unique tasks that need to be accomplished in order to move successfully to the next stage (Prochaska & DiClemente, 1992). However, the process of human intentional behavior change is dynamic. There are underlying processes of change and markers of change, such as decisional considerations and self-efficacy, that appear to increase and decrease in what seems to be a continuous fashion. Nevertheless, research data continue to demonstrate significant differences among groups of individuals in different stages of change. Moreover, there are complex interactions between the stages and other related variables. For example, self-efficacy correlates positively with processes of change activity in the earlier stages of change and correlates negatively with these same processes in the action and maintenance stages (DiClemente, Prochaska, & Gibertini, 1985). The stages represent parts of a process and not unrelated sets of tasks or goals. However, the more the stages become reified and are used as traitlike rather than statelike descriptions or labels for individuals, the more problematic will be the application of the stages. There is a flow to the process of change that is being artificially delineated by the stages. Thus, there will always be tension between the segments and the dynamic process. Movement back and forth between stages and the reality that stage-specific tasks are accomplished over very short as well as very long periods of time complicate the simplistic and inaccurate view of the stages as a static framework to track linear movement in a discrete, nonrecursive manner.

ASSESSING STAGES OF CHANGE

Assessment also plays a part in the continuous versus discrete debate. The stages have been operationalized in many different ways: Categorical algorithms; continuous ladders, lines, or rulers; continuous measures consisting of stage-specific subscales (URICA, SOCRATES, RTC*); and complex, multidimensional classifica-

---

*The URICA is the University of Rhode Island Change Assessment scale (McConnaughy, DiClemente, Prochaska, & Velicer, 1989); the SOCRATES is the Stages of Change and Treatment Eagerness Scale (Miller & Tonigan, 1996); and the RTC is the Readiness To Change questionnaire (Rollnick, Heather, Gold, & Hall, 1992).

tion systems have all been used to assess stages of change and categorize individuals and groups of individuals into stage-specific or stage-related subgroups.

Algorithms that discretely classify individuals into stages based on the individual's responses to specific questions (Are you seriously considering quitting smoking in the next six months?) have worked well in studies of smoking behavior that are community based. However, when individuals are entering a clinic for treatment of an addictive behavior, these types of measures have not worked as well (Rothfleisch, 1997), as there are demand characteristics that make affirmations of unwillingness to change or of ambivalence about change problematic for most clients. In situations in which there is no strong pressure to feign readiness, individuals can be assessed using even a single-item continuous measure that allows the individual to indicate readiness to change on a continuum from not at all ready to change to very ready to change or taking action. However, when the behaviors are illegal or there are perceived consequences for acknowledging lack of readiness, continuous measures of stage-specific attitudes and intentions have been more useful in finding subgroups of individuals classified according to the stages of change (Carney & Kivlahan, 1995; DiClemente & Hughes, 1990). It is important to note, however, that the various measures that have been developed to assess stages with multiple items and subscales tend to measure various aspects of the process of change somewhat differently. Stage-specific subscales of the SOCRATES have recently been shown to evaluate aspects of problem recognition, taking action, and ambivalence (Miller & Tonigan, 1996), whereas the subscales of the URICA have proven rather robust as correlated but identifiable subscales for precontemplation, contemplation, action, and maintenance (Carbonari, DiClemente, & Zweben, 1994). Researchers have typically used cluster analysis to create subgroups for the URICA subscales. Others, such as Rollnick, Heather, Gold, and Hall (1992), have used the highest single subscale score of the Readiness to Change (RTC) questionnaire in assessing stage. Staging individuals and creating stage subgroups requires care and, often, is difficult to do simply using single items or individual subscale scores. However, there may be a simpler way to assess stage status as readiness to change. Recently we have found that the subscales of the URICA that assess precontemplation, contemplation, action, and maintenance attitudes about change form a second-order factor and can be combined arithmetically (C + A + M − PC) to yield a continuous score that we have successfully used to assess readiness to change at entrance to treatment (Carbonari et al., 1994; Carbonari, DiClemente, Addy, & Pollack, 1996; Project MATCH Research Group, 1997).

There are clearly different ways of assessing readiness to change. As long as there is some assessment of attitudes and intentions toward a specific targeted behavior change and there is a clear definition of what behavior or behaviors constitute successful action (cessation of smoking, adherence to diet, reduction of drinking and driving) so that the preaction stages can be distinguished from the action and maintenance stages, the process of change can be divided into meaningful and useful parts. Whether assessed using a continuous measure or by specific stage or stage-related classifications, individuals earlier in the process differ from individuals in the later stages on measures of change process activity, decisional considerations, and self-efficacy, and these differences support the validity of the staging of the process of change. Measuring these stages in different behaviors has proved challenging but has been accomplished in the areas of smoking initiation and cessation, alcoholism, cocaine abuse, illegal drug use, condom use, exercise adoption, dietary consumption of fat and fiber, and a number of other behaviors.

STAGE INTERACTIONS WITH OTHER CONSTRUCTS

In a number of studies, individual processes of change and the larger set of experiential and behavioral processes have been reliably associated both with the stage status of individuals and with the movement of individuals through the stages (DiClemente *et al.,* 1991; Fitzgerald & Prochaska, 1989). In some current research we have found that shifting emphasis in process activity as individuals move from contemplation and preparation to action is related to successful outcome (Perz *et al.,* 1996). Understanding the interaction of stage and change process activity enables clinicians to target some particular change process with their interventions, evaluate whether these interventions are able to reliably instigate these processes, and ultimately assess whether these processes make the difference in successful change (DiClemente *et al.,* 1992; Snow, Prochaska, & Rossi, 1994). We have some exciting new data from research in progress that indicate that process activity is reliably related to initiating change and sustaining change both with pregnant smokers and with alcohol-dependent individuals engaging in alcoholism treatment.

Recent research has documented the importance of the interaction of stages and processes as doing the right thing at the right time (Perz *et al.,* 1996). Moreover, understanding this stage by process activity has yielded interesting experimental information about the lack of gender differences in smoking cessation (O'Connor, Carbonari, & DiClemente, 1996) and the external or imposed nature of the change in smoking of pregnant smokers who stop smoking for the pregnancy (Stotts, DiClemente, Carbonari, & Mullen, 1996). Similar interactions of stages with decisional balance and self-efficacy constructs have also yielded intriguing new information about the relationship of the process of change with these two important dimensions of the individual's self-evaluations with regard to his or her addictive behavior (DiClemente, Carbonari, Montgomery, & Hughes, 1993; DiClemente, Fairhurst, & Piotrowski, 1995; Prochaska, Velicer, *et al.,* 1994; Rossi *et al.,* 1996).

INTERVENTION PLANNING AND MATCHING

Let us turn to the application of the TTM model to see how it can be used to assist people with each of four important aspects of treatment planning and evaluation of interventions for the addictions. The four areas are recruitment, retention, progress, and outcomes.

RECRUITMENT

Too few studies have paid attention to one of the skeletons in the closet of professional treatment programs. The fact is that these programs recruit or reach too few people with addictions. Less than 25% of populations with lifetime *DSM-*

IV diagnoses of these disorders ever enter professional therapy programs (Veroff, Douvon, & Kulka, 1981a, 1981b). With smoking, the most deadly of addictions, less than 10% ever participate in professional programs (USDHHS, 1990). Given that the addictions are among the most costly of contemporary conditions, professionals must help many more people to participate in appropriate programs and can no longer be prepared to treat the addictions only on a reactive individual case basis. Treatment programs that are more proactive and can reach the addictions on a population basis must be designed and developed.

There are some government agencies and health care systems that are seeking to treat such costly conditions on a population basis. However, when they turn to the biggest and best clinical trials treating addictions on a population basis, they discover that trial after trial reports troubling outcomes (e.g., Commit Research Group, 1995; Ennett, Tabler, Ringwolt, & Fliwelling, 1994; Glasgow, Terborg, Hollis, Severson, & Boles, 1995; Luepker *et al.,* 1994; Sorenson *et al.,* 1996). Whether the trials were done with worksites, schools, or entire communities, the results are remarkably similar: little or no significant effect compared to the control conditions.

If we examine more closely one of these trials, the Minnesota Heart Health Study, we can find hints of what went wrong (Lando *et al.,* 1995; Lichtenstein, Lando, & Nothwehr, 1994). With smoking as one of their targeted behaviors, nearly 90% of the smokers in treated communities reported seeing media stories about smoking. But the same was true of smokers in the control communities. Only about 12% of smokers in the treatment and control conditions said their physicians talked to them about smoking in the past year. If we look at what percentage participated in the most powerful behavior change programs, clinics, classes, and counselors, we find only 4% of the smokers participated over the 5 years of planned interventions. Even when managed care offered free state-of-the-science cessation clinics, only 1% of smokers were recruited (Lichtenstein & Hollis, 1992).

Addiction professionals can move many more people with addictions to seek the appropriate help by changing paradigms and practices. There are two paradigms that these professionals need to contemplate changing. The first is an action-oriented paradigm that construes behavior change as an event that can occur quickly, immediately, discretely, and dramatically. Treatment programs that are designed to have people immediately quit abusing substances are implicitly or explicitly designed for the portion of the population who are in the preparation or action stages of change.

The problem is that across 15 unhealthy behaviors in 20,000 HMO members, we find that typically less than 20% are prepared to take action (Rossi, 1992). A rule of thumb in estimating stage distribution is 40, 40, 20: 40% in precontemplation, 40% in contemplation, and 20% in preparation, although these percentages can vary dramatically in different populations (Dijkstra *et al.,* 1996; Fava *et al.,* 1995). When programs offer action-oriented interventions, they are implicitly recruiting from less than 20% of the at-risk population. If our programs are to meet the needs of entire populations with addictions, then we must design interventions for the 40% in precontemplation and the 40% in contemplation.

By offering stage-matched interventions and applying proactive or outreach recruitment methods, we have been able to assist 80% to 90% of the smokers to enter our treatment programs in three large-scale clinical trials (Prochaska, Velicer, Fava, Rossi, & Tsoh, 1997; Prochaska, Velicer, Fava, Ruggiero, *et al.,* 1997). This is a substantial increase in our ability to reach and move many more people to take the action of starting therapy.

The second paradigm change that this more inclusive approach requires is movement from a passive-reactive approach to practice to a proactive one. Most professionals have been trained to be passive-reactive: to passively wait for patients to seek services and then react. The greatest problem with this approach is that the majority of people with addictions never seek such services. The passive-reactive paradigm is designed to serve populations with acute conditions. The pain, distress, or discomfort of such conditions can motivate people to seek the services of health professionals. But the major killers of our time are chronic conditions caused in large part by chronic lifestyle disorders such as the addictions, in which delay, indecision, and ambivalence interfere with help seeking.

If professionals are to intervene early to treat addictions, they need to reach out to entire populations and offer more stage-matched therapies. What happens if professionals change only one paradigm and proactively recruit entire populations to action-oriented interventions? This experiment has been tried in one of the United States's largest managed care organizations (Lichtenstein & Hollis, 1992). Physicians spent time with every smoker to get them to sign up for a state-of-the-art action-oriented clinic. If that didn't work, nurses spent up to 10 minutes to get them to sign up, followed by 12 minutes of health educators' time and a counselor's call to home. This most intensive recruitment protocol motivated 35% of smokers in precontemplation to sign up. But only 3% showed up, 2% finished, and none achieved significant cessation. From a combined contemplation and preparation group, 65% signed up, 15% showed up, 11% completed the treatment, and less than 10% achieved significant cessation. What can move a majority of people to engage in some type of professional treatment program for an addiction? One answer to that question would be professionals who are motivated and prepared to proactively reach out to entire populations and offer them interventions that match their current stage of change.

RETENTION

What motivates people to continue in therapy? Or conversely, what moves clients to terminate counseling quickly and prematurely as judged by their counselors? A metanalysis of 125 studies found that on average 50% of clients drop out of treatment (Wierzbicki & Pekarik, 1993). Across studies there were few consistent predictors of premature termination. There were indications that substance abuse, minority status, and lower education predicted greater dropout. Although important, these variables did not account for much of the variance in the prediction.

There are now several studies on dropouts from a stage model perspective on substance abuse, smoking, obesity, and a broad spectrum of psychiatric disorders (e.g., Medeiros & Prochaska, 1997; Prochaska, DiClemente, Velicer, Ginpil, & Norcross, 1985; Prochaska et al., 1992; Smith et al., 1995). These studies found that stage-related variables outpredicted demographics, type of problem, severity of problem, and other problem-related variables. Figure 2 presents the stage profiles of three groups of patients with a broad spectrum of psychiatric disorders. In this study transtheoretical variables were used to predict three groups: premature terminators, early but appropriate terminators, and continuers in therapy.

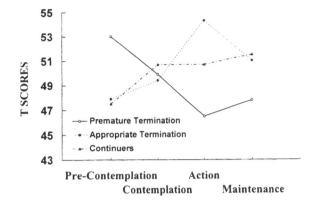

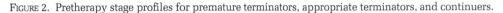

FIGURE 2. Pretherapy stage profiles for premature terminators, appropriate terminators, and continuers.

Figure 2 shows that the pretherapy profile on the URICA subscales of the entire group who dropped out quickly and prematurely (40%) was a profile of people in the precontemplation stage. The 20% who finished quickly but appropriately had a profile of patients who were in the action stage when entering therapy. Those who continued in longer-term treatment were a mixed group with the majority in the contemplation stage.

We cannot treat people in the precontemplation stage as if they are starting in the same place as those in the action stage and expect them to continue in therapy. If we try to pressure them to take action when they are not prepared, should we expect to retain them in therapy? Or do we drive them away and then blame them for not being motivated enough or not being ready enough for our action-oriented interventions?

Currently, we have four studies with stage-matched interventions in which we can examine retention rates of people entering interventions in the precontemplation stage (e.g., Prochaska et al., 1993; Prochaska, Velicer, Fava, Rossi, & Tsoh, 1997; Prochaska, Velicer, Fava, Ruggiero, et al., 1997; Velicer et al., 1997). It is clear that when treatment is matched to stage, people in precontemplation continue engagement at the same high rates as those who started in the preparation stage. This result held for clinical trials in which people were recruited proactively (we reached out to them to offer help) as well as in participants recruited reactively (they called us for help). Unfortunately, these studies have been done only with smokers. If the results hold up across addictions, a practical answer to the question, "What motivates people early in the process of change to engage and continue in therapy?" would be "receiving treatments that match their current stage of change."

PROGRESS

What moves people to progress in therapy and to continue to progress after therapy? In a number of studies we have found what can be called a stage outcome effect, when the amount of successful action taken during treatment and after treatment is proportionally related to the stage of change at the start of treatment (Prochaska et al., 1992). In the example in Figure 3, interventions with smokers

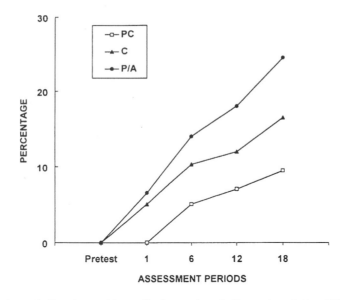

FIGURE 3. Percentage abstinent over 18 months for smokers in Precontemplation (PC), Contemplation (C), and Preparation (P/A) stages before treatment (N = 570).

in the three stages of precontemplation, contemplation, and preparation ended at 6 months. The group of smokers who started in the precontemplation stage show the least amount of effective action as measured by abstinence at each assessment point. Those who started in the contemplation stage made significantly more progress. And those who entered treatment already prepared to take action were most successful at every assessment.

The same type of stage effect has been found across a variety of problems and populations including rehabilitation for brain injury and recovery from anxiety and panic disorders following random assignment to placebo or active medication (Beitman *et al.,* 1994: Lam, McMahon, Priddy, & Gehred-Schultz, 1988). In the latter clinical trial the psychiatrist leading the trial concluded that patients need to be assessed for their stage of readiness to benefit from such medication and need to be helped through the stages so that they are well prepared prior to being placed on the medication.

One strategy for applying stage-sensitive interventions clinically is to set realistic goals for brief encounters with clients at each stage of change. A realistic goal is to help clients progress one stage in brief therapy. If clients move relatively quickly then we can help them progress two stages. The results of some longitudinal studies indicate that if clients progress one stage in 1 month they double the chances that they will be taking effective action by 6 months. If they progress two stages they increase their chances of taking effective action by three to four times (Prochaska, Velicer, Fava, Ruggiero, *et al.,* 1997). Setting realistic goals can enable many more people to enter therapy, continue in therapy, progress in therapy, and continue to progress after therapy.

The first results reported back from trainers and clinicians in Birmingham, England, where 4,000 health professionals have been trained in this approach to the addictions, are that there is a dramatic increase in the morale of these health professionals. They can now see progress with the majority of their patients where they once saw failure when immediate action was the only criteria of success. They are much more confident that they have treatments that can match the stages of all of their patients rather than only the 20% or so who are prepared to take immediate action.

OUTCOMES AND IMPACTS

What happens when all of these principles and processes of change are used to help patients and entire populations at each stage to move toward action on their addictions? A series of clinical trials applying stage-matched interventions can offer important lessons about the future of behavioral health care generally and treatment of the addictions specifically.

In an initial large-scale clinical trial of minimal interventions for smoking cessation, we compared four treatments: (1) one of the best home-based action-oriented cessation programs (standardized), (2) stage-matched manuals (individualized), (3) expert system computer reports plus manuals (interactive), and (4) counselors plus computers and manuals (personalized). Smokers ($N = 739$) were randomly assigned by stage to one of the four treatments (Prochaska *et al.*, 1993).

In the computer-generated feedback condition, participants completed by mail or telephone a series of questionnaires that were entered into our central computers and generated feedback reports. These reports informed participants about their stage of change, the pros and cons of change, and the use of change processes appropriate to their stages. At baseline, participants were given positive feedback on what they were doing correctly and guidance on the principles and processes they needed to apply more strongly in order to progress. In two progress reports delivered over the next 6 months, participants also received positive feedback on any improvement they made on any of the variables relevant to progressing. So, demoralized and defensive smokers could begin progressing without having to quit and without having to work too hard. Smokers in the contemplation stage could begin taking small steps, such as delaying their first cigarette in the morning for an extra 30 minutes. They could choose small steps that would increase their self-efficacy and help them become better prepared for quitting.

In the personalized condition, smokers received four proactive counselor calls over the 6-month intervention period. Three of the calls were based on the computer reports. Counselors reported much more difficulty in interacting with participants without any progress data. Without scientific assessments, it was much harder for both clients and counselors to tell whether any significant progress had occurred since their last interaction.

Figure 4 presents point prevalence abstinence rates for each of the four treatment groups over 18 months with treatment ending at 6 months. The two self-help manual conditions paralleled each other for 12 months. At 18 months, the stage-matched manual group moved ahead. This is an example of a *delayed action effect*, which often can be observed with stage-matched programs specifically and has been observed with self-help programs generally. It takes time for participants in early stages to progress all the way to action. Therefore, some treatment effects as measured by action will be observed only after considerable delay. However, it

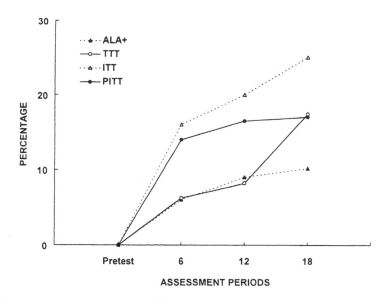

FIGURE 4. Point prevalence abstinence (%) for four treatment groups at pretest and at 6, 12, and 18 months. (ALA+ = standardized manuals; TTT = individualized stage-matched manuals; ITT = interactive computer reports; PITT = personalized counselor calls.)

is encouraging to find treatments producing therapeutic effects months and even years after treatment has ended.

The computer alone and computerized feedback plus counselor conditions paralleled each other for 12 months. Then, the effects of the counselor condition flattened out while the computer condition effects continued to increase. We can only speculate as to the delayed differences between these two conditions. Participants in the personalized condition may have become somewhat dependent on the social support and social control of the counselor's calling. The last call was after the 6-month assessment and benefits would be observed at 12 months. Termination of the counselors' calls could result in no further progress because of the loss of social support and control. The classic pattern in smoking cessation clinics is rapid relapse beginning as soon as the treatment is terminated. Some of this rapid relapse could well be due to the sudden loss of social support or social control provided by the counselors and other participants in the clinic.

The next test was to demonstrate the efficacy of the expert system when applied to an entire population recruited proactively. With more than 80% of 5,170 smokers who were reached by our recruitment participating and fewer than 20% of them in the preparation stage, the expert system of personalized feedback demonstrated significant benefit at each 6-month follow-up (Prochaska, Velicer, Fava, Rossi, & Tsoh, 1997). Furthermore, the advantages over proactive assessment alone increased at each follow-up for the full 2 years assessed. The implications are that expert system interventions in a population can continue to demonstrate benefits long after the intervention has ended.

Results of the expert system's efficacy were replicated in an HMO population of 4,000 smokers with 85% participation (Prochaska, Velicer, Fava, Ruggiero, *et al.*, 1997). In the first population-based study, the expert system was 34% more effective than assessment alone; in the second, it was 31% more effective. These replicated differences were clinically significant as well. Although working on a population basis, these studies were able to produce the level of success normally found only in intense clinic-based programs with low participation rates of much more selective samples of smokers. The implications are that once expert systems are developed and show effectiveness with one population, they can be transferred at much lower cost and produce replicable changes in new populations.

Enhancing Interactive Interventions

Recent research efforts have been attempting to create enhancements to our expert system to produce even better outcomes. In the first enhancement with an HMO population, a personal handheld computer designed to bring the behavior under stimulus control was added to the expert system feedback program (Prochaska, Velicer, Fava, Ruggiero, et al., 1997). This commercially successful innovation was an action-oriented intervention that did not enhance our expert system program outcomes. In fact, the expert system alone was twice as effective as the system plus the enhancement. There are two important potential implications of this result: More is not necessarily better, and providing interventions that are mismatched to stage can make outcomes markedly worse.

Counselor Enhancements

In the research with an HMO population, counselors plus expert system computers were outperforming expert systems alone at 12 months. But at 18 months the counselor enhancement outcomes had declined while the outcomes of the computer feedback alone had increased. Both interventions were producing identical outcomes of 23.2% point prevalence abstinence, which are excellent for a population intervention. Why did the effect of the counselor condition drop off after the intervention? It may be that once these social influences are withdrawn, people may do worse. The expert system computers, on the other hand, may maximize self-reliance. In a current clinical trial, counselors are being faded out over time as a method for dealing with dependency on the counselor. If fading is effective, it will have implications for how counseling should be terminated: gradually over time rather than suddenly.

We believe that the most powerful change programs will combine the personalized benefits of counselors and consultants with the individualized, interactive, and data-based benefits of expert system computers. But to date we have not been able to demonstrate that the more costly counselors, who had been our most powerful change agents, can actually add value over individualized computer feedback alone. If replicated, these findings would have clear implications for cost effectiveness of expert systems for entire populations needing behavioral health care programs.

Interactive versus Noninteractive Interventions

Another important aim of the HMO research project was to assess whether interactive interventions (computer-generated expert systems) are more effective than noninteractive communications (self-help manuals) when controlling for number of intervention contacts (Velicer *et al.,* 1997). At 6, 12, and 18 months for groups of smokers receiving a series of one, two, three, or six interactive versus noninteractive contacts, the interactive interventions (expert system) outperformed the noninteractive manuals in all four comparisons. In three of the comparisons (1, 2, and 3), the difference at 18 months was at least five percentage points, a difference between treatment conditions assumed to be clinically significant. These results clearly support the hypothesis that interactive interventions will outperform the same number of noninteractive interventions.

These results support our initial assumption that the most powerful health promotion programs for entire populations will be interactive. In the reactive clinical literature it is clear that interactive interventions such as behavioral counseling produce greater long-term abstinence rates (20% to 30%) than do noninteractive interventions such as self-help manuals (10% to 20%). It should be kept in mind that these traditional action-oriented programs were implicitly or explicitly recruiting for populations in the preparation stage. Results from the current research indicate that even with proactively recruited smokers with less than 20% in the preparation stage, the long-term abstinence rates can reach the 20% to 30% range for the interactive interventions and the 10% to 20% range for the noninteractive interventions. The implications are clear. Providing interactive interventions via computers is likely to produce greater outcomes than interventions relying on noninteractive communications, such as newsletters, media, or self-help manuals.

IMPLICATIONS AND ISSUES FOR THE FUTURE

The current research and applications of the TTM have important implications for addiction treatment and envision a number of shifts in thinking and practice for policymakers, health care providers, clinicians, and researchers (see Chapter 8, this volume). These implications are best summarized by examining application versus research needs, process versus outcome evaluations, proactive versus reactive approaches, and single versus multiple problems and approaches.

APPLICATION VERSUS RESEARCH NEEDS

There is growing desire to use the TTM in clinics and addiction treatment delivery systems. Although many individual practitioners and treatment systems have begun translating the concepts of the model into practice, the need for developing and evaluating assessment tools and the continued exploration for treatment strategies to engage the appropriate processes of change is critical. Assessment of stages and processes has become more psychometrically sophisticated over the past 15 to 20 years, but more attention and research are needed to understand how to accurately assess and track movement through the stages of change and to clarify process activities for target behaviors that differ greatly in intensity, frequency, and difficulty.

PROCESS VERSUS OUTCOME EVALUATIONS

Addiction treatment and research must focus not only on outcome but on the process of behavior change. Doing this requires longitudinal rather than simple cross-sectional research designs, greater attention to client-reported activities and processes, more assessment of during-treatment activities, and greater sophistication in measuring movement through the process of change. If movement and recycling through the stages represent progress, we need more sensitive and sensible outcomes with which to evaluate our interventions. If success is measured only by successful long-term change, then we will continue to be frustrated by our inadequacy to achieve substantial outcomes with one shot, action-oriented interventions.

We can envision both the initiation of addictions and the cessation of addictions as a process of change (Werch & DiClemente, 1994; DiClemente, in preparation). A process perspective is needed to help us understand how initiation and cessation are related and to develop prevention as well as treatment interventions that will address the needs of individuals vulnerable to initiation as well as those in need of cessation.

PROACTIVE VERSUS REACTIVE APPROACHES

If the process of change is dynamic, represented by stages of change, then the individual engaged in changing a behavior represents a moving target and not a static entity. There are solid indications that, when treatments are dynamically matched to the stages and processes of change, these interventions can be more effective. However, this requires individualizing the treatment process. Newer technologies, including computer-generated feedback, make it possible to create more individualized interventions.

We believe that the future of behavioral health care programs lies with stage-matched, proactive, and interactive interventions. Much greater impacts can be generated by proactive programs because of much higher participation rates, even if efficacy rates are lower. But we also believe that proactive programs can produce comparable outcomes to traditional reactive programs. It is counterintuitive to believe that comparable outcomes can be produced with people whom we reach out to help and with people who call us for help, but that is what informal comparisons strongly suggest. Unfortunately, there is no experimental design that could permit us to randomly assign people to proactive versus reactive recruitment programs. We are left with informal but provocative comparisons.

If these results continue to be replicated, therapeutic programs will be able to produce significant impacts with entire populations. We believe that such effects would require scientific and professional shifts:

1. from an action paradigm to a stage paradigm,
2. from reactive to proactive recruitment,
3. from expecting participants to match the needs of our programs to having our programs match their needs,
4. and from completely clinic-based to population-based individualized and interactive programs.

SINGLE VERSUS MULTIPLE PROBLEMS AND APPROACHES

In addition to the stages and processes of change for a single behavior, research is needed on the reality of multiple problems and how change in one is related to change in others in order to see whether sequential, simultaneous, or some combination of approaches is most effective. As the field of addictions begins to focus more on dually diagnosed individuals, polydrug users, and the multiple psychosocial problems that exist in the lives of the addicted individuals that either predated or arrived subsequent to the addiction, the need to understand the process of change for all these interrelated problems increases. These additional, complicating problems have important implications for the process of change (Emmons *et al.*, 1994; McLellan *et al.*, 1993; Velasquez, 1997). Before we can create the most effective interventions for the addicted, multiproblemed individuals, we must learn more about how readiness to change and barriers to change interact for these individuals.

As managed care organizations move to briefer and briefer therapies for the addictions and other disorders even with the most complicated of cases, there is a danger that most health and addiction professionals will feel pressured to produce immediate action and results. If this pressure is then transferred to patients who by and large are not prepared for such action, interventions will repeat past problems: not reaching most patients and not retaining most patients. Addiction professionals can help move a majority of patients to progress in relatively brief encounters only if they set realistic goals for their clients and for themselves. Otherwise, they risk demoralizing and demotivating both client and counselor.

The treatment situation becomes more complicated as we begin to use various social and environmental forces to produce individual change. The impact of social influences on the process of change is clearly demonstrable in the case of smoking cessation, in which more than 40 million Americans have successfully achieved sustained cessation over the past 30 years (USDHHS, 1990). However, this outcome has not occurred without the efforts of each individual smoker who quit. The fascinating interaction of social forces and the process of individual change demands additional, innovative, and process-oriented research.

CONCLUSION

The transtheoretical model includes the interaction of stages, processes, and levels of change and continues to provide a useful heuristic with which to examine the process of addictive behavior change. Understanding this process and how to intervene most effectively has advanced enormously over the past 15 years and there are dramatic implications of these discoveries for treatment and research. Research results support the existence and applicability of the basic constructs of the TTM. However, the process of intentional human behavior change is a complex one requiring continued efforts to gain a complete understanding of the entire process of change with addictive behaviors.

REFERENCES

Abrams, D. B., Orleans, C. T., Niaura, R. S., Goldstein, M. G., Prochaska, J. O., & Velicer, W. (1996). Integrating individual and public health perspectives for treatment of tobacco dependence under managed health care: A combined stepped-care and matching model. *Annals of Behavioral Medicine, 18,* 290–304.

Beitman, B. D., Beck, N. C., Deuser, W., Carter, C., Davidson, J., & Maddock, R. (1994). Patient stages of change predicts outcome in a panic disorder medication trial. *Anxiety, 1,* 64–69.

Belding, M., Iguchi, M., & Lamb, R. J. (1996). Stages of change in methadone maintenance: Assessing the convergent validity of two measures. *Psychology of Addictive Behaviors, 10,* 157–166.

Bowen, A., & Trotter, R. (1995). HIV risk in intravenous drug users and crack cocaine smokers: Predicting stage of change for condom use. *Journal of Consulting and Clinical Psychology, 63,* 238–248.

Carbonari, J., DiClemente, C., & Zweben, A. (1994, Nov.). A readiness to change scale: Its development, validation and usefulness. *Discussion symposium: Assessing critical dimensions for alcoholism treatment.* Presented at the 28th annual convention of the Association for the Advancement of Behavioral Therapy, San Diego.

Carbonari, J., DiClemente, C., Addy, R., & Pollack, K. (1996, March). *Alternate Short Forms of the Readiness to Change.* Poster presented at the Fourth International Congress on Behavioral Medicine, Washington, DC.

Carney, M. M., & Kivlahan, D. R. (1995). Motivational subtypes among veterans seeking substance abuse treatment: Profiles based on stages of change. *Psychology of Addictive Behaviors, 9,* 1135–1142.

Commit Research Group. (1995). The Community Intervention Trial of Smoking Cessation (COMMIT): Summary of cohort results. *American Journal of Public Health, 85,* 183–193.

DiClemente, C. C. (1978). *Perceived processes, change on the cessation of smoking and the maintenance of that change.* Unpublished doctoral dissertation, University of Rhode Island, Kingston.

DiClemente, C. C. (1991). Motivational interviewing and the stages of change. In W. R. Miller & S. Rollnick (Eds.), *Motivational interviewing: Preparing people to change addictive behavior* (pp. 191–202). New York: Guilford.

DiClemente, C. C. (1993). Changing addictive behaviors: A process perspective. *Current Directions in Psychological Science, 2*(4), 101–106.

DiClemente, C. C. (1994). If behaviors change, can personality be far behind? In T. Heatherton & J. Weinberger (Eds.), *Can personality change?* (pp. 175–198). Washington, DC: American Psychological Association.

DiClemente, C. C. (in preparation). *Addiction and change.* New York: Guilford.

DiClemente, C. C., & Hughes, S. O. (1990). Stages of change profiles in alcoholism treatment. *Journal of Substance Abuse, 2,* 217–235.

DiClemente, C. C., & Scott, C. W. (1997). Stages of change: Interactions with treatment compliance and involvement. In L. S. Onken, J. D. Blaine, & J. J. Boren (Eds.), *Beyond the therapeutic alliance: Keeping the drug-dependent individual in treatment.* (NIDA Research Monograph 165). Washington, DC: U.S. Department of Health and Human Services.

DiClemente, C. C., Prochaska, J. O., & Gibertini, M. (1985). Self-efficacy and the stages of self-change smoking. *Cognitive Therapy and Research, 9*(2), 181–200.

DiClemente, C. C., Prochaska, J. O., Fairhurst, S., Velicer, W. F., Velasquez, M., & Rossi, J. (1991). The process of smoking cessation: An analysis of Precontemplation, Contemplation & Preparation. *Journal of Consulting and Clinical Psychology, 59*(2), 295–304.

DiClemente, C. C., Carbonari, J. P., & Velasquez, M. M. (1992). Alcoholism treatment mismatching from a process of change perspective. In R. R. Watson (Ed.), *Treatment of drug and alcohol abuse* (pp. 115–142). Totowa, NJ: Humana.

DiClemente, C. C., Carbonari, J. P., Montgomery, R., & Hughes, S. (1993). The Alcohol Abstinence Self-Efficacy Scale. *Journal of Studies on Alcohol, 55,* 141–148.

DiClemente, C. C., Fairhurst, S. K., & Piotrowski, N. A. (1995). The role of self-efficacy in the addictive behaviors. In J. Maddux (Ed.), *Self-efficacy, adaptation and adjustment: Theory, research and application* (pp. 109–142). New York: Plenum.

DiClemente, C. C., Carbonari, J. C., Addy, R., & Rothfleisch, J. (1996, March). *Structure and function of the processes of change.* Poster presented at the Fourth International Congress on Behavioral Medicine, Washington, DC.

Dijkstra, A., DeVries, H., & Bakker, M. (1996). Pros and cons of quitting, self-efficacy, and the stages of change in smoking cessation. *Journal of Consulting and Clinical Psychology, 64,* 758–763.

Donovan, D. M., & Marlatt, G. A. (Eds.). (1988). *Assessment of addictive behaviors.* New York: Guilford.

Emmons, K. M., Marcus, B. H., Linnan, L., Rossi, J. S., & Abrams, D. B. (1994). Mechanisms in multiple risk factor interventions: Smoking, physical activity, and dietary fat intake among manufacturing workers. *Preventive Medicine, 23,* 481–489.

Ennett, S. T., Tabler, N. S., Ringwolt, C. L., & Fliwelling, R. L. (1994). How effective is drug abuse resistance education? A meta-analysis of Project DARE outcome evaluations. *American Journal of
Public Health, 84,* 1394–1401.

Farkas, A. J., Pierce, J. P., Zhu, S-H., Rosbrook, B., Gilpin, E. A., Berry, C., & Kaplan, R. M. (1996) Addiction versus stages of change models in predicting smoking cessation. *Addiction, 91*(9),
1271–1280.

Fava, J. L., Velicer, W. F., & Prochaska, J. O. (1995). Applying the Transtheoretical Model to a representative sample of smokers. *Addictive Behaviors, 20,* 189–203.

Fitzgerald, T. E., & Prochaska, J. O. (1989). Nonprogressing profiles in smoking cessation: What keeps
people refractory to self-change? *Journal of Substance Abuse, 2,* 93–111.

Glasgow, R. E., Terborg, J. R., Hollis, J. F., Severson, H. H., & Boles, S. M. (1995). Take Heart: Results
from the initial phase of a work-site wellness program. *American Journal of Public Health, 85,*
209–216.

Glynn, T. J., Boyd, G. M., & Gruman, J. C. (1990). Essential elements of self-help/minimal intervention
strategies for smoking cessation. *Health Education Quarterly, 17*(3), 329–345.

Grimley, D. M., Riley, G. E., Bellis, J. M., & Prochaska, J. O. (1993, December). Assessing the stages of
change and decision-making for contraceptive use for the prevention of pregnancy, sexually trans-
mitted diseases, and Acquired Immunodeficiency Syndrome. *Health Education Quarterly, 20*(4),
455–470.

Heather, N., Rollnick, S., & Bell, A. (1993). Predictive validity of the Readiness to Change Questionnaire, *Addiction, 88,* 1667–1677.

Isenhart, C. (1994). Motivational subtypes in an inpatient sample of substance abusers. *Addictive Behaviors, 19,* 463–475.

King, T., & DiClemente, C. C. (1993, Nov.). *A decisional balance measure for assessing and predicting
drinking behavior.* Poster presented at the 26th annual convention of the Association for the Advancement of Behavior Therapy, Atlanta.

Lam, C. S., McMahon, B. T., Priddy, D. A., & Gehred-Schultz, A. (1988). Deficit awareness and treatment performance among traumatic head injury adults. *Brain Injury, 2*(3), 235–241.

Lando, H. A., Pechacek, T. F., Pirie, P. L., Murray, D. M., Mittelmark, M. B., Lichtenstein, E., Nothwehyr,
F., & Gray, C. (1995). Changes in adult cigarette smoking in the Minnesota Heart Health Program.
American Journal of Public Health, 85, 201–208.

Lichtenstein, E., & Hollis, J. (1992). Patient referral to smoking cessation programs: Who follows
through? *Journal of Family Practice, 34,* 739–744.

Lichtenstein, E., Lando, H. A., & Nothwehr, F. (1994). Readiness to quit as a predictor of smoking
changes in the Minnesota Heart Health Program. *Health Psychology, 13,* 393–396.

Luepker, R. V., Murray, D. M., Jacobs, D. R., Mittelmark, M. B., Bracnt, N., Carlaw, R., Crow, Elmer, P.,
Finnegan, J., Folsom, A. R., Grimm, R., Hannan, P. J., Jeffrey, R., Pirie, P., Sprafra, J. M., Weisbrod, R.,
and Blackburn, H. (1994). Community education for cardiovascular disease prevention: Risk factor
changes in the Minnesota Heart Health Program. *American Journal of Public Health, 84,* 1383–1393.

Marcus, B. H., Rossi, J. S., Selby, V. C., Niaura, R. S., & Abrams, D. B. (1992). The stages and processes
of exercise adoption and maintenance in a worksite sample. *Health Psychology, 11*(6), 386–395.

Martin, R., Rossi, J., Rosenhow, D., Monti, P., & Rosenbloom, D. (1994, Nov.). *Stages of change profiles
for quitting cocaine.* Poster presented at the 28th annual convention of the Association for the Advancement of Behavior Therapy, San Diego.

Martin, R. A., Velicer, W. F., & Fava, J. I. (1996). Latent transition analysis to the stages of change for
smoking cessation. *Addictive Behaviors, 21,* 67–80.

McConnaughy, E. A., DiClemente, C. C., Prochaska, J. O., & Velicer, W. F. (1989). Stages of change in
psychotherapy: A follow-up report. *Psychotherapy: Theory, Research and Practice, 4,* 494–503.

McLellan, A., Arndt, I., Metzger, D., Wooky, G., & O'Brien, C. (1993). The effects of psychosocial services in substance abuse treatment. *Journal of the American Medical Association, 269*(15),
1953–1959.

Medeiros, M. E., & Prochaska, J. O. (1997). *Predicting termination and continuation status in psychotherapy using the Transtheoretical Model.* Manuscript under review.

Miller, W. R., & Rollnick, S. (1991). *Motivational interviewing: Preparing people to change addictive behavior.* New York: Guilford.

Miller, W. R., & Tonigan, J. S. (1996). Assessing drinkers' motivation for change: The stages of change
readiness and treatment eagerness scale (SOCRATES). *Psychology of Addictive Behaviors, 10,*
81–89.

Miller, W. R., Zweben, A., DiClemente, C. C., & Rychtarik, R. G. (1992). *Motivational Enhancement Therapy manual: A clinical research guide for therapists and individuals with alcohol abuse and dependence.* Rockville, MD: National Institute on Alcohol Abuse and Alcoholism.

Norcross, J. C., Prochaska, J. O., & DiClemente, C. C. (1995). The stages and processes of weight control: Two replications. In A. P. Simopoulous & T. B. Vanitalie (Eds.), *Obesity: New directions in assessment and management* (pp. 172–184). Philadelphia: Charles Press.

O'Connor, E., Carbonari, J. P., & DiClemente, C. C. (1996). Gender and smoking cessation: A factor structure comparison of processes of change. *Journal of Consulting and Clinical Psychology, 64,* 130–138.

Perz, C. A., DiClemente, C. C., & Carbonari, J. P. (1996). Doing the right thing at the right time? Interaction of stages and processes of change in successful smoking cessation. *Health Psychology, 15,* 462–468.

Piotrowski, N., Delucchi, K., Presti, D., Tunis, S., & Young, M. (1995, August). *Stage of change, alcohol dependent inpatients, and early treatment response.* Poster presented at the 103rd annual convention of the American Psychological Association, New York.

Prochaska, J. O. (1979). *Systems of psychotherapy: A transtheoretical analysis.* Homewood, IL: Dorsey.

Prochaska, J. O., & DiClemente, C. C. (1982). Transtheoretical therapy: Toward a more integrative model of change. *Psychotherapy: Theory, Research and Practice, 19*(3), 276–288.

Prochaska, J. O., & DiClemente, C. C. (1984). *The transtheoretical approach: Crossing the traditional boundaries of therapy.* Malabar, FL: Krieger.

Prochaska, J. O., & DiClemente, C. C. (1986). Toward a comprehensive model of change. In W. R. Miller & N. Heather (Eds.), *Treating addictive behaviors: Processes of change* (pp. 3–27). New York: Plenum.

Prochaska, J. O., & DiClemente, C. C. (1992). Stages of change in the modification of problem behavior. In M. Hersen, R. Eisler, & P. M. Miller (Eds.), *Progress in behavior modification* (Vol. 28, pp. 184–214). Sycamore, IL: Sycamore.

Prochaska, J. O., DiClemente, C. C., Velicer, W. F., Ginpil, S., & Norcross, J. C. (1985). Predicting change in smoking status for self-changers. *Addictive Behaviors, 10,* 395–406.

Prochaska, J. O. Velicer, W. F., DiClemente, C. C. & Fava, J. S. (1988). Measuring the processes of change: Applications to the cessation of smoking. *Journal of Consulting and Clinical Psychology, 56,* 520–528.

Prochaska, J. O., Velicer, W. F., Guadagnoli, J. O., Rossi, J. S., & DiClemente, C. C., (1991). Patterns of change: Dynamic typology applied to smoking cessation. *Multivariate Behavioral Research, 26,* 83–107.

Prochaska, J. O., DiClemente, C. C., & Norcross, J. C. (1992). In search of how people change: Applications to the addictive behaviors. *American Psychologist, 47,* 1102–1114.

Prochaska, J. O., DiClemente, C. C., Velicer, W. F., & Rossi, J. S. (1993). Standardized,individualized, interactive and personalized self-help programs for smoking cessation. *Health Psychology, 12,* 399–405.

Prochaska, J. O., Norcross, J. C., & DiClemente, C. C. (1994). *Changing for good.* New York: Morrow.

Prochaska, J. O., Velicer, W. F., Rossi, J. S., Goldstein, M. G., Marcus, B. H., Rakowski, W., Fiore, C., Harlow, L. L., Redding, C. A., Rosenbloom, D., & Rossi, S. R. (1994). Stages of change and decisional balance for twelve problem behaviors. *Health Psychology, 13*(1), 39–46.

Prochaska, J. O., Velicer, W. F., Fava, J., Rossi, J., & Tsoh, J. (1997). *A stage matched expert system intervention with a total population of smokers.* Manuscript under review.

Prochaska, J. O., Velicer, W. F., Fava, J., Ruggiero, L., Laforge, R., & Rossi, J. (1997). *Counselor and stimulus control enhancements of a stage matched expert system for smokers in a managed care setting.* Manuscript under review.

Project MATCH Research Group. (1997). Matching alcoholism treatments to client heterogeneity: Project MATCH post-treatment drinking outcomes. *Journal of Studies on Alcohol, 58*(1), 7–29.

Rollnick, S., Heather, N., & Bell, A. (1992). Negotiating behaviour change in medical settings: The development of brief motivational interviewing. *Journal of Mental Health, 1,* 25–39.

Rollnick, S., Heather, N., Gold, R. E., & Hall, W. (1992). Development of a short "Readiness to Change Questionnaire" for use in brief, opportunistic interventions among excessive drinkers. *British Journal of Addiction, 87,* 743–754.

Rossi, J. S. (1992, March). *Stages of change for 15 health risk behaviors in an HMO population.* Paper presented at the 13th annual meeting of the Society for Behavioral Medicine, New York.

Rossi, J. S., Martin, R. A., Redding, C. A., Rosenbloom, D., Rohsenow, D. J., & Monti, P. M. (1996). Decisional balance and stages of change for cocaine use. *Journal of Consulting and Clinical Psychology* (under review).

Rothfleisch, J. (1997). Assessing different measures of stages of change with cocaine dependent clients. Unpublished doctoral dissertation, University of Houston, Houston, TX.

Rychlak, J. (1968). *A philosophy of science for personality theory.* Boston: Houghton Mifflin.

Sewell, M. S., Carbonari, J. P., & DiClemente, C. C. (1994, August). *A Markov analysis of stages of change in smoking cessation.* Paper presented at the annual convention of the American Psychological Association, Los Angeles.

Shaffer, H. J. (1992). The Psychology of stage change: The transition from addiction to recovery. In J. H. Lowison, P. Ruiz, R. B. Millman, & J. G. Langrod (Eds.), *Substance abuse: A comprehensive textbook* (2nd ed., pp. 100–105). Baltimore: Williams & Wilkins.

Smith, K. J., Subich, L. M., & Kalodner, C. (1995). The Transtheoretical Model's stages and processes of change and their relation to premature termination. *Journal of Counseling Psychology, 42,* 34–39.

Snow, M., Prochaska, J., & Rossi, J. (1994). Processes of change in Alcoholics Anonymous: Maintenance factors in long-term sobriety. *Journal of Studies on Alcohol, 55,* 362–371.

Sorenson, G., Thompson, B., Glanz, K., Feng, Z., Kinne, S., DiClemente, C. C., Emmons, K., Heimendinger, J., Probart, C., Lichtenstein, E., & Working Well Trial. (1996). Worksite-based cancer prevention: Primary results from the Working Well Trial. *American Journal of Public Health, 86*(7), 939–947.

Stotts, A., DiClemente, C. C., Carbonari, J. P., & Mullen, P. (1996). Pregnancy smoking cessation: A case of mistaken identity. *Addictive Behaviors, 21,* 459–471.

Strecher, V. T., & Rimer, B. (1987). *Freedom from smoking for you and your family.* New York: American Lung Association.

Tsoh, J. (1995). *Stages of change, drop-outs and outcome in substance abuse treatment.* Unpublished doctoral dissertation, University of Rhode Island, Kingston.

U.S. Department of Health and Human Services. (1990). *The health benefits of smoking cessation: A report of the Surgeon General* (DHHS Publication No. CDC 90-8416). Washington, DC: U.S. Government Printing Office.

Velasquez, M. (1997). *Psychiatric severity and behavior change in alcoholism: The relation of the transtheoretical model variables to psychiatric distress in dually diagnosed patients.* Unpublished doctoral dissertation, University of Texas School of Public Health, Houston, TX.

Velicer, W. F., Prochaska, J. O., Bellis, J. M., DiClemente, C. C., Rossi, J. S., Fava, J. L., & Steiger, J. H. (1993). An expert system intervention for smoking cessation. *Addictive Behaviors, 18,* 269–290.

Velicer, W. F., Prochaska, J. O., Fava, J. L., Laforge, R. G., & Rossi, J. S. (1997). *Interactive versus noninteractive interventions and dose-response relationships for stage matched smoking cessation programs in a managed care setting.* Manuscript under review.

Veroff, J., Douvan, E., & Kulka, R. A. (1981a). *The inner America.* New York: Basic Books.

Veroff, J., Douvan, E., & Kulka, R. A. (1981b). *Mental health in America.* New York: Basic Books.

Werch, C. E., & DiClemente, C. C. (1994). A multi-component stage model for matching drug prevention strategies and messages to youth stage of use. *Health Education Research: Theory and Practice, 9,* 37–46.

Wierzbicki, M., & Pekarik, G. (1993). A meta-analysis of psychotherapy dropout. *Professional Psychology: Research and Practice, 29,* 190–195.

2

The Transtheoretical Model

A Critical Overview

ROBIN DAVIDSON

INTRODUCTION

Some years ago models that charted apparently discrete stages of emotional, attitudinal, or behavioral change were very influential in clinical and social psychology. For example, Kübler-Ross (1969) described stages in an individual's emotional response to terminal illness, Parkes (1972) wrote about the phases of grief, and social psychologists Hall, Cross, and Freedle (1972) classified attitudinal change in terms of discrete stages. In subsequent years much was written about stage models, but it has been suggested that stage theories may be undergoing a dignified burial in psychology (Bandura, 1998).

The story of the waxing and waning, the popularity, and arguably the demise of stage models over the years is strikingly similar in the various literatures. Indeed, it could be said that the reaction of practitioners and researchers to stage models can in itself be characterized by the stages of uncritical acceptance, guarded and sympathetic commentary, downright hostility, and finally archival status: that is, good to have around for reference purposes but not particularly useful. Older readers will recall the criticism of Kübler-Ross's stage model. Not everyone facing death experiences the five stages of denial, anger, bargaining, depression, and acceptance. Some people oscillate between stages. There are individual differences in stage sequencing according to age, background, and personality and perhaps it is really a continuum rather than discrete categories. Almost three decades later clinicians would say that the precise details of the

---

ROBIN DAVIDSON • Department of Psychology, Belvoir Park Hospital, Belfast BT8 8JR, Northern Ireland.

Treating Addictive Behaviors, 2nd ed., edited by Miller and Heather. Plenum Press, New York, 1998.

Kübler-Ross model do not really matter much but would concede that it has made a contribution in terms of its face validity for patients and has helped some understand their fluctuating emotions when facing death (Smith, 1993).

The current popular response to the transtheoretical model is illustrative of these phases, with the possible exception of the archival state. After Prochaska and DiClemente (1983) first described the model, it enjoyed universal popularity in the addiction field. It was variously hailed as intuitively appealing and making good sense (Saunders & Allsop, 1991), as giving expression to a profound truth about the process of changing drug-using behavior (Stockwell, 1992) and even as a Kuhnian paradigm shift that cast the process of change in an entirely new mold (Orford, 1992). The first mild, almost self-conscious critique appeared nearly a decade after the model was first enunciated (Davidson, 1992). This was followed in the succeeding years by rather more animated and detailed criticism, culminating in Bandura's (1998) pronouncement.

A contemporary version of the transtheoretical model of change has been detailed in Chapter 1 (this volume). It describes the stages, processes, and levels of change but it is the stage component which has caught the imagination of addiction specialists over the years. The stage aspect of the model has evolved as its key component; therefore, the discussion here focuses primarily on this component. Most of the work on validating the transtheoretical model has been produced by James Prochaska's research group at the University of Rhode Island where the model originated. This review emphasizes independent research carried out by workers unconnected with the Rhode Island group and highlights issues surrounding the construct validity of the model itself rather than the efficacy of stage-matched manuals or computer-generated systems. This is a sympathetic review that outlines some of the observations made about the model over recent years, but it should be interpreted against this author's continued enthusiasm about its use.

While the transtheoretical model of change has been by far the most influential in the addiction literature, it was not the first. The prototypical stage model was that of Glatt (1972), whose U-shaped curve adorned most alcohol workers' walls during the seventies. Later Tuchfeld (1976) articulated a two-stage model based on his excellent qualitative study of more than 50 recovered problem drinkers. Essentially he argued that when defensive avoidance becomes untenable, a commitment to change is made. This is followed by a maintenance stage during which time the person develops coping strategies to reduce the possibility of relapse. Kanfer and Grimm (1980) also defined a number of what they called critical transition points in the motivational and behavioral phases of change. It was against this backdrop that the transtheoretical model of change emerged.

OPERATIONALIZING THE STAGES

A fundamental observation about all stage models in psychology is that stages are an artificial segmentation of a naturally occurring continuum of change. Human behavioral and attitudinal change is too complex to be simplified into discrete phases, stages, or categories.

Bandura (1998) argued that the transtheoretical model describes pseudo-stages as if they were genuine transitions. He cited Piaget's work as one of the few genuine stage models in which an individual permanently evolves from one stage to a qualitatively different one. For example, preoperational thought is genuinely and qualitatively distinct from its successor, operational thought. It is a transition from caterpillar to butterfly rather than from a small caterpillar to a somewhat larger one. In order to elaborate on this we must examine how the stages are operationalized.

A number of staging algorithms have been described for the transtheoretical model but all include a time component. Precontemplation, contemplation, and preparation are arbitrary differences in degree of *intention.* Essentially, a precontemplator has no stated intention to stop drug use in the next 6 months. Someone in the preparation stage is actively planning to quit within 30 days and has made at least one attempt to stop in the past year. Contemplators intend to quit somewhere between 30 days and 6 months.

Action and maintenance are arbitrary divisions on a *behavioral* continuum. Having quit less than 6 months ago is said to represent the action stage while abstinence for longer than 6 months is said to indicate maintenance. In other words, a person can evolve through some stages simply with the passage of time but with no real alteration in psychological state. Sutton (1996b) and Bandura (1998) make the same point. The stages are not grounded in transformational change and the cutoff points are arbitrary. Why not 20 rather than 30 days? Why not 9 months instead of 6 months? Furthermore, if an individual is required to have made at least one recent quitting attempt before qualifying as a preparer, logically he or she cannot go through the preparation stage during a first successful change attempt. Pierce, Farkas, Zhu, Berry, and Kaplan (1996) comment that the stage classification system, which is the foundation on which the transtheoretical model is built, fails the test for basic requirements of scientific measurement.

Besides this type of chronological algorithm, the authors of Chapter 1 argue that there are other methods for successfully isolating stages—for example, the University of Rhode Island Change Assessment scale (URICA). This is a psychometrically sound, 32-item questionnaire with subscales corresponding to the stages. Using cluster analysis on individuals presenting with a range of addiction problems, clear profiles corresponding to the predicted stages have emerged with considerable consistency. The standardization rigor of URICA cannot be disputed, but it should be acknowledged that a scale may have excellent psychometric credentials yet be trivial because of the way the questions are framed. A scale will, for example, have almost perfect internal validity if there is semantic overlap between the questions. In other words, if each item means the same as the other items, they will share specific variance as well as common factor variance. If the same item is phrased in several different ways, this will result in large interitem correlations that will inflate the reliability coefficients. It will also lead to a spurious factor structure. This problem of semantic overlap between scale items was described by Cattell (1971) as a "bloated specific," but has been largely ignored over the years by psychometricians in their quest for psychometric perfection at the expense of assessing something meaningful (Cooper, 1997). A few examples of URICA items which may help clarify this are outlined in Table 1. The key question that supersedes any issues about psychometric excellence is whether, for the average questionnaire completer, there is any real distinction between the items. That is to say, does the response to the first item of any pair logically determine the response to the second item? The reader can make this decision from the example items illustrated in Table 1, but it is possible that we have here a psychometrically sound

TABLE 1
Sample Items from URICA

PRECONTEMPLATION
(1) As far as I'm concerned I don't have any problems that need changing.
(2) I guess I have faults but there is nothing that I really need to change.

CONTEMPLATION
(1) I have a problem and I really think I should work on it.
(2) I've been thinking that I want to change something about myself.

ACTION
(1) I am doing something about the problems that have been bothering me.
(2) Anyone can talk about change, I am actually doing something about it.

MAINTENANCE
(1) It worries me that I might slip back on a problem I have already changed and I am here to seek help.
(2) I am here to prevent myself from having a relapse of my problem.

scale with categories that are no more than bloated specifics. The same criticism can be leveled at other scales, such as the Readiness to Change questionnaire (RTC; Rollnick, Heather, Gold, & Hall, 1992), that are explicitly based on the trans-theoretical model.

TRANSITION ACROSS STAGES

Some time ago Davidson (1992) commented that it is not at all clear what pro-portion of people who successfully deal with an addiction do so by progressing in an orderly way through the stages. In response to this, Prochaska, DiClemente, Velicer, and Rossi (1992) made two important observations. First, they reiterated a previous finding that this is a spiral rather than a circular model in that people generally tend to recycle through the stages until some eventually achieve main-tenance. Only a small minority demonstrate a strictly linear pattern. Second, they suggested that successful individuals must pass through each stage, as they had not found anyone who successfully omitted a stage in the personal change pro-cess. Strictly speaking, as noted previously, there is a certain lack of internal logic about this second observation inasmuch as people who successfully quit the first time cannot by definition have passed through the preparation stage, as it requires one previous quit attempt. There is some evidence that would indicate successful noncontemplative change among heavy drinkers admitted to general medical wards (Orford, Somers, & Daniels, 1992). For those admittedly few drug users who seem to stop abruptly as a result of sudden and personally significant life events (Tuchfeld, 1976), there does not seem to be an inevitable progression through stages. More significantly, the original Prochaska, Velicer, Guadagnoli, Rossi, and DiClemente (1991) data have been reanalyzed in order to clarify movement through the stages (Sutton, 1996a). Subjects were smokers and only 16% showed a stable progression over 2 years from one stage to the next in the sequence. Apparently *none* of the sample of 544 self-changers showed a stable progres-sion through three or more stages. In other words, stable progression across two stages is the maximum and over one third of the sample remained in the same stage over the 2-year period. Members of the Rhode Island group (McConnaughy, DiClemente, Prochaska, & Velicer, 1989) and others have argued that the so-called simplex structure of the model means that there are significantly higher correlations between adjacent than between nonadjacent stages. Sutton's reanalysis of the data cast some doubt on this finding; it seemed that nonadjacent stages were almost as highly correlated as adjacent ones.

In the light of the Sutton findings, Budd and Rollnick (1996) reanalyzed some of the original data used to validate the RCQ. Through the use of structural equation modeling, these authors addressed questions that relate to the simplex structure of the stages and whether the data could best be modeled by a single continuous variable or discrete stages. The original sample consisted of 174 men the majority of whom showed low to moderate alcohol dependence. Essentially it was found that the stages or factors were highly intercorrelated and the best fit was a single variable that represented a continuum of readiness to change. Bandura (1998) put this another way when he claimed that we cannot substitute a categorical approach for a process model of human adaptation and change. In addition, the Budd and Rollnick (1996) data did not fit the simplex structure proposed by McConnaughy and colleagues (1989). The implication of these results is that it is very difficult in practice to classify people into discrete categories; this raises questions about the model's internal validity.

Based on current findings it is premature to conclude that good quality change will occur only if an individual proceeds through each stage of change, as no one showed a stable progression through more than two stages. Furthermore, it may be best to construe the change process as a continuous variable rather than a series of discrete stages.

PREDICTIVE VALIDITY

The litmus test for any clinical model is its usefulness in specifying the conditions under which future change will occur and the extent and direction of that change. Clinicians are primarily interested in the unique contribution of stage membership over other, better established predictors of outcome variance associated with behavioral improvement. This is a correlational rather than a causal question, inasmuch as the stage system is simply a taxonomy and the error of tautological interpretation of stages as causes rather than descriptions of behavior change is well known. An individual does not stop drug use simply because he or she moves from preparation to action. Nonetheless, it is valid to inquire about the relationship between current stage and future substance use.

Farkas and colleagues (1996) noted that, because of the absence of multivariate analyses of predictors, we cannot draw conclusions about the relative importance of stage membership predicting future behavior. These authors attempted to remedy this situation in their analysis of longitudinal data from a large cohort of more than 2,000 Californian smokers by examining the proposition that stage membership would add significantly to addiction-related variables in the prediction of future smoking cessation. They argued that traditional addiction-type variables include the number and type of cigarettes smoked daily, the latency of the first cigarette in the day, and the duration of the most recent quit attempt. The outcome measure was smoking status at between 1- and 2-year follow-up; this was treated as a binary variable. Because of the way outcome was assessed, a logistic regression analysis was employed to untangle the relative and combined predictive power of the stage and addiction variables. The authors found that the former did not add to the predictive power of the overall model. In other words, the best predictors of future cessation were the so-called addiction variables, particularly the duration of the most recent quit attempt and the number of cigarettes smoked per day. Farkas and colleagues (1996) went on to question the utility of stage membership as an independent, stand-alone predictor of future smoking behavior. Although these findings are substance specific, it is argued that they have clear and far-reaching implications for the treatment and prevention of all addictive behavior.

This is a unique and important piece of work that is highly relevant to any discussion about deployment of the stage model of change, but it is not without its problems. The stage allocation algorithm used may have been an oversimplification, in that it was based on only two questions. The first was "Are you planning to quit smoking in the next 30 days?" Those smokers who answered "no" were asked a further question, "Are you contemplating quitting smoking in the next 6 months?" Those who answered "yes" to the first question were assigned to preparation; those who answered "yes" to the second were assigned to contemplation, and two negative responses signaled precontemplation. Stockwell (1996) disagreed with the assumption that a single question is adequate for allocating a person to a subtle psychological construct such as motivational stage. Furthermore, multiple addiction variables were pitted against a single stage variable, so they inevitably have a greater possibility of accounting for a higher proportion of the outcome variance, and follow-up time was not accurately specified. The study, to some extent, may also be comparing unlike constructs: what is essentially a measure of intention is pitted against measures of current smoking behavior. The only outcome variable was smoking cessation, so the study does not tell us anything about other important future behavior such as uptake or attrition from treatment programs that may be more related to current intention. The relationship between the model and process variables such as recruitment into treatment and subsequent retention has been fully discussed in Chapter 1.

A conceptual rather than a methodological criticism was made by Hughes (1996), who questioned the value of comparing models in a "first past the post takes all fashion" (p. 1284) and emphasized the importance of how they interrelate rather than merely their relative power. The Rhode Island group (Prochaska *et al.*, 1994) also takes exception to this horse race approach to scientific endeavor. The group has always been keen on cooperation rather than competition and would say that it is more apt to examine how one model can integrate empirically with the core constructs of another. The group eloquently wrote that this integrative approach can "take us beyond the parochial pairing of partisan theories towards a more comprehensive approach to behavior change" (p. 44). On the other hand, some would argue that, even if models agree on behavior change but are incompatible with regard to etiology, they offer contrary prescriptions on how to change behavior and apparent integration is nothing more than woolly-minded eclecticism.

Despite these shortcomings, the study by Farkas and colleagues (1996) does represent an important first step in the demonstration that addiction variables can outperform stage categorization in the prediction of smoking cessation in the relatively long term.

INTENTION AND BEHAVIOR

As noted previously, the stage model describes a simple, quantitative, chronological relationship between intention and behavior. This notion of intention or preparedness to change is central to our understanding of eventual cessation of addictive behavior. Although Farkas and colleagues (1996) emphasize the overriding importance of so-called quitting history in determining future success, the importance of aspiration, motivation, or intention to change popularized by the transtheoretical model should not be underestimated. Stockwell (1996), in a response to Farkas and colleagues' findings noted that "preparedness to change matters greatly and should be central to the design and delivery of interventions" (p. 1283).

Some other stage models are perhaps more systematic in their integration of intention and behavior and incorporate determinants explicitly derived from social learning theory. These series of models have been used primarily to inform research on health behavior decision making and they emphasize cognitive processes as crucial determinants in the adoption of health beneficial behavior. Of late they have been increasingly cited in the addiction literature and have been summarized elsewhere (Davidson, 1997; Sutton, 1996c). The health belief model (Becker, 1974) was superseded by the Theory of Reasoned Action (Ajzen & Fishbein, 1980) and then came the Theory of Planned Behaviour (Ajzen, 1988). Of interest in the present discussion is that the latter model detailed a number of variables which predicted intention and tightly specified the relationship between intention and behavior. The most recent addition to this family of models is the Health Action Process Approach (HAPA) developed by Ralph Schwarzer (1992). This model will be discussed briefly to highlight some of the overlap and contrasts with the transtheoretical model.

Schwarzer (1992) commented quite legitimately that traditional relapse prevention approaches like that of Marlatt and Gordon (1985) have focused on the maintenance stage and more or less ignored change strategies in what he called the motivational and action stages. In the motivational phase an individual forms an intention to decrease risky behavior in favor of more adaptive behaviors. The action phase is an attempt to explain the relationship between intention and subsequent behavior, with emphasis placed on what are termed action control and action plans. Estimates of the relative proportion of outcome variance explained by predictors of intention have been drawn from a variety of sources. For example, outcome beliefs and subjective normative influences contribute to about one half of the variance in intention to stop smoking. However, stated intention to quit accounts for only some 20% to 25% of the variance in actual observed long-term smoking abstention. When beliefs about self-efficacy are added to the model its explanatory power increases substantially both at the intention and behavioral change levels. Schwarzer (1992) and others would now argue that self-efficacy expectation, which is the belief that addictive behavior can be changed by mobilizing personal resources, is the most powerful predictor of intention and subsequent behavioral control. For example, Kok, De Vries, Mudde, and Strecher (1990) demonstrated that efficacy expectation alone could account for over two thirds of the variance in smoking intention and subsequent abstinence. The reason for briefly alluding to HAPA is that it could be seen as a tightly specified model that describes the stages of intention and behavioral change, not in terms of some temporal sequence, but rather in terms of efficacy and outcome beliefs and particularly the relative contribution of self-efficacy at all points in the change process. It also introduces the ideas of action planning and control in bridging the gap between intention and behavior.

The Rhode Island group has, over the years, attempted to identify factors that may correlate with stage membership or facilitate movements through the stages. The remainder of this chapter summarizes some of the evidence on matching stage with change processes and expectations. The integrative view would be that, if individuals in different stages also differ on etiologically relevant variables drawn from other related theories, this could be interpreted as support for the idea of distinct stages. In other words, as noted in Chapter 1, these should be stage-specific, unique tasks that need to be successfully accomplished in order to move forward.

STAGE AND PROCESS

The stage component of the transtheoretical model is a temporal organizational structure that tells us something about when people change but nothing about how or why they change. It is a taxonomy of dispositional states and is at best descriptive rather than explanatory. Unlike the approach of Schwarzer (1992), which specifically links social learning theory constructs with intention and behavior change, the ten processes of the transtheoretical model are essentially interventions drawn from a range of diverse behavioral, cognitive, existential, and psychodynamic theories that have been retrospectively grafted onto the stage system. Rather than using the term transtheoretical, Davidson (1992) called the model atheoretical inasmuch as it does not systematically integrate a description of behavioral change with psychological determinants of that change. The stages are simply categorical sequelae of these underlying factors, some of which are incompatible with others in terms of their etiological significance. Bandura (1998) also noted that this menagerie of interventions is not transtheoretical, which implies an "overreaching integration of apparent diversity," and that the link between the stage and process is loose and debatable, with one not being explicitly derived from the other.

Nonetheless, as outlined in Chapter 1, the Rhode Island group has produced some evidence to suggest that there is matching between stage and process. It has been suggested (Davidson, 1991) that individuals in contemplation are more likely to benefit from consciousness-raising strategies, whereas maintainers, for example, tend more toward behavioral strategies such as counterconditioning and stimulus control. Prochaska, DiClemente, and Norcross (1992) put it more simply by saying that good quality change depends on people "doing the right things [processes] at the right time [stages]" (p. 1110). There is some independent evidence for this position from other centers for different populations of drug users.

Belding, Iguchi, and Lamb (1996) examined the relationship between stage and process for a cohort of patients on a methadone maintenance program. They derived four process scales and found that the match between process and stage was largely consistent with predictions of the transtheoretical model. In a group of heavy drinkers, Heather, Rollnick, Bell, and Richmond (1996) found that for precontemplators and contemplators a brief motivational interview was relatively more beneficial than a skills-based intervention. It could be argued that motivational interventions lean more heavily toward self-reevaluation and consciousness raising while a skills-based, more behavioral approach places emphasis on processes such as stimulus control and contingency management.

Project MATCH (Project MATCH Research Group, 1997) is undoubtedly the largest treatment trial ever mounted in the field of alcohol addiction. This multicenter project sought a match of a variety of client characteristics with each of three treatment modalities, namely, motivational enhancement therapy, twelve-step facilitation, and cognitive behavior therapy. Meticulous attention was paid to all aspects of the trial design although some problems associated with the interpretation of results have been highlighted elsewhere (Davidson, in press). The motivation hypothesis of Project MATCH is relevant to the present discussion. As noted previously, each treatment modality could be said to emphasize different processes and the motivational measure was a subset of the URICA scale. The prediction was that subjects lower in motivation would respond relatively better to motivational enhancement therapy than cognitive behavior therapy. On a percentage days abstinence outcome measure and contrary to expectation, less motivated outpatients in the cognitive behavioral condition in fact did relatively better in the short term. This effect, however, was reversed in the expected direction at 15-month follow-up when the less motivated subjects gained more from motivational therapy. There was no matching effect for more highly motivated subjects. The authors drew a tentative conclusion about the possible delayed effect of motivational enhancement therapy for those initially less motivated subjects.

These treatment studies are essentially cross-sectional designs in that they relate current stage membership to the optimal benefit of the deployment of a particular process profile. Weinstein, Rothman, and Sutton (in press) noted that the key test of the model is the identification of factors that produce *transitions* between adjacent stages. Sutton (1996a) made the same point and noted that specific strategies that cause people to move from one stage to the next stage in the sequence are currently not well defined. In other words, are different processes employed more frequently by people who progress from one stage to the succeeding one than by those who remain static? Herzog, Abrams, Emmons, Linnan, and Shadel (1997) was the first reported study that specifically attempted to address this question. Using a series of logistic regression analyses, they found that the pattern of processes employed by a group of problem drinkers failed to predict movement from each stage to the adjacent one. These authors concluded that individual processes of change do not predict progressive stage movement. There was, however, some evidence that processes predicted movement *within* the contemplation stage.

The Herzog and colleagues (1997) study awaits replication. However, based on current evidence it may be premature to draw firm conclusions about the role of particular processes in helping individual drug users progress from one stage to

the next. Although we can say with some assurance, for example, that contemplators may employ different processes than preparers, we cannot yet conclude that
the contemplator who progresses to preparation has a different process profile
than the contemplator who remains static.

STAGE AND EXPECTATION

Besides examining the link between stage and process, the Rhode Island
group, in its quest for integration, has attempted to explore the relationship between the stage schema and cognitive constructs. This work has primarily taken
account of a type of outcome expectation (perceived pros and cons of smoking)
and efficacy expectations as one progresses through the stages.

The relationship between decisional balance or outcome expectations and
stage of change has been examined for behaviors ranging from smoking and cocaine cessation to sunscreen use and radon gas exposure (Prochaska *et al.*, 1994).
The decisional balance is a balance sheet of comparative expected gains and losses
accruing from anticipated behavioral change. For example, the pros of smoking
could be its pleasurable or subjective anxiolytic effects and the cons could include
negative health consequences or disapproval from others. The cons can be thought
of as facilitators of change and the pros can be seen as barriers to change. The general findings from the Rhode Island group are that during precontemplation the
pros of smoking will be judged to outweigh the cons, whereas the opposite will be
the case in the action stage. Crossover is said to occur during the preparation and
contemplation stages. Velicer *et al.* (1985) have demonstrated that those in the
contemplation stage are high on both, whereas the preparation stage is rather like
action, namely, high cons and low pros. Furthermore, it has been noted that an increase in the cons is more important than a decrease in the pros if an individual
is to successfully negotiate the stages. Kraft, Sutton, and McCreath (in press) have
attempted to replicate these findings in a sample of Norwegian smokers by testing
the hypothesis of discontinuity patterns between pros and cons across stages.

Details of the statistical analysis employed by Kraft and his colleagues are not
described here. Suffice it to say that they were able to replicate the Rhode Island
findings to some extent in that they demonstrated a relationship between the decisional balance construct and stage of change in the predicted direction. They concluded that this discontinuity pattern appears to partially support the idea of
qualitatively different stages but with the caveat that no distinction can be drawn
between preparers and contemplators. In other words, they would say that there are
really only two intentional stages, that is, precontemplators and the rest. However
the data could also be interpreted as supporting a model in which an underlying
continuous variable has been divided into a number of ordered categories. The results from this cross-sectional study can be seen as providing some, albeit tentative,
support for the proposition that the comparative weighting of pros and cons depends on the individual's stage of change. However, Herzog and colleagues (1997)
examined the power of the pros and cons balance to predict evolution from one
stage to the next in the sequence and found that the pros and cons of smoking did
not significantly predict progressive stage movements. These results may indicate
that although people at different stages utilize different outcome expectations,

changes in such expectations are not well identified for people who move from one stage to the succeeding one.

The Rhode Island group has also related stage membership to efficacy expectations. For smokers it was argued that a large difference between low self-efficacy and degree of temptation during precontemplation narrows through contemplation and preparation. Efficacy beliefs were said to increase quite substantially at the action stage. Bandura (1998) rather dismissively commented that it hardly requires the encumbrance of stage theorizing to tell us that precontemplators do not have what it takes to succeed. This may be a slight oversimplification. For example, an interesting relationship is said to exist between efficacy, process, and stage. High efficacy scores in early stages are correlated with more change process activity and at the later stages high efficacy is correlated with decreased change process activity. In summary, however, the Rhode Island work suggests that efficacy evaluation is a solid predictor in the later stage transitions but less important in moving people from precontemplation to contemplation. This is in part supported by the work of De Vries and Backbier (1994) who found, in a cohort of pregnant smokers, that the key significant difference in self-efficacy was between the action and the earlier intentional stages.

In their group of smokers, Kraft and colleagues (in press) also attempted to replicate the Rhode Island findings by hypothesizing that there would be no difference in efficacy evaluation between precontemplation and contemplation but that this would become significant between contemplation and preparation. Efficacy was defined in terms of the subjective probability of succeeding when a quit attempt is made. The hypothesis was not supported, in that they found no significant differences in efficacy estimates among any of the intentional stages. These authors concluded that, as far as this criterion variable was concerned, the results failed to support the view that contemplation and preparation can be distinguished as qualitatively separate stages. As was the case with outcome expectations, Herzog and colleagues (1997) found that self-efficacy did not predict progressive stage movement. Clearly, further work needs to be done to specify the nature of the relationship between efficacy, stage, and process and indeed Prochaska *et al.* (1992) would themselves counsel caution in the interpretation of efficacy self-evaluations with individuals from different stages of change.

CONCLUSION

It is clear from this review that stage theories, at least within addiction, are far from requiring burial. The extent of ongoing work drawn from a variety of centers and stimulated by the transtheoretical model is a testament to its continued heuristic value and longevity. Unlike theories, models cannot be falsified and pertain more to the context of discovery than to the context of justification. They do wax and wane but clearly the transtheoretical model continues, for the time being, to suggest new hypotheses and connections. It has also been practically useful, for example, in the development of the individualized, tailored intervention programs summarized in Chapter 1. Stage-matched manuals for smokers are consistently and considerably better than more standardized self-help programs. The model has clear implications for the design and implementation of future effective interventions. More generally, it has caught the imagination of workers in the addiction field because of its obvious pansubstance application. It synthesizes diverse treatment methods and appeals to workers from a variety of theoretical orientations. It also places motivational interviewing in a context important to many practitioners.

The work reviewed in this chapter, however, has highlighted a number of ongoing problems with the model, including the following:

1. There are significant deficiencies in the chronological algorithms and psychometric instruments employed for stage allocation.
2. Many of the data taken as supporting the stage approach are arguably more consistent with a continuum model of health behavior change.
3. Most studies that relate stage to process have been cross-sectional designs in that particular processes are matched with stage membership. There has as yet been no demonstration of processes or beliefs that facilitate stage progression in a systematic way. This is the key test for any stage model.
4. Progression may not occur in either a spiral or cyclical fashion if the best maximum forward movement is limited to only two adjacent stages.

Stockwell (1992) noted that perhaps the precise details of the model do not really matter much. Rather, it is important that, along with other health behavior decision-making models, the transtheoretical model has given expression to the importance of intention and motivation in the treatment of addictive behavior. Despite its shortcomings this model shows no signs of easing gracefully into senility. This volume is an ample demonstration that the model continues to challenge our understanding of the process of change.

REFERENCES

Ajzen, I. (1988). *Attitudes, personality and behaviour.* Milton Keynes, England: Open University Press.

Ajzen, I., & Fishbein, M. (1980). *Understanding attitudes and predicting social behavior.* Englewood Cliffs, NJ: Prentice Hall.

Bandura, A. (1998). Health promotion from the perspective of social cognitive theory. *Psychology and Health, 13,* 4.

Becker, H. M. (1974). *The health belief model and personal health behavior.* Thorofare, NJ: Slack.

Belding, M. A., Iguchi, M. Y., & Lamb, R. J. (1996). Stages of change in methadone maintenance: Assessing the convergent validity of two measures. *Psychology of Addictive Behaviors, 10*(3), 157–166.

Budd, R., & Rollnick, S. (1996). The structure of the Readiness to Change questionnaire: A test of Prochaska & DiClemente's transtheoritical model. *British Journal of Health Psychology, 1,* 365–376.

Cattell, R. (1971). *Personality and mood by questionnaire.* San Francisco: Jossey Bass.

Cooper, C. (1997). *Individual differences.* London: Arnold.

Davidson, R. (1991). Facilitating change in problem drinkers. In R. Davidson, S. Rollnick, & I. MacEwan, I. (Eds.) *Counselling problem drinkers.* London: Routledge.

Davidson, R. (1992). Prochaska and DiClemente's model of change: A case study. *British Journal of Addiction, 87,* 821–822.

Davidson, R. (1997). Motivational issues in the treatment of addictive behavior. In G. Edwards and C. Dare (Eds.), *Psychotherapy, psychological treatments, and the addictions* (pp. 173–188). Cambridge: Cambridge University Press.

Davidson, R. (in press). The treatment of substance abuse and dependence. In P. Salkovskis (Ed.), *Comprehensive clinical psychology.* Oxford, England: Elsevier Science.

De Vries, H., & Backbeir, E. (1994). Self-efficacy as an important determinant of quitting among pregnant women who smoke: The O-pattern. *Preventive Medicine, 23*, 176–174.

Farkas, A. J., Pierce, J. P., Zhu, S-H., Rosbrook, B., Gilpin, E. A., Berry, C., & Kaplan, R. M. (1996). Addiction versus stages of change models in predicting smoking cessation. *Addiction, 91*(9), 1271–1280.

Glatt, M. M. (1972). *The alcoholic and the help he needs.* London: Priory Press.

Hall, W., Cross, W., & Freedle, R. (1972). Stages in the development of black awareness: An exploratory investigation. In R. Jones (Ed.), *Black psychology* (pp. 101–113). New York: Harper & Row.

Heather, N., Rollnick, S., Bell, A., & Richmond, R. (1996). Effects of brief counselling among male heavy drinkers identified on general hospital wards. *Drug and Alcohol Review, 15*(1), 29–38.

Herzog, T. A., Abrams, D. B., Emmons, K. M., Linnan, L., & Shadel, W. (1997). *Do processes of change predict stage movements?* San Francisco: Society of Behavioural Medicine.

Hughes, J. R. (1996). My dad can predict better than your dad: So what? *Addiction, 91*(9), 1284–1285.

Kanfer, F. H., & Grimm, G. L. (1980). Managing clinical change: A process model of therapy. *Behaviour Modification, 4*, 419–444.

Kok, G., De Vries, H., Mudde, A., & Strecher, V. (1990). Planned health education and the role of self efficacy: Dutch research. *Health Education Research, 5*, 157–168.

Kraft, P., Sutton, S., & McCreath (in press). *Psychology and health.*

Kübler-Ross, E. (1969). *On death and dying.* New York: Macmillan.

Marlatt, G. A., & Gordon, J. R. (1985). *Relapse prevention: Maintenance strategies in the treatment of addictive behavior.* New York: Guilford.

McConnaughy, E. A., DiClemente, C. C., Prochaska, J. O., & Velicer, W. (1989). Stages of change in psychotherapy: A follow-up report. *Psychotherapy, 26*, 494–503.

Orford, J. (1992). Davidson's dilemma. *British Journal of Addiction, 27*, 832–833.

Orford, J., Somers, M., & Daniels, V. (1992). Drinking amongst medical patients: Level of risk and models of change. *British Journal of Addiction, 87*(12), 1691–1703.

Parkes, C. M. (1972). *Bereavement: Studies of grief in adult life.* New York: International Universities Press.

Pierce, J. P., Farkas, A., Zhu, S., Berry, C., & Kaplan, R. M. (1996). Should the stage of change model be challenged? *Addiction, 91*(9), 1290–1293.

Prochaska, J. O., & DiClemente, C. C. (1983). Stages and processes of self-change of smoking: Toward an integrated model of change. *Journal of Consulting and Clinical Psychology, 51*, 390–395.

Prochaska, J. O., DiClemente, C. C., & Norcross, J. (1992). In search of how people change: Applications to addictive behaviors. *American Psychologist, 7*, 1102–1114.

Prochaska, J. O., DiClemente, C. C., Velicer, F., & Rossi, J. S. (1992). Criticisms and concerns of the transtheoretical model in light of recent research. *British Journal of Addiction, 87*(6), 825–828.

Prochaska, J. O., DiClemente, C. C., Velicer, F., & Rossi, J. S. (1993). Standardized, individualized, interactive and personalised self-help programmes for smoking cessation. *Health Psychology, 12*, 399–405.

Prochaska, J. O., Velicer, W. F., Guadagnoli, E., Rossi, J. S., & DiClemente, C. C. (1991). Patterns of change: Dynamic typology applied to smoking cessation. *Multivariate Behavioral Research, 26*, 83–107.

Prochaska, J. O., Velicer, W. F., Rossi, J. S., Goldstein, M. G., Marcus, B. H., Rakowski, W., Fiore, C., Harlow, L. L., Redding, C. A., Rosenbloom, D., & Rossi, S. R. (1994). Stages of change and decisional balance for 12 problem behaviours. *Health Psychology, 13*, 39–46.

Project MATCH Research Group. (1997). Matching alcoholism treatments to client heterogeneity. Project MATCH post treatment drinking outcomes. *Journal of Studies on Alcohol, 58*, 7–29.

Rollnick, S., Heather, N., Gold, R., & Hall, W. (1992). Development of a short 'readiness to change' questionnaire for use in brief opportunistic interventions among excessive drinkers. *British Journal of Addiction, 87*, 743–754.

Saunders, B., & Allsop, S. (1991). Helping those who relapse. In R. Davidson, S. Rollnick, & I. McEwan (Eds.), *Counselling problem drinkers.* London: Routledge.

Schwarzer, R. (1992). Self efficacy in the adoption and maintenance of health behaviours: Theoretical approaches and a new model. In R. Schwarzer (Ed.), *Self efficacy: Thought control of action* (pp. 84–104). New York: Hemisphere.

Smith, R. (1993). *Psychology.* Los Angeles: West.

Stockwell, T. (1992). Models of change, heavenly bodies and weltanschauungs. *British Journal of Addiction, 87*(6), 830–832.

Stockwell, T. (1996). Interventions cannot ignore intentions. *Addiction, 91*(9), 1283–1284.

Stockwell, T., Murphy, D., & Hodgson, R. (1983). The severity of alcohol dependence questionnaire: Its use reliability and validity. *British Journal of Addiction, 78*, 145–155.

Sutton, S. (1996a). Can 'stages of change' provide guidance in the treatment of addictions? A critical examination of Prochaska and DiClemente's model. In G. Edwards & C. Dare (Eds.), *Psychotherapy, psychological treatments and the addictions*, pp. 189–205. Cambridge, England: Cambridge University Press.

Sutton, S. (1996b). Further support for the stages of change model? *Addiction, 91*(9), 1287–1289.

Sutton, S. (1996c). Transtheoretical model of behaviour change. In A. Baum, C. McManus, S. Newman, J. Weinman, & R. West (Eds.), *Cambridge handbook of psychology, health and medicine* (pp. 240–242). Cambridge: Cambridge University Press.

Tuchfeld, B. (1976). *Changes in the patterns of alcohol use without the aid of formal treatment*. Research Triangle Park, NC: Research Triangle Institute.

Velicer, W. F., DiClemente, C. C., Prochaska, J. O., & Brandenburg, N. (1985). Decisional balance measure for assessing and predicting smoking status. *Journal of Personality and Social Psychology, 48*, 1279–1289.

Weinstein, N., Rothman, A., & Sutton, S. (in press). *Health psychology*.

3

Comments, Criteria, and Creating Better Models

In Response to Davidson

JAMES O. PROCHASKA AND CARLO C. DICLEMENTE

INTRODUCTION

We have appreciated Davidson's (Chapter 2, this volume) reviews and critiques of the transtheoretical model. His approach provides a balanced perspective between the strengths and weaknesses of the model and conceptual, empirical, and practical concerns. Nevertheless, we need to make clear how we differ from Davidson's interpretations and applications of the model (Prochaska & Velicer, 1997).

Whether change is best represented as a continuous process or by discrete stages is an ongoing debate. Bandura (1997) suggests that science is rejecting discrete stage models. Others, including the Nobel prize–winning physicist Prigogine (Prigogine & Stengers, 1989) and the organizational theorist Gersick (1991), view discrete models as a means of comparing and understanding discontinuous changes across such diverse disciplines as cosmology, evolution, and organizational and individual development.

Fortunately, we are not forced to make an either/or decision as to whether change is best assessed by discrete or continuous variables. In the transtheoretical model we can use both discrete variables such as stages and continuous variables such as the pros and cons of change that have predictable patterns of

JAMES O. PROCHASKA • Department of Psychology, University of Rhode Island, Kingston, Rhode Island 02881. CARLO C. DICLEMENTE • Department of Psychology, University of Maryland Baltimore County, Baltimore, Maryland 21250.

Treating Addictive Behaviors, 2nd ed., edited by Miller and Heather. Plenum Press, New York, 1998.

relationships to the stages of change. It is only when individuals focus on a single variable in the transtheoretical model that concerns arise about continuous versus discrete representations of change. One reason that the debate over change as continuous versus discrete will continue is that both perspectives are useful. And both can be included in a more comprehensive approach to change.

The stages of change segment the process of change in order to identify specific and clearly differentiated tasks and markers related to how individuals go about changing specific behaviors. Coping activities such as the processes of change, decision-making attitudes, and efficacy evaluations vary significantly by stage of change (DiClemente, Prochaska, & Gibertini, 1985; DiClemente et al., 1991). Moreover, these continuous variables do not shift in a linear fashion over time (which would argue against stages) but change over time in a curvilinear and quadratic manner, making the case for a complex multifaceted process and more discrete stages. Movement through the stages also argues against a more primitive, linear process of change. This movement includes progression, regression, and cycling through the stages. Thus, the stages have provided the framework for integrating a number of more continuous variables from social learning, decision making, and health attitudes arenas into a larger, more dynamic perspective that can complement these other models.

Operationalizing stages is a more practical and empirical concern. Staging algorithms have a practical advantage in population-based programs because they are simple and short, while having had remarkable construct and predictive validity across most studies. The URICA instrument, on the other hand, is longer but has the advantage of being more subtle and less susceptible to misreporting in contexts such as intensive clinics where people may feel pressured to report that they are more prepared to take action. It is not well known, but clients with alcohol addictions can be assessed in the precontemplation stage even though they mildly disagree with each of the eight items in the precontemplation scale. Measurement of the stages is critical and continues to be a work in progress. The URICA subscales have been replicated in several studies by investigators not associated with the development of the model. The reality is that individuals who are at any point in the process of change can experience many of the attitudes in the URICA subscales at the same time. That is why we have used cluster analysis rather than the more simplistic approach of classifying individuals solely based on which subscale score is the highest. Clear intake profiles that represent precontemplation, contemplation, and preparation stages differ in hypothesized ways on other variables (Carney & Kivlahan, 1995; DiClemente & Hughes, 1990). There are no perfect ways to measure constructs in human behavior change. However, at least two methods have been able to divide the process of change into meaningful segments or stages. Multimethod assessment with significant differences on important continuous variables further supports a stage perspective.

Davidson's concern about "bloated specifics" in the URICA measure cannot be answered by selecting the two of eight items in a scale that have the greatest similarity. This question has to be answered statistically by seeing whether measurement models using LISREL-type methods require correlated error residuals for an adequate fit. Such analyses have not needed such residuals; thus, Davidson's concerns about "bloated specifics" are not supported.

Davidson is mistaken in stating that *none* of our sample of 544 self-changers showed a stable progression through three or more stages. Of 180 smokers who started in the contemplation stage, 9 progressed to maintenance without relapsing (Prochaska, DiClemente, & Norcross, 1992). Figure 1 presents the pattern of change process used for this most successful group. We have hypothesized that one of the reasons so few find their way through this maze is that self-changers rely on trial and error learning. Such learning is known to be highly inefficient and ineffective. This is one of the key reasons that we have employed expert systems as a means of providing guided learning, which has proven to be more efficient and effective. However, even with the best methods, the process of change is not a linear one for most changers.

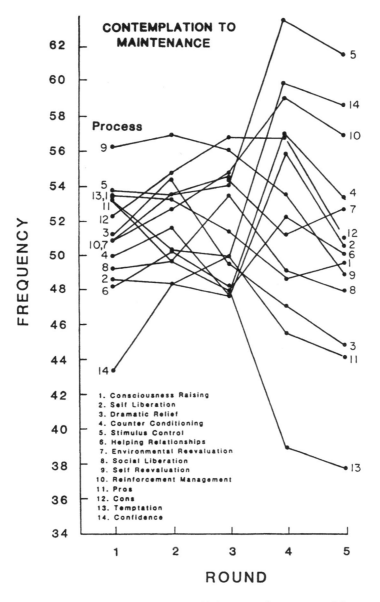

FIGURE 1. Process variables (T scores) for nine self-changers who progressed from contemplation to maintenance across five rounds over 2 weeks.

Furthermore, many of the 544 self-changers could not progress through three stages. About half of the sample were in the action and maintenance stages at the start of the 2 years. Those in action could progress only one stage and those in maintenance could not progress further. Furthermore, there is the reality of no change in status. If over one third of the sample remained in the same stage, then any future progression would have occurred beyond the time frame of the study. The longitudinal patterns over time—stable, progressing, and regressing—have played an important role in our development of stage-based expert systems that are proving to be effective with entire populations of smokers. This important data set should be seen as supporting rather than challenging the stage model. Furthermore, it is not clear why a lack of stable progressing patterns would support a continuous variable more than a discontinuous variable such as stages.

Davidson repeats Bandura's criticism that we cannot substitute a categorical approach for a process model of human adaptation and change. But, we do not substitute stage categories for continuous processes (Prochaska & Velicer, 1997). We use discrete stages as a method to integrate and match continuous processes. This criticism occurs when the stage variable is taken to equal the transtheoretical model.

Davidson reviews alternative criticisms of the stage variable that appear to contradict each other. Is it past and current behavior that best account for behavior change (e.g., Farkas, 1995; Pierce, 1995)? Or is it future intentions (e.g., Ajzen, 1998; Becker, 1974)? Or is it self-efficacy (e.g., Bandura, 1997; Schwarzer, 1992). Farkas and colleagues as well as others make an untenable assumption when they attempt to rely only on stage status as a long-term outcome predictor. Taking current stage status and trying to predict outcomes two years down the road fails to take into account the reality of recycling. Current stage status can influence outcomes and certainly does, as we have shown in numerous studies. In fact, most recently among outpatients in Project MATCH, a readiness to change variable based on the stages of change was one of the most robust predictors of drinking status through the 1-year follow-up (Project MATCH Research Group, 1997). However, individuals do move around through the stages and only a small minority of any group of smokers and other addicted individuals attempting to quit reach maintained change even after 2 years (Sewell, Carbonari, & DiClemente, 1994). Thus there is stage progression, stage regression, and stage stagnation. We must understand this movement and lack of movement through the stages of change rather than try to pit predictors against one another as Farkas and colleagues have done.

Davidson also points to the potential power of self-efficacy as a predictor that is possibly more potent than the stages. However, in our research we have clearly demonstrated that efficacy varies in its function and predictive ability depending on stage of change (DiClemente et al., 1985; DiClemente, Fairhurst, & Piotrowski, 1995). Efficacy is most important during the action and maintenance stages of change, although it can have a role in earlier transitions. Efficacy among a group of precontemplators is a different phenomenon than efficacy in a group of maintainers. One of the advantages of an integrative model like TTM is that we do not have to choose between such important variables. Instead, we seek to integrate these variables and to assess the stages at which particular processes, principles, and variables are most important as predictors and determinants of progress.

Herzog, Abrams, Emmons, Linnan, and Shadel (1997) is not the first reported study that specifically attempts to address this question (Are different processes employed more frequently by people who progress from one stage to the succeeding one than by those who remain stuck?). Our first predictive study of this type was published 12 years before Herzog's presentation (Prochaska, DiClemente, Velicer, Ginpil, & Norcross, 1985).

Herzog and colleagues (1997) failed to recognize the curvilinear relationship between variables such as pros and cons and change processes and the stages of change. Lumping all of these variables into one large analysis assumed a linear relationship between these variables, while previous research clearly indicates curvilinear relationships. It is critical for evaluation of the stages and other elements of the model to make sure that the application of the constructs is done in as accurate a manner as possible. It is impossible to conclusively prove any theory. A number of articles have purported to evaluate the model but have used poor assessments, limited numbers of subjects, and an inadequate understanding of the model constructs and the process of behavior change. Metanalysis that first defines the basic evaluation criteria needed for inclusion and reaches across behaviors is needed to make the case for or against the constructs of the transtheoretical model.

Davidson claims that the ten processes of the transtheoretical model "have been retrospectively grafted onto the stage system" (p. 32). The transtheoretical model began with the processes of change abstracted from across leading theories of therapy and behavior change (Prochaska, 1978). The stages were discovered afterward while empirically studying how different processes from divergent theories related to successful smoking cessation (DiClemente, 1978). Further empirical studies demonstrated systematic relationships between the stages and processes of change (DiClemente *et al.*, 1991; Prochaska & DiClemente, 1983). None of these discoveries had to do with "retrospective grafting." They had to do with attempting to understand how ordinary people applied change processes at different stages to progress toward quitting.

Like Bandura, Davidson has problems with the fact that these processes were "drawn from a range of diverse behavioral, cognitive, existential, and psychodynamic theories" (p. 32). They prefer the purity of linking constructs drawn only from social learning theory. Davidson suggests that some of the TTM factors "are incompatible with others in terms of their etiological significance." Theorists who prefer the purity of single systems tend to assume that integration of processes across systems is theoretically impossible. But self-changers have taught us that such processes in practice can be compatible when applied at the appropriate stages. Fortunately such folks do not let purity get in the way of practicality.

Perhaps the most promising approach to constructing a more comprehensive model of behavior change is to abstract the best that alternative models have to offer. Then searching and researching for systematic methods for integrating more constructs drawn from diverse theories can help advance an integrative transtheoretical model of change. This has been the spirit of the science and service of our transtheoretical model.

Of course the transtheoretical model is open to criticism. Absolutely. But models are not meant to be assessed by absolute criteria. For us a key question for criticism is how well the transtheoretical model performs relative to any other leading theories. Davidson compares TTM to one variable from one particular theory and then another variable from a different theory, as if the TTM should be able to perform better than all other theories combined.

We simply do not know another model of intentional human behavior change that has resulted in such practical and multiple predictions, such as who will sign up for therapy, who will show up, who will finish, and who will end up better off after treatment has ended. We do not know any alternative that has been able to demonstrate a consistent pattern of relationships among multiple variables (five stages and pros and cons of change) across 12 different behaviors and 12 different populations. We do not know any model that has led to practical methods for dramatically increasing recruitment, retention, and progress with entire populations with addictions. If Davidson could direct us to a model that can outperform TTM on such a range of relatively critical criteria, we hope we would have the wisdom to change our minds and our methods. After all, our mission is to enhance the quality and quantity of life of as many people as possible who are plagued by such problems as the addictions. For now the transtheoretical model offers us the richest heuristic perspective on change for fulfilling that mission. We will leave it to readers to judge for themselves whether the transtheoretical model can help them in their clinical and scientific endeavors.

REFERENCES

Ajzen, J. (1988). *Attitudes, personality, and behaviour.* Milton Keynes: Open University Press.

Bandura, A. (1997a). The anatomy of Stages of Change [Editorial]. *American Journal of Health Promotion, 12,* 8–10.

Bandura, A. (1997b). *Self-efficacy: The exercise of control.* New York: W. H. Freeman.

Becker, H. M. (1974). *The health belief model and personal health behaviour.* Thorofare, NJ: Slack.

Carbonari, J., DiClemente, C., & Zweben, A. (1994). A readiness to change scale: Its development, validation and usefulness. *Discussion symposium: Assessing critical dimensions for alcoholism treatment.* Presented at the 28th annual convention of the Association for the Advancement of Behavioral Therapy.

Carney, M. M., & Kivlahan, D. R. (1995). Motivational subtypes among veterans seeking substance abuse treatment: Profiles based on stages of change. *Psychology of Addictive Behaviors, 9,* 1125–1142.

DiClemente, C. C. (1978). *Processes of change in smoking cessation.* Unpublished doctoral dissertation, University of Rhode Island, Kingston.

DiClemente, C. C., & Hughes, S. O. (1990). Stages of change profiles in alcoholism treatment. *Journal of Substance Abuse, 2,* 217–235.

DiClemente, C. C., & Prochaska, J. O. (1982). Self-change and therapy change of smoking behavior. A comparison of processes of change in cessation and maintenance. *Addictive Behaviors, 7,* 133–142.

DiClemente, C. C., Prochaska, J. O., & Gibertini, M. (1985). Self-efficacy and the stages of self-change of smoking. *Cognitive Therapy and Research, 9,* 181–200.

DiClemente, C. C., Prochaska, J. O., Fairhurst, S., Velicer, W. F., Velasquez, M., & Rossi, J. S. (1991). The process of smoking cessation: An analysis of precontemplation, contemplation and preparation stages of change. *Journal of Consulting and Clinical Psychology, 59,* 259–304.

DiClemente, C. C., Fairhurst, S. K., & Piotrowski, N. A. (1995). The role of self-efficacy in the addictive behaviors. In J. Maddux (Ed.), *Self-efficacy, adaptation and adjustment: Theory, research and application.* New York: Plenum.

Farkas, A. J., Pierce, J. P., Zhu, S-H., Rosbrook, B., Gilpin, E. A., Berry, C., & Kaplan, R. M. (1996). Addiction versus stages of change models in predicting smoking cessation. *Addiction, 91*(9), 1271–1280.

Gersick, C. J. (1991). Revolutionary change theories: A multilevel exploration of the punctuated equilibrium paradigm. *Academy of Management Review, 16,* 10–36.

Herzog, T. A., Abrams, D. B., Emmons, K. M., Linnan, L., & Shadel, W. (1997, March). *Do processes of change predict stage movements?* San Francisco, CA: Society of Behavioural Medicine,

Pierce, J. P., Farkas, A., Zhu, S-H., Berry, C., & Kaplan, R. M. (1996). Should the stage of change model be challenged? *Addiction, 91*(9), 1290–1293.

Prigogine, L., & Stengers, I. (1989). *Order out of chaos: Man's new dialogue with nature.* New York: Bantam.

Prochaska, J. O. (1978). *Systems of psychotherapy: A transtheoretical analysis* (2nd ed., 1984; 3rd ed., 1993). Pacific Grove, CA: Brooks-Cole.

Prochaska, J. O. (1996). A revolution in health promotion: Smoking cessation as a case study. In R. J. Resnick & R. H. Rozensky (Eds.), *Health psychology through the lifespan: Practice and research opportunities.* Washington, DC: American Psychological Association.

Prochaska, J. O., & DiClemente, C. C. (1983). Stages and processes of self-change of smoking: Toward an integrative model of change. *Journal of Consulting and Clinical Psychology, 51,* 390–395.

Prochaska, J. O., & Norcross, J. C. (1994). *Systems of psychotherapy: A transtheoretical analysis* (3rd ed.). Pacific Grove, CA: Brooks-Cole.

Prochaska, J. O., & Velicer, W. F. (1997). Response: Misinterpretations and misapplications of the transtheoretical model. *American Journal of Health Promotion, 12,* 11–12.

Prochaska, J. O., DiClemente, C. C., Velicer, W. F., Ginpil, S. E., & Norcross, J. C. (1985). Predicting change in smoking status for self-changers. *Addictive Behaviors, 10,* 395–406.

Prochaska, J. O., DiClemente, C. C., & Norcross, J. C. (1992). In search of the structure of change. In J. D. Fisher, J. M. Chensky, & A. Nadler, (Eds.), *Initiating self-changes: Social psychological and clinical perspectives.* New York: Springer-Verlag.

Project MATCH Research Group. (1997). Matching alcoholism treatments to client heterogeneity: Project MATCH post-treatment drinking outcomes. *Journal of Studies on Alcohol, 58*(1), 1–29.

Schwarzer, R. (1992). Self-efficacy in the adoption and maintenance of health behaviors: Theoretical approaches and a new model. In R. Schwarzer (Ed.), *Self-efficacy: Thought control of action.* New York: Hemisphere.

Sewell, K. B. (1993). *The identification of Markovian processes in the transtheoretical "Stages of Change" model of smoking cessation.* Unpublished doctoral dissertation, University of Houston, Houston, TX.

Sewell, M. S., Carbonari, J. P., & DiClemente, C. C. (1994, August). *A Markov analysis of stages of change in smoking cessation.* Paper presented at the annual convention of the American Psychological Association, Los Angeles.

II

Understanding Change

Five Perspectives

The transtheoretical model provides a useful description of stages and processes of change, but has been less focused on a clear explanatory or causal account. By its very nature it is, in fact, compatible with a broad range of theoretical perspectives regarding the determinants of change. It is in this context that Part II offers a menu of perspectives on the *why* of change. Stephen Rollnick kindly took up our challenge to comment on critical conditions or prerequisites for change. His Chapter 4 provides some seasoned observations on three underlying elements reflected in the natural language of "ready, willing, and able." He also offers a provocative perspective on the idea of matching treatment interventions to clients' stages of change. In Chapter 5, Janice Brown explores self-regulation theory as a way of conceptualizing cognitive and learning mechanisms in behavior change. This was itself the subject of another international conference and volume on the treatment of addictive behaviors (Heather, Miller, & Greeley, 1991). The seven-component model of self-regulation that she describes, building on the work of Frederick Kanfer, offers some informative parallels with the stages of change.

As already seen in Part I, positive and negative drug use expectancies have been widely discussed in relation to the transtheoretical model of change. Positive and negative expectancies appear to shift in levels of importance over the course of the development and resolution of addictive behavior problems. Barry Jones and John McMahon summarize this body of research in Chapter 6 and consider its implications for research and practice. They also offer an interesting integration of what have seemed to be contradictory findings on expectancies.

Useful insights often follow when old problems are viewed through the lens of emerging fields and different disciplines. In Chapter 7, Rudy Vuchinich and Jalie Tucker offer a behavioral economics perspective on addictive behaviors, in an intriguing combination of analytic approaches from economics and radical behaviorism. Their discussion moves the conception of addictions past the individual behavior level, incorporating contextual analysis. Katherine Horgen and Kelly Brownell take this a step further in the final chapter of Part II, exhorting readers to think bigger about both causes and change strategies. They bring a public policy perspective to the addictive behaviors, giving specific examples of applications to smoking, obesity, and alcohol disorders. They remind those of us engaged in the day-to-day business of pulling victims out of the river that it is vital to work upstream as well. Their public health perspective also urges us to be mindful of the harm caused by addictive behaviors in the population at large, and not merely the more obvious victims of that harm who present for treatment. When read together, these five chapters offer a stimulating array of approaches for understanding not only the *how* but also the *why* of change in addictive behaviors.

REFERENCES

Heather, N., Miller, W. R., & Greeley, J. (Eds.). (1991). *Self-control and the addictive behaviours*. Sydney, Australia: Maxwell Macmillan.

4

Readiness, Importance, and Confidence

Critical Conditions of Change in Treatment

STEPHEN ROLLNICK

INTRODUCTION

It is no exaggeration to suggest that a crisis pervades the understanding of the critical conditions of change in the treatment of addictive behaviors. How and why people use treatment often does not match the way in which it is conceptualized, provided, and studied. The clients in Project MATCH, for example, largely evaded the most thoughtful and meticulous attempts of clinicians and researchers to understand what kind of treatment they respond best to and why (Project MATCH Research Group, 1997). The case for recommending different forms of treatment has, as a result, been left somewhat threadbare. Inevitably, in seeking to resolve this crisis, attention must turn to processes common across treatments.

This chapter addresses the following question: What are the critical psychological processes that promote behavior change? It is argued that if the treatment experience is unpacked, freed from the shackles of being labeled as a dose of this or that technical intervention, then common elements emerge that more readily match theory to practice, whether the latter involves a brief 10-minute discussion or more prolonged therapy. The chapter unashamedly uses accounts of clinical experience in addition to theory and research on behavior change. The aim is not to provide a comprehensive and definitive account of common processes, or to

STEPHEN ROLLNICK • Department of General Practice, University of Wales College of Medicine, Llanedeyrn, Cardiff CF3 7PN, Wales.

Treating Addictive Behaviors, 2nd ed., edited by Miller and Heather. Plenum Press, New York, 1998.

review the undoubtedly useful attempts of others to carry out this task. Inevitably, attention is focused on some concepts and processes at the expense of others.

The chapter begins with the concept of readiness and a critical examination of the alluring idea that treatments can be matched to the stage of change of the individual. It will be argued that matching should be more loosely defined as a process of maintaining congruence in a consultation with the person's feelings and perceptions of change. Doing this in practice often leads to questions such as, "Why do people say they are at a particular stage of change?" and "What topic should I focus on?" In answer to these questions I point to two general themes: the perceived *importance* of change and the perceived *confidence* to achieve it. The relevance of these two constructs varies across stages. They are well grounded in current models of behavior change, and they are discusssed in most forms of treatment. Their enhancement does, I believe, promote behavior change. Taken together, the three concepts of readiness, importance, and confidence provide a framework for understanding the critical conditions of change in treatment.

The question of natural recovery and the environmental forces that so often hinder or precipitate change (Orford, 1986) is not reviewed in this chapter (see Chapter 14, this volume). However, it will be seen that the concepts of readiness, importance, and confidence are likely to be the psychological channel through which social and other forces outside treatment act on the individual to trigger change.

READINESS

One of the most striking features of the stages of change model is its potential for matching clients to treatment. Attempts to compare a stage-matched intervention package with a nontailored one, mostly using computers and self-help manuals, have met with mixed success (Ashworth, 1997). Another line of recent research has examined the more specific hypothesis that a motivational intervention is best suited to clients at earlier stages of change, and a skills-building one is best suited to those at later stages of change. The evidence that has emerged from this effort can only be described as tantalizingly slender. There might be something in this idea, but why are the findings not stronger? Heather, Rollnick, Bell, and Richmond (1996) found that heavy drinkers who were *less ready* did better with a form of brief motivational interviewing than with a skills-based approach, but the other half of the matching hypothesis was not confirmed: those *more ready* to change did not do better with the skills-based approach. This study was unfortunately bedeviled by small cell sizes. In the more ambitious Project MATCH, a similar matching effect was observed among *less motivated* clients, but only in the outpatient arm of the study, and only toward the end of a long follow-up period. The other half of the matching hypothesis, as in the Heather and colleagues (1996) study, was not confirmed (Project MATCH Research Group, 1997). We might tentatively conclude that at earlier stages of change, some clients appear to benefit more from examining the costs and benefits of change than from talking about matters of action. At later stages, it appears to make less difference.

Some of this confusion might have arisen because of a tendency to oversimplify the link between stages and particular interventions. It is often said, for example, that clients in the precontemplation and contemplation stages have problems with motivation (i.e., the perceived costs of change still outweigh the benefits), hence the need for motivational interviewing; those in the preparation stage, more concerned with their ability to change, need a skills-based approach (Annis, Schober, & Kelly, 1996). Although both of these matching studies appear to have made this assumption, it could be seen as oversimplified. Clients in the preparation and action stages might still be confused about costs and benefits; those in the contemplation stage, or even the precontemplation stage, might be concerned about matters of confidence. The treatments themselves might also have been too narrowly conceptualized to fit into this kind of stage–dose thinking. Motivational interviewing, for example, was never restricted entirely to problems of ambivalence about costs and benefits. It also focused on helping people make action plans (Miller & Rollnick, 1991). Most hazardous of all, however, is the assumption that motivational problems somehow do not arise when it comes to talking about action plans around the preparation stage, as if making decisions about what to do is somehow free of doubt and struggle. To think that all that people need is some form of motivation-free, skills-based action plan could be a serious mistake.

One way of resolving these difficulties is to view matching not as a process of giving a discrete type of treatment to someone apparently in a particular stage of change but as an ongoing task of matching the topic of conversation, or strategy being used, to the shifting needs and readiness to change of the client. This is quite compatible with the way clinicians view the stages of change model. Its popularity is probably not because it allows them to match a well-defined form of treatment with a stage of change, but because of its prospects for maintaining congruence with clients more generally, often by avoiding too much action talk when clients are not ready for it.

This more flexible view of matching can be justified by the observation that clients sometimes appear to shift stages within a single session, or even within the space of a minute or two, as if they have different voices in their minds, capable of expression in words that place them in more than one stage of change. Some attempts to measure stages have encountered the same problem; that is, people can have positive scores in more than one stage of change (see Rollnick, Heather, Gold, & Hall, 1992). Under these circumstances, matching with stage-specific interventions is fraught with danger.

Conceived thus, matching is surely not just a matter of *what* is talked about, but also of *how* the client is spoken to. Speak about the "right" subject but in the "wrong" way and the outcome could be resistance. For example, argue forcefully for the benefits of change with a contemplator and the person will slip back and give voice to the world of a precontemplator.

The sensitivity of clients to the way they are spoken to is not sufficiently well understood. Certainly, the critical conditions of accurate empathy, genuineness, and respect are important and have survived the test of over 30 years of research effort (Bergin & Garfield, 1994). It is less clear however, what the role of *directiveness* should be for maintaining congruence and good treatment outcome. This term can mean many things. If it means being confrontational, as illustrated in the previous example about arguing forcefully with a contemplator, then it is probably dysfunctional, evidence for which can be gleaned from the study of therapeutic style by Miller, Benefield, and Tonigan (1993). This is likely to apply across all stages of change, including among those ready to change: Adopt an instructional tone and the outcome could be resistance, not because the topic of conversation is inappropriate, but because the way the client is spoken to generates defensiveness. However, directiveness might also mean providing structure and direction to a discussion, something that could be perfectly compatible with client-centeredness (Rollnick, Mason, & Butler, in press). Clients vary in how much direction of this kind they want. It probably depends on the person and the topic under discussion. It might also depend on the stage of change in ways yet to be fully understood.

In summary, the stages of change model could provide a useful guideline for maintaining congruence with clients. The idea that specific interventions can be matched to particular stages might be oversimplified and incompatible with the ever-shifting nature of readiness to change in the consulting room. Rather, the topic of conversation needs to be matched to readiness, using a therapeutic style compatible with Rogerian counseling. How much direction and structure different clients want is an issue yet to be clarified.

Unanswered thus far is the question, What topic of conversation is suited to people who vary in their readiness to change? How do people's needs vary across stages? We know that talk in treatment covers topics that range from fundamental questions about where to go in life, to more specific matters like the costs and benefits of change and one's confidence to achieve it. Additional concepts are clearly required in order to understand clients' needs at different stages of change.

IMPORTANCE AND CONFIDENCE

If, instead of making assumptions about clients' needs, we asked them about this more directly, what would they say? For example, would people identified as contemplators say that they were concerned about costs and benefits of change rather than action plans and their competence to achieve them? We decided to ask this kind of question of smokers in a primary care clinic, with the aim of using their observations to build a framework for brief intervention based on the stages of change model (Rollnick, Butler, & Stott, 1997). Patients identified where they saw themselves on a readiness to change continuum, and were then asked a series of scaling questions such as, "Why are you here, and not there (another point on the continuum)?" Their answers were compatible with familiar models of behavior change and associated treatment methods. Some talked about the *personal value* of change, its importance to them, or the costs and benefits of change, while others spoke about their *ability* to achieve it. With "contemplators" (i.e., people with marks midway along the line), for example, a variety of needs emerged: Some had little doubt about the importance of change but lacked confidence to achieve it, while others felt they could stop smoking if they wanted to but did not feel it was a priority at that time.

CONCEPTUAL MATTERS

The discussion of these two concepts, importance and confidence, pervades much of the literature on behavior change. The distinction served as the basis for self-efficacy theory (outcome versus efficacy expectations), although Bandura (1994) has tended to highlight the role of efficacy expectations as a predictor of behavior change. In contrast, value expectancy theories (e.g., reasoned action theory) and models of health behavior change (e.g., the health belief model) have tended to focus on expectations of the value or outcome of change. In the addictions field, a similar pattern can be discerned between models that focus on self-efficacy (relapse prevention) and those that emphasize the process of resolving the conflict between the perceived benefits and costs of change (e.g., Orford, 1985, 1986). It is worth noting that more recent models have tended to combine these as predictors of behavior change (e.g., Schwartzer & Fuchs, 1996). This move toward integration matches clinical experience of addictive problems: Clients move within and between these two domains when talking about change, as illustrated by our survey of smokers.

It seems reasonable to conclude that a critical process in changing addictive behavior has to do with asking and resolving these two questions (Is change worthwhile? and Can I succeed?) in addition to the question about readiness (Is now the right time?). Discussion of these two issues cuts across stages of change and different forms of treatment, including experiential, cognitive-behavioral, motivational interviewing, and 12-step approaches. They also arise outside treatment. Most of the theories of behavior change (e.g., self-efficacy, reasoned action), it should be recalled, do not focus on treatment but on the ingredients and predictors of change in everyday life.

Knowing someone's stage of change is thus a useful first step toward understanding their needs. This state of readiness will be influenced to varying degrees by the person's perceptions of importance and confidence. The relationship between these three concepts (importance, confidence, and readiness) is discussed toward the end of this chapter. Attention now focuses on the clinical challenges posed in talking about importance and confidence matters with clients.

CLINICAL PROCESSES

Importance

The examination of this issue can take a quite simple form. This usually has been conceived as helping the client to articulate the benefits and costs of the behavior in question, of change, or both, a strategy that has formed a central part of some applications of motivational interviewing among drug users (Saunders, Wilkinson, & Phillips, 1995) and heavy drinkers (Heather *et al.*, 1996; Rollnick, Heather, & Bell, 1992). Other intervention studies unfortunately have not studied this particular strategy in sufficient detail to reach any conclusions about its relevance.

EXAMPLE

A woman came for help with a compulsive shopping problem. There was apparently no room in the house free of bags of secondhand clothing and her husband was threatening to leave her. She said that this problem was dominating their lives. When asked about the benefits of cutting back on shopping, she said this was very important but mainly to please her husband. Shopping relieved a feeling of oppressive boredom. She would value change more if she could find other stimulating things to replace the hunt for cheap clothing. Treatment, which consisted of two brief sessions of about 30 minutes each, involved looking at the boredom issue and her need for stimulation and interest. Follow-up some months later revealed that she was doing a language teaching course. She had experienced little difficulty in controlling her urges to shop. When asked how she had done it, she replied: "I'm a determined person, that's how I acquired such good shopping bargains in the first place. All I did was use my determination in the opposite direction!"

This relatively brief intervention could have been sidetracked by the issue of competence to resist shopping urges. However, the client succeeded in articulating her main concern, the personal value or perceived importance of change, thereby effecting behavior change and preventing a family breakup.

The examination of importance can be much more complex. In the following example, the client is not only "stuck" but brings to the counselor a deeply personal, even existential or spiritual problem.

EXAMPLE

A 40-year-old man was asked about his feelings about coming off tranquilizers. It emerged that he had deep-seated fears about getting better, that the personal value of change was far from clear. He said that whatever the costs of his dependence, he nevertheless felt surrounded by a shell of security, that he had no vision of himself as anything other than living the way he did. In fact, he feared change and did not see it as a simple matter of getting "better." His levels of confidence in his ability to achieve this change were understandably low, although it became apparent that he had not thought much about this. Why then, he was asked, had he come for help? The answer revolved around hope.

Brief contact with this person might or might not help, depending on what other forces outside the consulting room are holding sway over his well-being. A critical part of the change process, however, may well be taking stock of what he wants to get out of life, whether this is done with or without the help of a counselor. If the contemplation stage was a continuum, he would probably place himself at the early contemplator end of this line. It is not difficult to imagine how any of a number of traditional treatment methods might be of help. We can also note that talk about improving competence, as guided by a skill-based treatment, would probably not be matched to his needs at this point. One hypothesis worth considering is that this man will consider change when his substance use is felt to be incompatible with his more deeply held values. It is for this reason that the term *importance* has been used in this chapter, rather than a range of other alternatives (e.g., "pros and cons"): It focuses attention on the *personal value* of change.

Confidence

People with addictive problems are often overwhelmed by a lack of confidence to cope with craving, feelings of depression, social encounters, celebrations, and so on. The predictive importance of high self-efficacy has been confirmed in numerous studies of behavior change (Bandura, 1994) and there is no shortage of strategies and manuals in the addictions field for working with clients to build confidence to overcome difficult and tempting situations (e.g., Monti, Abrams, Kadden, & Cooney, 1989). In contrast, outcome research has not emerged with consistently strong evidence for the *specific* value of confidence-building strategies, whether these have a behavioral basis or are combined with a cognitive element (Miller *et al.*, 1995). For some reason(s), this clarity of explanation about what to do with clients (i.e., build self-efficacy) does not match what happens in the consulting room. If it did, the evidence would be stronger and clinicians much more enthusiastic. Many a well-meaning counselor has complained with frustration about clients simply not seeming to come to grips with making the necessary changes. This seems to be a critical process, but how does one assist clients with it? It is probably time to move away from simple answers to this question such as, Use treatment "x" or treatment "y."

One appealing explanation for this paradox is that a sizable proportion of clients are not ready for action talk; they are more concerned with the costs and benefits of change. Those who are ready will respond to a skills-based or cognitive-behavioral treatment. Unfortunately, this hypothesis was not confirmed in either Project MATCH (Project MATCH Research Group, 1997) or the study by Heather and colleagues (1996). Another possibility is that the problem of skill building is too narrowly conceptualized as a technical matter, when, in fact, the consultation is bogged down with motivational problems about competence that counselors need to come to terms with. The way in which clients are spoken to might be critical. Here one can open up a number of unanswered questions: Do clients react against an advice-giving approach? Is it critical for them to come up with the goals and targets themselves? Is it a good idea to tackle easiest problems first? What needs to be in place before people increase their efforts to make specific changes?

EXAMPLE

A 25-year-old woman maintained a job, but only just. She lived in what her primary care physician describes as a multiple-problem family. She was grossly obese and dealt with feelings of depression with bouts of compulsive eating. She had been investigated medically over many years in search of explanations for high blood pressure, dizziness, and headache. Eventually, her family physician reported that she had begun to accept that a medical explanation would not be forthcoming, and that she would like to make changes in her lifestyle. On referral to treatment she said that she did not know where to begin. She remained in a state of helplessness for 9 months, resisting many well-meant attempts to structure weight reduction and recreational activities. One Saturday evening a friend coerced her into going dancing. She enjoyed herself a lot. She began to feel that she might be able to control her life a little more. She became more active and responded more favorably in the consulting room to target setting for weight reduction.

Our understanding of building confidence or self-efficacy might be improved if we do not conceptualize this process too narrowly as a technical matter. In the example just mentioned, low self-efficacy across different behavior changes were clearly manifestations of a more pervasive lack of self-esteem and feeling of helplessness.

It proved necessary, for example, to talk about how poorly this person valued herself. Finally, an explanation favored by Bandura (1994) calls for humility about what we can achieve. Clients need to practice; it is in the world of doing rather than talking that most progress will be made. This raises the possibility that face-to-face treatment has a limited role to play in helping people enhance their confidence in their ability to change.

In conclusion, it appears that we might be some way from knowing how to help people with confidence building. The proliferation of different forms of skills-based interventions might have resulted in a premature focus on matters of treatment technique, to the neglect of both deeply personal matters for the client and interpersonal matters in the consulting room.

READY, WILLING, AND ABLE

CONCEPTUAL MATTERS

Three concepts have been used to examine behavior change in this chapter: readiness, importance, and confidence. One way of thinking about the links between them is to view readiness as a state of mind that reflects the person's feelings about importance and confidence. Thus, if someone says, "I am definitely ready to change," and you ask this person why this is the case, reference will be made to importance and confidence, for example, "I value this change and feel able to do it." This is what happened when we spoke to smokers about their feelings of readiness. The stages of change model, with its focus on readiness, is useful precisely because it provides a general impression of how close someone is to making a change. At this level of generality, expressed readiness can be viewed as equivalent to motivation (see Miller & Rollnick, 1991, p. 14).

The phrase "ready, willing, and able" is widely used in everyday language to embrace the prerequisites for action. Its components correspond to the three concepts discussed in this chapter. The terms "willing" and "able" appear to correspond to the underlying constructs of importance and confidence, respectively. Thus, if individuals believe that change is important, they are likely to say that they are willing to do it, that they want, desire, or value this change. If people feel confident about achieving the change, they are likely to say they feel able to do it.

Importance and confidence, as noted previously, have clear reference points in models of behavior change and have also been used in analyses of the language of commitment (Amrhein, 1996). The confidence construct would appear to be the most distinct of the three, with its focus on the world of action, technique, and competence (self-efficacy). The distinction between readiness and importance is more subtle. However, examination of any number of behavior change scenarios appears to confirm the usefulness of the distinction, and the proposal that readiness is best viewed as the more general expression of the other two. Someone might be very keen on skydiving and have a strong sense of its personal value or importance. This person might also have the confidence and ability to achieve this task. Readiness, however, is that state of mind reflected in the almost inevitable wavering that occurs in the buildup to the final leap into the atmosphere. Similarly, the tranquilizer user described previously will be ready to change when at least two critical decision-making tasks are resolved: It will be personally valuable to enter a new phase of life without tranquilizers (importance), and it will be possible to cope with the demands of withdrawal, anxiety, and sleeplessness without recourse to this substance (confidence).

Attempts have been made by stages of change researchers to examine the links between these three concepts, albeit by using slightly different terminology. Hence the question, What happens to perceptions of self-efficacy (confidence) and perceptions of the pros and cons of change (importance) as people move through the stages of change? Although based largely on cross-sectional analyses, some of the findings have emerged with striking consistency across different health behaviors: Perceived costs and benefits (or pros and cons) appear to be more favorable in the later than in earlier stages (see Rollnick, Morgan, & Heather, 1996; Velicer, DiClemente, Prochaska, & Brandenberg, 1985); a *crossover* effect can also be observed across a wide range of behaviors in which the pros of change appear more important than the cons, mostly during the contemplation stage (Prochaska *et al.,* 1994). Prochaska (1994) has even identified what is termed a "strong principle," in which the benefits of behavior change are apparently more important than the perceived costs in the progression through stages. Analyses of the second concept, confidence or self-efficacy, are unfortunately less clear. While those in the action or maintenance stages have higher levels of self-efficacy, no consistent pattern emerges in earlier stages (DiClemente, Prochaska, & Gilbertini, 1985).

Finally, one might ask the question, If readiness can be thought of in stages or on a continuum, why not the other two as well? The conceptual and psychometric issues involved are likely to cover terrain similar to those encountered with the stages of change model (see Chapters 1–3). From a clinical point of view, however, there might be some value in developing this idea.

CLINICAL IMPLICATIONS

We used two continua representing importance and confidence in training physicians to conduct a quick assessment of the patient's feelings about behavior change. Although we initially made the mistake of using the more general term *motivation* instead of *importance* (Rollnick *et al.,* 1997), the value of this exercise was threefold. First, it ensured that the clinician did not focus on importance if the patient's concerns revolved around confidence, and vice versa. They were able to match the topic of conversation to what was salient for the patient. Second, the notion of a continuum gave patient and practitioner a realistic sense of how far the person was from decision making. Third, the assessment provided a rational and concrete framework for deciding what strategy to use next. In this context, strategy simply refers to a way of structuring the conversation around a particular topic so as to maximize participation and exploration by the patient (see Rollnick *et al.,* in press).

When all three concepts are assessed, the variety of patterns across people and health behaviors is more striking than the consistency. Many smokers who describe themselves as precontemplators emerge with high levels of importance but feel lacking in confidence to succeed with change. With many heavy-drinking precontemplators, the reverse often applies: They do not lack confidence but are unconvinced about the importance of change. We also encountered two smoking contemplators with a similar disparity in their needs: One felt desperate to quit, suffering from a very serious lung condition, but lacked confidence; the other, an international sports person, expressed no concerns about succeeding in quitting but said that she enjoyed her smoking and would probably quit when she decided the time was right. We inferred from these observations that stage-based interventions that focus on either importance or confidence but not both are likely to flounder.

The discussion thus far has been decidedly narrow, with a focus on three dimensions across a single behavior. When, as is often the case, clinicians come across multiple, interrelated behaviors, one has to engage in a more complex discussion (see Chapter 13, this volume).

EXAMPLE

A 45-year-old father, increasingly fearful of a range of things, used alcohol "to calm his nerves." If he smoked when he was too anxious, this could make him nauseous. Nausea led to panic and sometimes a drink. After a conversation about changes in alcohol use and smoking that focused on what this client felt able and willing to do, he said that he would like to increase his smoking, particularly in the evening, and stay relaxed enough to avoid entering a spiral of nausea, anxiety, and alcohol use.

This is a fairly unusual scenario, in which an increase in a problem behavior is pursued. However, the observation of delicate interconnectedness between different behaviors is common, and requires one to keep closely to what the client is ready, willing, and able to do. A major task facing clinicians is to set an agenda so that both parties agree about what changes to talk about (Stott, Rollnick, Rees, & Pill, 1995). Eating and exercise, gambling and alcohol, cocaine and ecstasy—clinicians need an ability to tolerate the complex and seemingly illogical relationships between changes in health behaviors and other activities. Understanding how people feel about readiness, importance, and confidence can help to clarify matters for both parties.

SUMMARY AND CONCLUSION

The amount of time and effort put into developing and evaluating specific addiction treatments unfortunately has not been matched by a detailed study of exactly what happens in counseling sessions. As a result, we have been left with a dizzying array of treatments (Miller *et al.*, 1995) with little idea of which one to use with which client. The search for the best *match* has focused on measurable pretreatment characteristics of the client or some globally defined form of treatment. In this chapter it was suggested that the best match probably lies in a closer examination of how the counselor maintains congruence with the readiness to change of the client in the treatment session. Using this as a starting assumption, a search for the critical processes in treatment has led to the discussion of two further concepts, the perceived importance of change and the person's confidence to achieve it, the enhancement of which should predict behavior change both across different treatments and in the natural environment. They could serve as a more sensitive criterion for matching research.

Helping people with addiction problems raises special issues and tensions, none more so than the delicate dance around the subject of whether change is worthwhile, how it can be achieved, and whether the person feels ready to take action. It is quite possible that a study of how these issues are tackled in treatment could lead to the construction of a single broad model or method of treatment in which counselors match their contributions or strategies to the client's feelings and perceptions of change.

REFERENCES

Amrhein, P. (1996). *The psycholinguistics of addiction: An analysis of verbal commitments in therapist–client interaction.* Paper presented to the National Institute of Drug Abuse, Washington, DC.

Annis, H., Schober, R., & Kelley, E. (1996). Matching addiction outpatient counseling to client readiness for change: The role of structured relapse prevention counseling. *Experimental and Clinical Psychopharmacology, 4,* 37–45.

Ashworth, P. (1997). Breakthrough or bandwagon? Are interventions tailored to stage of change more effective than non-tailored interventions? *Health Education Journal, 56,* 166–174.

Bandura, A. (1994). *Self-efficacy: The exercise of control.* New York: Freeman.

Bergin, A., & Garfield, S. (1994). Overview, trends and future issues. In A. Bergin & S. Garfield (Eds.), *Handbook of psychotherapy & behavior change* (4th ed., pp. 821–830). New York: Wiley.

DiClemente, C., Prochaska, J., & Gilbertini, M. (1985). Self-efficacy and the stages of change of smoking. *Cognitive Therapy and Research, 9,* 181–200.

Heather, N., Rollnick, S., Bell, A., & Richmond, R. (1996). Effects of brief counselling among heavy drinkers identified on general hospital wards. *Drug & Alcohol Review, 15,* 29–38.

Miller, W., Benefield, R., & Tonigan, S. (1993). Enhancing motivation for change in problem drinking: A controlled comparison of two therapist styles. *Journal of Consulting and Clinical Psychology, 61,* 455–460.

Miller, W., Brown, J., Simpson, T., Handmaker, N., Bien, T., Luckie, L., Montgomery, H., Hester, R., & Tonigan, S. (1995). In R. Hester & W. Miller (Eds.), *Handbook of alcoholism treatment approaches* (2nd ed., pp. 12–44). Boston: Allyn and Bacon.

Miller, W. R., & Rollnick, S. (1991). *Motivational interviewing: Preparing people to change addictive behaviour.* New York: Guilford.

Monti, P., Abrams, D., Kadden, R., & Cooney, N. (1989). *Treating alcohol dependence: A coping skills training guide.* London: Cassell.

Orford, J. (1985). *Excessive appetites. A psychological view of addiction.* Chichester, England: Wiley.

Orford, J. (1986). Critical conditions for change in the addictive behaviours. In J. Prochaska & C. DiClemente (Eds.), *Treating addictive behaviours: Processes of change).* New York: Plenum.

Prochaska, J. (1994). Strong and weak principles for progressing from precontemplation to action on the basis of twelve problem behaviors. *Health Psychology, 13*(1), 47–51.

Prochaska, J., Velicer, W., Rossi, J., Goldstein, M., Marcus, B., Rakowski, W., Fiore, C., Harlow, L., Redding, C., Rosenbloom, D., & Rossi, S. (1994). Stages of change and decisional balance for 12 problem behaviours. *Health Psychology, 13*(1), 39–46.

Project MATCH Research Group. (1997). Matching alcoholism treatments to client heterogeneity: Project MATCH posttreatment drinking outcomes. *Journal for Studies on Alcohol, 58,* 7–29.

Rollnick, S., Heather, N., & Bell, A. (1992). Negotiating behaviour change in medical settings: The development of brief motivational interviewing. *Journal of Mental Health, 1,* 25–37.

Rollnick, S., Heather, N., Gold, R., & Hall, W. (1992). Development of a short 'readiness to change' questionnaire for use in brief opportunistic interventions among excessive drinkers. *British Journal of Addiction, 87,* 743–754.

Rollnick, S., Morgan, M., & Heather, N. (1996). The development of a scale to measure outcome expectations of reduced consumption among excessive drinkers. *Addictive Behaviours, 21*(3), 377–387.

Rollnick, S., Butler, C., & Stott, N. (1997). Helping smokers make decisions: The enhancement of brief intervention for general medical practice. *Patient Education & Counselling, 31,* 191–203.

Rollnick, S., Mason, P., & Butler, C. (in press). *Health behavior change: A guide for practitioners.* Edinburgh, Scotland: Churchill Livingstone.

Saunders, W., Wilkinson, C., & Phillips, M. (1995). The impact of a brief motivational intervention with opiate users attending a methadone program. *Addiction, 90,* 415–424.

Schwartzer, R., & Fuchs, R. (1996). Self-efficacy and health behaviors. In M. Conner & P. Norman (Eds.), *Predicting health behavior: Research and practice with social cognition models* (pp. 163–195). Buckingham, England: Open University Press.

Stott, N., Rollnick, S., Rees, M., & Pill, R. (1995). Innovation in clinical method: Diabetes care and negotiating skills. *Family Practice, 12*(4), 413–418.

Velicer, W., DiClemente, C., Prochaska, J., & Brandenberg, N. (1985). A decisional balance measure for assessing and predicting smoking status. *Journal of Personality and Social Psychology, 48,* 1279–1289.

5

Self-Regulation and the Addictive Behaviors

JANICE M. BROWN

INTRODUCTION

Clearly substance abuse problems do not occur in isolation. Rather, they are often part of a cluster of other problems, many of which are associated with poor impulse control (i.e., increased risk-taking behavior) and vary over time and from individual to individual. Numerous studies of individuals with substance abuse problems have reported findings concerning increased aggression and antisocial personality (Jaffe, Babor, & Fishbein, 1988), more frequent negative social consequences (e.g., arguments with a spouse, loss of employment, encounters with law enforcement officers; Hilton, 1991), and family interaction problems (Jessor & Jessor, 1977). What is missing is an organizing theme for explaining the relationship between substance abuse and the problems with impulse control reported in the literature. The construct of self-regulation provides such a conceptual basis for understanding the etiology and maintenance of addictive behaviors.

Kanfer (1986) described self-control or self-regulation as controlling responses that reduce the probability of a behavior that is momentarily attractive. In the larger context of societal relations, self-regulatory processes are those in which individual needs are subordinated to the larger goal of the survival of the group. It is the control of these acts that are aimed at immediate satisfaction that forms part of the social contract. But many behaviors (i.e., alcohol abuse, eating disorders, sexual disorders) are not easily preventable by the social or physical environment.

JANICE M. BROWN • Department of Psychology, University of Arkansas, Fayetteville, Arkansas 72701.

Treating Addictive Behaviors, 2nd ed., edited by Miller and Heather. Plenum Press, New York, 1998.

Thus, self-regulation is seen as a result of the interplay between urges, opportunities, and social demands (Kanfer, 1977).

Although most people believe that change occurs without much thought or planning, the actual process includes carefully chosen and well-organized steps. A variety of mechanisms are used to initiate change. Theoretically, self-change is motivated by both commitment and feedback, and is most likely to be permanent if seen to be under the individual's control (Kolb, Winter, & Berlew, 1968). According to Donovan and O'Leary (1979), if individuals are in control of both internal and external sources of stress, their behavior is considered to be self-directed. It is when they have a limited repertoire of coping skills that they experience perceptions of helplessness and their behavior may become impulsive. Researchers have consistently found that disinhibition, or the lack of self-regulation, is significant in discriminating heavy substance use from light use in both men and women (Kammeier, Hoffman, & Loper, 1973; Knowles & Schroeder, 1990; Nixon, Tivis, & Parsons, 1995). This chapter discusses self-regulation theory as it relates to addictive behaviors. The chapter begins with a brief overview of self-regulation and two important issues in addictions research—delay of gratification and mechanisms of self-change. Research support for self-regulation theory is provided, the processes of self-regulation are outlined, and guidelines for prevention and treatment interventions using a self-regulatory approach are included.

SELF-REGULATION

Self-regulation is a construct encompassing developmental, personality, and social determinants of individual decisions and behavior. Self-regulation is defined as the capacity to plan, guide, and monitor one's behavior flexibly in the face of changing circumstances (Miller & Brown, 1991). The capacity for self-regulation involves, therefore, the ability to act according to a self-formulated plan even in the absence of external support structures or reward contingencies. The extent of self-regulatory control varies for a given individual across behaviors, for a given behavior across individuals, and for a given individual and behavior across time.

THE DEVELOPMENT OF SELF-REGULATION

Self-regulatory capacities originate in the context of adult–child interactions (Luria, 1961; Vygotsky, 1986). The child's performance and behavior are first controlled by the verbal instructions and reactions of external agents (e.g., parents). Children then begin to regulate some of their own actions through audible self-talk. These self-statements gradually become covert and expand their regulatory influence. It is through the use of language for self-regulatory purposes that children begin to internalize the parental regulating role and to exercise flexible and adaptive control over their own behavior. It is possible to chart the development of self-regulation, therefore, proceeding from a phase of dyadic regulation, in which the child is other-regulated, to a phase in which the child plans and directs his or her own activity in a self-regulatory fashion (Diaz, 1986; Diaz & Fruhauf, 1991). As children develop regulation of their own behavior, they become increasingly independent from external control and directives.

This perspective is consistent with social learning theory, which emphasizes that behavior is influenced by both its *actual* consequences and by *cognitive representations* of those consequences (Mischel, 1968; Rotter, 1954). Kanfer (1986, 1987) distinguished between two models of cognitive functioning: automatic and controlled. *Automatic* processing requires little dedicated attention and is seen in behaviors that are carried out with little conscious control (e.g., eating, walking, and many routine tasks of one's occupation). *Controlled* processing, on the other hand, occurs during engagement in unfamiliar behaviors or disengagement from and modification of an established automatic behavior sequence. Self-regulation, in this model, is specifically associated with controlled processing. When automatic processing occurs, self-regulation is bypassed.

CONCEPTUALIZATIONS OF SELF-REGULATION

The fundamental contributions to self-regulation theory were made by Kanfer (1970a, 1970b) who proposed a three-stage model of self-regulation. The first process involves *self-monitoring* wherein one observes and records behavior. Information regarding one's present state is a crucial element for triggering change (Bandura & Cervone, 1983; Miller, 1985). The requisite information may be received by intentional focus on one's behavior or through external sources. A fundamental process for self-regulation is the ability to recognize and monitor relevant behaviors and internal states (Kopp, 1982) and such intentional observation has been found to lead to short-term behavior changes (Bellack, Rozensky, & Schwartz, 1974; McFall & Hamman, 1971). Second is *self-evaluation*, in which the observed behavior is compared to one's personal internal criterion or norm, and the degree of discrepancy is noted. The detection of a discrepancy between one's goal and one's current state is a second prerequisite for adequate self-regulation. Finally, during the third process, *self-reinforcement*, one uses verbalizations or external rewards as a means of motivation. The processes occurring here are much broader than reinforcement, and amount to the cognitive, affective, and behavioral reactions to the self-evaluation. If little or no status or goal discrepancy is noted, motivation favors maintenance of the current behavior; a discrepancy initiates change.

Kanfer's model of change suggested that individuals develop new behaviors by using techniques ranging from strengthening controlled information processing to establishing contingencies. *Self-control* situations are defined as those in which the person engages in or stops behaviors that are initially less motivating (or less enjoyable) than the more easily carried out "automatic acts." That is, the person must override immediate gratification through controlled processing, by making decisions and generating their own incentives. Kanfer asserted that individuals whose biological and psychological makeup leave them dependent on external messages (rather than their own internal feedback cues) for guidance may be particularly vulnerable to substance abuse (Kanfer, 1986).

DELAY OF GRATIFICATION

One reported commonality of the addictive behaviors is the choice of short-term gratification at the expense of long-term detriment to the individual, society, or both (Funder, Block, & Block, 1983; Miller, 1980; Wagner, 1993). The immediate reinforcing properties of alcohol and drugs are weighed against the longer-term negative consequences of substance use. Delay of gratification is developmentally associated with the emergence of self-regulation (Kopp, 1982) and may be compromised in individuals whose self-regulation processes are disrupted. Related to this, Fingarette (1988) suggested that the choice to use drugs depends on situational factors and on the rewards and consequences the individual believes will ensue. According to Fingarette, it is the *perception* of the pattern of positive and negative reinforcers that affects the choice. For example, substance use may be motivated by the desire both to increase socialization and to remove negative affect. This interpretation suggests that choice depends, at least partially, on the accurate evaluation of those reinforcers. Indeed, the alcohol expectancy literature consistently indicates that there is a relationship between heavy use or problems and positive outcome expectancies (Chapter 6, this volume).

SPONTANEOUS REMISSION

Several studies have examined the life course of untreated alcoholism, indicating that alcohol problems can remit over time. Some common factors leading to a resolution of alcohol problems without treatment include identification with a negative role model, a personally humiliating event, the onset of serious health problems, a sudden religious experience, or exposure to educational information about alcohol misuse (Kendell & Stanton, 1966; Lemere, 1953; Tuchfeld *et al.*, 1978). The major components appear to be recognition of a need to change, disengagement from the addiction, and, ultimately, behavior change—processes that are consistent with a self-regulation theory of the process of change.

Research on both self-changers and therapy-changers has indicated common stages of change that people experience in the course of quitting addictive behaviors (DiClemente & Prochaska, 1982). Although particular processes are emphasized within each change stage, the importance of these processes lies in developing strategies for intervening across multiple levels of change. Individuals with self-regulatory deficits may well lack the ability to bring about changes in themselves and their behavior and may require varying degrees of intervention in order to initiate change. Self-regulation theory suggests specific intervention approaches that can be applied at each stage in the change process.

BUILDING ON EARLY CONCEPTUALIZATIONS OF SELF-REGULATION THEORY

Kanfer's model is complicated by the presence of additional factors that may enter during self-reinforcement: attributional factors (i.e., believing change is beyond one's control), self-efficacy (the availability of a feasible response), and the costs and benefits of changing or not changing. Given this complexity of self-reinforcement, Miller and Brown (1991) elaborated on Kanfer's model to clarify multiple processes involved, particularly those subsumed in self-reinforcement. There is evidence that deficits may be present in each of these processes in those with alcohol or drug problems or both (Miller & Brown, 1991). The model has diagnostic implications for ascertaining where self-regulation deficits may be, and points to specific strategies for intervention.

Miller and Brown (1991) have proposed a model of self-regulation that encompasses several component processes for successful behavior change. The first process of self-regulation involves *informational input.* The process of self-monitoring, or intentionally focusing on one's behavior, is central here, and is one source of information. External cues also provide information to the individual. The ability to integrate various sources of information and to make use of previous experience determine the effectiveness of an individual's capacity for coping with situational demands and are essential for initiating effective self-regulatory control (Abrams & Niaura, 1987).

The effective use of informational input triggers a recognition that current behaviors are not working, and that a change is required. This "recognition" may come from internal or external cues and involves an awareness of one's behavior that may not occur during automatic processing. With recognition, the second component of the model, *self-evaluation,* is instigated. Self-evaluation involves the comparison of informational input with a goal or norm after which the degree of discrepancy is noted. For any homeostatic system, the detection of a discrepancy is a critical feature for initiating change. When a detected discrepancy is above threshold, the third process, *instigation to change,* occurs, triggering a shift from automatic to controlled processing and the consideration of a change goal.

If the self-evaluation process yields a perceived discrepancy and an instigation to change, the individual begins to *search* for alternatives to reduce the discrepancy. This fourth process of self-regulation also involves self-efficacy (Bandura, 1982) because if the person finds an alternative that is perceived to be both efficacious and possible (high self-efficacy) that behavior is more likely to be performed. Low-efficacy estimations may result in failure to initiate change and deployment of defensive cognitive strategies to reduce the perceived dissonance (Janis & Feshbach, 1953; Orford, 1985). The identification of at least one alternative that is efficacious and feasible leads to the next process of self-regulation: *planning.* The best course of action is chosen after weighing the pros and cons of available alternatives. Planning also involves deriving specific strategies for carrying out the action and may include specific rules for behavior, coping strategies, and alternatives for increasing the repertoire of actions.

Having a plan does not ensure adherence, no matter how well-formulated and specified the plan. Once a course of action is decided on, another set of regulatory skills may be engaged to conform behavior to the plan. *Implementation* may incorporate other behavior changes as aids to compliance (Miller & Brown, 1991). This is the point at which Kanfer's conceptualization applies: the selection and practice of specific "controlling" behaviors to influence the occurrence of other target behaviors (Kanfer & Gaelick, 1986; Karoly & Kanfer, 1982). Finally, the process is cyclical as the individual evaluates progress toward the goal in a process of *plan evaluation.* Ongoing feedback is obtained (informational input), and is compared with the standard or goal (self-evaluation).

Large individual differences exist in the capacity for each of these self-regulatory processes. In individuals with attentional problems, for example, minimal distractions may overtax their attentional systems, resulting in an overreliance on external structures or a failure to engage in controlled information processing. Others may have sufficient capacity for self-evaluation or planning but may not have learned effective implementation strategies for overriding prior patterns.

Self-regulation has been applied as a conceptual basis for understanding the development of addictive behaviors (Kanfer, 1986; Miller & Brown, 1991), for guiding effective prevention efforts (Agostinelli, Brown, & Miller, 1995), and for developing effective treatment interventions (Baer, Kivlahan, Fromme, & Marlatt, 1991; Brown & Miller, 1993). Recognized addictive behaviors such as eating disorders, drug and alcohol abuse, and pathological gambling appear to share a common set of underlying psychological characteristics that may manifest differently across situations, ages, and cultures (Diaz & Fruhauf, 1991; Orford, 1985). These characteristics can be understood as deficits in the component processes of self-regulation.

SELF-REGULATORY DEFICITS AS RISK FACTORS FOR ADDICTIONS

In addictive behaviors, a maladaptive response is chosen over a more adaptive one to provide immediate gratification rather than long-term benefits. The addictive behaviors may be thought of as breakdowns in self-regulatory processes that normally exert a corrective or protective influence (Miller & Brown, 1991). The following discussion briefly considers specific deficits in self-regulatory capacity at each component process, and corresponding intervention strategies that can be considered as elements of treatment and prevention of addictive behaviors.

Informational Input

Self-regulation can break down at the very first step. There are several mechanisms by which individuals may fail to receive information regarding their current status or the adverse effects of drug use. For example, both alcoholics and obese individuals have been found to be relatively insensitive to internal cues that trigger termination of consumption (Lipscomb & Nathan, 1980). Positive expectancies for the effects of alcohol may result in differential recall of, and selective attention to, positive effects. Persons may set up their environment in such a way as to minimize discrepant sources of information, essentially allowing them to continue maladaptive behaviors without triggering the recognition of a need to change (e.g., spending time with others who drink heavily). With the best of intentions, significant others may also shield the person from adverse feedback of effects ("enabling").

Interventions for increasing the likelihood of change at this stage may include training significant others to provide objective feedback and not to interfere with negative consequences (Chapter 11, this volume). Self-monitoring of use and urges also shows a consistent initial suppressing effect; instructing individuals to direct attention to specific details of their use (i.e., times, amounts, places) is likely to impact this early process of self-regulation. A number of brief interventions designed to trigger initial self-regulatory processes have demonstrated significant suppression of alcohol use. These brief interventions which include the Drinker's Check-up (Miller, Sovereign, & Krege, 1988), education about the adverse effects of substance use and other feedback interventions (Agostinelli *et al.*, 1995) appear to disrupt automatic processing and put in motion a sequence of controlled processing (Miller & Brown, 1991).

Self-Evaluation

Once adequate information is flowing, self-evaluation, the comparison of that information to personal standards or goals, normally occurs. The detection of a discrepancy is a prerequisite for triggering a shift from automatic to controlled processing and may be inhibited by defective processing of cues. Heilbrun, Tarbox, and Madison (1979) found that alcoholics rely less on internal scanning and engage less in comparing input with previous experience or possible consequences; they suggested that these individuals may not make the necessary comparisons to detect discrepancies. Alternatively, a discrepancy may be noted, but the individual may choose to continue substance use because the perceived benefits of the addictive behavior and the costs of change outweigh the perceived benefits of change and costs of continuing. Finally, the *false consensus effect,* in which individuals incorrectly perceive their behavior to be common and normal, may mitigate change.

Providing clear, objective feedback may be insufficient without also giving the individual some reference point for comparison. Brief interventions that include a comprehensive risk assessment with *norm-referenced* feedback have been shown to be effective for suppressing alcohol use in adult (Bien, Miller, & Tonigan, 1993; Brown & Miller, 1993) and college (Agostinelli *et al.*, 1995) populations and in reducing tobacco use (Russell, Merriman, Stapleton, & Taylor, 1983). Interventions that challenge erroneous positive expectancies that individuals have for substance use have also been shown to be useful for reducing substance use (Botvin, Baker, Renick, Filazzola, & Botvin, 1984; Darkes & Goldman, 1993; Marlatt, Baer, & Larimer, 1995; Smith & Goldman, 1994).

Instigation to Change

Normally, the perception of a discrepancy between current behavior and a goal state serves to instigate change. However, one of the puzzles of addiction is that individuals often fail to respond to this discrepancy, continuing the addictive behavior despite evidence of harmful effects. What interferes with the shift from automatic to controlled processing to change behavior? Defensive cognitive processing appears to inhibit adaptive behavior change. When an individual perceives his or her personal freedom is threatened, for example, psychological reactance may occur, increasing both the attractiveness and probability of the threatened behavior (Brehm, 1966). Neuropsychological studies of alcoholics have reported a common pattern of perseverative responses, or the failure to shift response strategies when informational input indicates an earlier response is no longer adaptive (Miller & Saucedo, 1983). This inflexibility may result in establishing simplistic rules for governing behaviors that are highly resistant to change.

An important clinical point here is that the experiencing of a significant discrepancy is typically unpleasant, evoking negative emotions. It is here that people may go one of two ways: using *risk reduction* strategies which include changing addictive behaviors, or *fear reduction* techniques involving cognitive processes such as denial, rationalization, or other defensive strategies to decrease the discrepancy. Motivational enhancement approaches have been shown to be effective in instigating behavior change at this point, increasing the likelihood of choosing risk reduction rather than defensiveness (Miller, 1995; Miller & Rollnick, 1991).

Search

Instigation to change activates a cognitive search to identify alternative responses. If individuals have a perceived or actual narrow repertoire of responses, fewer alternatives will be identified. It is also here that low self-efficacy may result in the perception that no viable (efficacious) coping response exists, favoring fear reduction (defensiveness) rather than behavior change. Strategies that serve to increase efficacy expectations and strengthen coping responses may be effective during this process. Encouraging individuals to identify other areas in which they have demonstrated efficacy (e.g., beginning an exercise program, studying for a test) may generalize to support perceived efficacy for change in the addictive behavior. Presenting a menu of effective approaches from which to choose can also be useful here.

Planning

Selecting strategies, deriving guidelines, and adopting a goal are all features of the planning process. Individuals choose from available alternatives and develop specific steps for behavior change. Impairments in both decision-making and planning abilities may compromise successful engagement in these processes. Neuropsychological testing of alcoholics shows a common pattern of cognitive deficits, particularly implicating the frontal lobes (Beatty, Katzung, Moreland, & Nixon, 1995; Miller & Saucedo, 1983; Tarter & Ryan, 1983). Such impairment compromises cognitive flexibility and planned behavior change, disrupts self-monitoring, and can produce attitudes of unconcern (Miller & Brown, 1991).

Effective strategies at this step would include helping individuals develop concrete goals and providing assistance evaluating alternatives for reaching those goals. Individuals with deficient planning abilities often need guidance in selecting appropriate options and may well benefit from the use of a menu of alternative choices or options. Planning processes may be disabled by deficits in decision making and problem solving. The use of problem-solving techniques is a key element for weighing alternatives and choosing options (Goldstein, 1976; Janis & Mann, 1977).

Implementation

Once a plan has been developed, an individual conforms behavior to that plan, a process that requires sustained controlled cognitive processing. Difficulties arise for individuals with attentional problems, distractability, and a high level of reactivity when exposed to salient drug cues. Dietary restraint theory (Ruderman, 1986) may be relevant for this process. According to this theory, individuals differ widely in the degree of subjective restraint necessary to sustain moderation. High-restraint individuals experience a constant need to exercise restraint to avoid overindulgence. For these individuals, a pattern of disinhibition may result from alternating between periods of dieting and indulgence. In a study of drinking behavior, Curry, Southwick, and Steele (1987) found that individuals with external styles of controlling their drinking produced high scores on a measure of drinking restraint. These individuals, who relied less on internal self-regulation, also showed a heightened responsiveness to drinking cues. Finally, cognitions may be at issue here as well. Marlatt described a *rule violation effect,* where a single slip from planned restraint triggers cognitions that precipitate full-blown relapse (Cummings, Gordon, & Marlatt, 1980). Implementing a plan requires modifying behavior flexibly and adherence may be compromised by such rigid beliefs.

Treatment approaches for individuals evidencing difficulties implementing their plans may include those which emphasize compensatory external control strategies such as cue exposure training, self-control strategies, external cues (blood alcohol concentration tables), and behavior contracting. Each of these approaches attempts to teach the individual to respond to changing situations and does so by reinforcing the use of external control strategies. Social skills training and stress management techniques, by providing specific strategies to rely on, could also be useful for those who demonstrate impaired control in specific situations. For some, the addition of drug antagonists and disulfiram may prove to be most useful. In particular, individuals with impaired control *and* high levels of restraint may benefit more from approaches stressing abstinence rather than moderation.

Plan Evaluation

As mentioned earlier, flexible adherence to a plan requires continued self-monitoring and self-evaluation. A continued (or enlarged) discrepancy signals the need for a plan adjustment or a change in strategies (Miller & Brown, 1991). Processes important here are similar to those of the first two components of self-regulation, demonstrating that these capacities are represented as an ongoing loop rather than a linear process. Plan evaluation also involves self-reinforcement for goal attainment. Including significant others in treatment planning and implementation may help in the process of identifying reinforcers and evaluating progress toward goals. Structured, scheduled follow-up interviews for assessing progress may also assist individuals who are impaired in this component process.

SUMMARY

The study of addictions benefits from the development of integrating concepts, rather than picking and choosing among the data for responses or causes that are believed to be explanatory. This chapter has provided a context for understanding the development and maintenance of addictive behaviors. If self-regulation is an accurate model of the causal processes underlying addictive behaviors, then effective prevention and treatment strategies should be those that strengthen normal self-regulatory processes, compensate for self-regulation deficits that predispose individuals to addictive behaviors, or both (Miller & Brown, 1991).

Ideas concerning the development of addictive behaviors are important in deciding what measures are necessary for both treatment and prevention. Brief interventions may induce an enduring behavior change for individuals with relatively intact self-regulation capacities. Self-evaluation approaches and interventions designed to trigger self-management may be sufficient to instigate change for some subsets of individuals (Brown & Miller, 1993). Others may benefit from more focused strategies to impact later self-regulation processes such as planning or implementation. Deficits related to these later processes may be more effectively addressed through more focused treatment approaches (e.g., cue exposure training, behavioral marital therapy, community reinforcement approach). Knowledge of self-regulation impairments may be helpful in individualizing prevention and intervention efforts for specific individuals and populations.

In the alcohol treatment literature, a variety of approaches have been supported as having specific efficacy (Hester & Miller, 1989, 1995). The modalities receiving reasonable support include behavior contracting, behavioral self-control training, brief interventions, community reinforcement, covert sensitization, disulfiram, and social skills training, the components of which are quite sensible from a self-regulation perspective. Whether explicitly teaching self-control (behavioral self-control), modifying external contingencies (behavioral contracting, community reinforcement approach), decreasing the attractiveness of the behavior (covert sensitization), or providing new coping skills (social skills training), each is consistent with processes in the model.

Another critical feature of self-regulation theory involves clarifying *normal* processes of behavioral control. It is clearly the case that substance problems can occur in individuals without generalized deficits in self-regulation. Instead, the dyscontrol is circumscribed; self-control breaks down only in relation to specific behaviors, and often in particular circumstances (Miller & Brown, 1991). Self-regulation theory can guide primary prevention approaches in this broader arena. From this perspective, one task in preventing problem emergence is to induce, within the general population, a shift from automatic processing to controlled processing (i.e., triggering the need for vigilance and change) at relatively low and early levels of risk and problem development. For example, Prochaska and DiClemente (1982) determined that one difficulty in the prevention of substance abuse among college students is the failure of these individuals to perceive a problem. Primary prevention programming, then, could seek to signal problem recognition and engage normal change instigation and self-regulatory processes that would restrain individuals from alcohol and other drug abuse. Although it is easiest to identify substance abuse in those most severely affected, the more difficult, and perhaps more important, challenge is to identify those individuals early in their substance use involvement.

REFERENCES

Abrams, D. B., & Niaura, R. S. (1987). Social learning theory. In H. T. Blane & K. E. Leonard (Eds.), *Psychological theories of drinking and alcoholism* (pp. 131–178). New York: Guilford.
Agostinelli, G., Brown, J. M., & Miller, W. R. (1995). Effects of normative feedback on consumption among heavy drinking college students. *Journal of Drug Education, 25,* 31–40.

Baer, J. S., Kivlahan, D. R., Fromme, K., & Marlatt, G. A. (1991). Secondary prevention of alcohol abuse with college student populations: A skills-training approach. In N. Heather, W. R. Miller, & J. Greeley (Eds.), *Self-control and the addictive behaviours* (pp. 339–356). Sydney, Australia: Maxwell Macmillan.

Bandura, A. (1982). Self-efficacy mechanism in human agency. *American Psychologist, 37,* 122–147.

Bandura, A., & Cervone, D. (1983). Self-evaluative and self-efficacy mechanisms governing the motivational effects of goal systems. *Journal of Personality and Social Psychology, 45,* 1017–1184.

Beatty, W. W., Katzung, V. M., Moreland, V. J., & Nixon, S. J. (1995). Neuropsychological performance of recently abstinent alcoholics and cocaine abusers. *Drug and Alcohol Dependence, 37,* 247–253.

Bellack, A. S., Rozensky, R., & Schwartz, J. (1974). A comparison of two forms of self-monitoring in a behavioral weight reduction program. *Behavior Therapy, 5,* 523–530.

Bien, T. H., Miller, W. R., & Tonigan, J. S. (1993). Brief interventions for alcohol problems: A review. *Addiction, 88,* 315–336.

Botvin, G. J., Baker, E., Renick, N. L., Filazzola, A. D., & Botvin, E. M. (1984). A cognitive-behavioral approach to substance abuse prevention. *Addictive Behaviors, 9,* 137–147.

Brehm, J.W. (1966). *A theory of psychological reactance.* New York: Academic Press.

Brown, J. M., & Miller, W. R. (1993). Impact of motivational interviewing on participation and outcome in residential alcoholism treatment. *Psychology of Addictive Behaviors, 7,* 211–218.

Cummings, C., Gordon, J. R., & Marlatt, G. A. (1980). Relapse: Prevention and prediction. In W. R. Miller (Ed.), *The addictive behaviors: Treatment of alcoholism, drug abuse, smoking, and obesity* (pp. 291–321). Oxford, England: Pergamon.

Curry, S., Southwick, L., & Steele, C. (1987). Restrained drinking: Risk factor for problems with alcohol? *Addictive Behaviors, 12,* 73–77.

Darkes, J., & Goldman, M. S. (1993). Expectancy challenge and drinking reduction: Experimental evidence for a mediational process. *Journal of Consulting and Clinical Psychology, 61,* 344–353.

Diaz, R. M. (1986). The union of thought and language in children's private speech. *Quarterly Newsletter of the Laboratory of Comparative Human Cognition, 8,* 90–97.

Diaz, R. M., & Fruhauf, A. G. (1991). The origins and development of self-regulation: A developmental model on the risk for addictive behaviours. In N. Heather, W. R. Miller, & J. Greeley (Eds.), *Self-control and the addictive behaviours* (pp. 83–103). Sydney, Australia: Maxwell Macmillan.

DiClemente, C. C., & Prochaska, J. O. (1982). Self-change and therapy change of smoking behavior: A comparison of processes of change in cessation and maintenance. *Addictive Behaviors, 7,* 133–142.

Donovan, D. M., & O'Leary, M. R. (1979). Control orientation among alcoholics: A cognitive social learning perspective. *American Journal of Drug and Alcohol Abuse, 44,* 487–499.

Fingarette, H. (1988). *Heavy drinking: The myth of alcoholism as a disease.* Berkeley, CA: University of California Press.

Funder, D. C., Block, J. H., & Block, J. (1983). Delay of gratification: Some longitudinal personality correlates. *Journal of Personality and Social Psychology, 44,* 1198–1213.

Goldstein, G. (1976). Perceptual and cognitive deficit in alcoholics. In G. Goldstein & C. Neuringer (Eds.), *Empirical studies of alcoholism* (pp. 115–151). Cambridge, MA: Ballinger-Lippincott.

Heilbrun, A. B., Jr., Tarbox, A. R., & Madison, J. K. (1979). Cognitive structure and behavioral regulation in alcoholics. *Journal of Studies on Alcohol, 40,* 387–400.

Hester, R. K., & Miller, W. R. (1989). *Handbook of alcoholism treatment approaches: Effective alternatives.* New York: Pergamon.

Hester, R. K., & Miller, W. R. (1995). *Handbook of alcoholism treatment approaches: Effective alternatives* (2nd ed.). Boston: Allyn & Bacon.

Hilton, M. E. (1991). The demographic distribution of drinking problems in 1984. In W. B. Clark & M. E. Hilton (Eds.), *Alcohol in America: Drinking practices and problems* (pp. 87–101). Albany: State University of New York Press.

Jaffe, J. H., Babor, T. F., & Fishbein, D. H. (1988). Alcoholics, aggression and antisocial personality. *Journal of Studies on Alcohol, 49,* 211–218.

Janis, I. L., & Feshbach, S. (1953). Effects of fear-arousing communications. *Journal of Abnormal and Social Psychology, 48,* 78–92.

Janis, I. L., & Mann, L. (1977). *Decision-making: A psychological analysis of conflict, choice, and commitment.* New York: Free Press.

Jessor, R., & Jessor, S. L. (1977). *Problem behaviors and psychosocial development: A longitudinal study of youth.* Orlando, FL: Academic Press.

Kammeier, M. K., Hoffman, H., & Loper, R. G. (1973). Personality characteristics of alcoholics as college freshmen and at time of treatment. *Quarterly Journal of Studies on Alcohol, 34,* 390–399.

Kanfer, F. H. (1970a). Self-monitoring: Methodological limitations and clinical applications. *Journal of Consulting and Clinical Psychology, 35,* 148–152.

Kanfer, F. H. (1970b). Self-regulation: Research, issues, and speculations. In C. Neuringer & J. L. Michael (Eds.), *Behavior modification in clinical psychology* (pp. 178–220). New York: Appleton-Century-Crofts.

Kanfer, F. H. (1977). The many faces of self-control, or behavior modification changes is focus. In R. B. Stuart (Ed.), *Behavioral self-management* (pp. 1–48). New York: Brunner/Mazel.

Kanfer, F. H. (1986). Implications of a self-regulation model of therapy for treatment of addictive behaviors. In W. R. Miller & N. Heather (Eds.), *Treating addictive behaviors: Processes of change* (pp. 29–47). New York: Plenum.

Kanfer, F. H. (1987). Self-regulation and behavior. In H. Heckhausen, P. M. Gollwitzer, & F. E. Weinert (Eds.), *Jenseits des Rubikon* (pp. 286–299). Heidelberg, Germany: Springer-Verlag.

Kanfer, F. H., & Gaelick, L. (1986). Self-management methods. In F. H. Kanfer & A. P. Goldstein (Eds.), *Helping people change* (3rd ed., pp. 283–345). New York: Pergamon.

Karoly, P., & Kanfer, F. H. (1982). *Self-management and behavior change: From theory to practice.* New York: Pergamon.

Kendell, R. W., & Stanton, M. C. (1966). The fate of untreated alcoholics. *Quarterly Journal of Studies on Alcohol, 27,* 30–41.

Knowles, E. E., & Schroeder, D. A. (1990). Personality characteristics of sons of alcohol abusers. *Journal of Studies on Alcohol, 51,* 142–147.

Kolb, D. A., Winter, S. K., & Berlew, D. E. (1968). Self-directed change: Two studies. *Journal of Applied Behavioral Science, 4,* 453–471.

Kopp, C. B. (1982). Antecedents of self-regulation: A developmental perspective. *Developmental Psychology, 18,* 199–214.

Lemere, F. (1953). What happens to alcoholics? *American Journal of Psychiatry, 109,* 674–676.

Lipscomb, T. R., & Nathan, P. E. (1980). Blood alcohol level discrimination: The effects of family history of alcoholism, drinking pattern, and tolerance. *Archives of General Psychiatry, 37,* 571–576.

Luria, A. R. (1961). *The role of speech in the regulation of normal and abnormal behavior.* New York: Basic Books.

Marlatt, G. A., Baer, J. S., & Larimer, M. (1995). Preventing alcohol abuse in college students: A harm-reduction approach. In G. M. Boyd, J. Howard, & R. A. Zucker (Eds.), *Alcohol problems among adolescents: Current directions in prevention research* (pp. 147–172). Hillsdale, NJ: Erlbaum.

McFall, R. M., & Hamman, C. L. (1971). Motivation, structure, and self-monitoring: Role of nonspecific factors in smoking reduction. *Journal of Consulting and Clinical Psychology, 37,* 80–86.

Miller, W. R. (Ed.). (1980). *The addictive behaviors: Treatment of alcoholism, drug abuse, smoking, and obesity.* Oxford, England: Pergamon.

Miller, W. R. (1985). Motivation for treatment: A review with special emphasis on alcoholism. *Psychological Bulletin, 98,* 84–107.

Miller, W. R. (1995). Increasing motivation for change. In R. K. Hester & W. R. Miller (Eds.), *Handbook of alcoholism treatment approaches: Effective alternatives* (2nd ed., pp. 89–104). Needham Heights, MA: Allyn & Bacon.

Miller, W. R., & Brown, J. M. (1991). Self-regulation as a conceptual basis for the prevention and treatment of addictive behaviours. In N. Heather, W. R. Miller, & J. Greeley (Eds.), *Self-control and the addictive behaviours* (pp. 3–79). Sydney, Australia: Maxwell Macmillan.

Miller, W. R., & Rollnick, S. (1991). *Motivational interviewing: Preparing people to change addictive behavior.* New York: Guilford.

Miller, W. R., & Saucedo, C. F. (1983). Assessment of neuropsychological impairment and brain damage in problem drinkers. In C. J. Golden, J. A. Moses, Jr., J. A. Coffman, W. R. Miller, & F. D. Strider (Eds.), *Clinical neuropsychology: Interface with neurologic and psychiatric disorders* (pp. 141–195). New York: Grune & Stratton.

Miller, W. R., Sovereign, R. G., & Krege, B. (1988). Motivational interviewing with problem drinkers: II. The Drinker's Check-up as a preventive intervention. *Behavioural Psychotherapy, 16,* 251–268.

Mischel, W. (1968). *Personality and assessment.* New York: Wiley.

Nixon, S. J., Tivis, R., & Parsons, O. A. (1995). Behavioral dysfunction and cognitive efficiency in male and female alcoholics. *Alcoholism: Clinical and Experimental Research, 19,* 577–581.

Orford, J. (1985). *Excessive appetites: A psychological view of alcoholism.* New York: Wiley.

Prochaska, J. O., & DiClemente, C. C. (1982). Transtheoretical therapy: Toward a more integrative model of change. *Psychotherapy: Theory, Research, and Practice, 19,* 276–288.

Rotter, J. B. (1954). *Social learning and clinical psychology.* Englewood Cliffs, NJ: Prentice-Hall.

Ruderman, A. J. (1986). Dietary restraint: A theoretical and empirical review. *Psychological Bulletin, 99,* 247–262.

Russell, M. A. H., Merriman, R., Stapleton, J., & Taylor, W. (1983). Effect of nicotine chewing gum as an adjunct to general practitioner's advice against smoking. *British Medical Journal, 287,* 1782–1785.

Smith, G. T., & Goldman, M. S. (1994). Alcohol expectancy theory and the identification of high-risk adolescents. *Journal of Research on Adolescence, 4,* 229–247.

Tarter, R. E., & Ryan, C. M. (1983). Neuropsychology of alcoholism: Etiology, phenomenology, process, and outcome. In M. Galanter (Ed.), *Recent developments in alcoholism* (Vol. 1, pp. 449–469). New York: Plenum.

Tuchfeld, B. S., Simuel, J. B., Schmitt, M. L., Reis, J. L., Kay, D. L., & Waterhouse, G. L. (1978). Changes in patterns of alcohol use without the aid of formal treatment: An exploratory study of former problem drinkers. *Journal of Studies on Alcohol, 39,* 638.

Wagner, E. F. (1993). Delay of gratification, coping with stress, and substance use in adolescence. *Experimental and Clinical Psychopharmacology, 1,* 27–43.

Vygotsky, L. S. (1986). *Thought and language.* Cambridge, MA: MIT Press.

6

Alcohol Motivations as Outcome Expectancies

BARRY T. JONES AND JOHN MCMAHON

INTRODUCTION

A better understanding of the cognitive processes surrounding alcohol consumption should provide new directions for more effective alcohol education, problem prevention, and treatment. Such an understanding would be easier if the cognitive processes underpinning alcohol use were not qualitatively different from those underpinning misuse and abuse (and even dependence) and if they could be represented in a common framework. Common frameworks are considered more elegant than several qualitatively different frameworks because they predicate on fewer assumptions with wider application (Occam's razor). More pragmatically, though, it would permit the extrapolation of knowledge about alcohol cognitions from any one point on the continuum of use-misuse-abuse to any other point. This would deliver two advantages. First, a larger body of collaborated knowledge would be generated than would otherwise be the case. Second, different points along the continuum should provide glimpses of different (but related) aspects of the process and a more complete picture should be revealed. Social learning theory (Rotter, Chance, & Phares, 1972) has provided one contending common framework within which behavior (alcohol consumption) is explained by individuals having expectations of particular reinforcing effects as the outcome of behavior performance (drinking). Such expectations, or *alcohol outcome expectancies,* derive from memory structures resulting from both direct and indirect experience

BARRY T. JONES • Department of Psychology, University of Glasgow, Glasgow, G12 8QQ, Scotland. JOHN McMAHON • Centre for Alcohol and Drug Studies, University of Paisley, Paisley PA2 6BY, Scotland.

Treating Addictive Behaviors, 2nd ed., edited by Miller and Heather. Plenum Press, New York, 1998.

with alcohol. Alcohol motivation (Chapter 9, this volume) is at the center of much of contemporary thinking on alcohol consumption and alcohol outcome expectancy is one plausible representation of this central construct.

ALCOHOL OUTCOME EXPECTANCIES AND EXPECTANCY QUESTIONNAIRES

During the 1980s, alcohol expectancy researchers principally sought to explore the statistical associations between whatever expectancies individuals held and the amount of alcohol they normally consumed. From this exploration emerged considerable speculation that variation in alcohol consumption might be explained by variation in expectancies held and that an understanding derived from basic science might transfer to the applied domain. To explore associations between expectancies held and consumption researchers needed to generate comprehensive lists of expectancies and to deliver the lists in "alcohol expectancy questionnaire" format. Armed with a drinking details questionnaire and an alcohol expectancy questionnaire, researchers would be able to explore the possible association and evaluate the speculation that expectancy might have an important role in alcohol education, problem prevention, and treatment. There has been, however, considerable disagreement about what the item-content of population expectancy assessment questionnaires should be and a wide range of different expectancy questionnaires have been independently constructed and variously used. This diversity of structure and process has not helped the emergence of consistency in alcohol expectancy research. Two major issues stalled progress.

POSITIVE AND NEGATIVE ALCOHOL EXPECTANCIES

The first major issue has been the relative contribution that positive and negative expectancies might make to alcohol decisions and the extent to which they should each be represented in expectancy questionnaires. Example positive expectancies are "I would expect to be more relaxed upon drinking" or "be more sociable"; example negative expectancies are "I would expect to be belligerent upon drinking" or "get into debt."

Early researchers appeared to be of the view that only positive expectancies were of importance in understanding consumption and, indeed, the most widely used and influential questionnaire of the 1980s (Alcohol Expectancy Questionnaire [AEQ]; Brown, Goldman, Inn, & Anderson, 1980) consisted of only positive items. By contrast, a 1990s questionnaire (Negative Alcohol Expectancy Questionnaire [NAEQ]; Jones & McMahon 1994b; NIAAA, 1995) represented only negative expectancies. While still recognizing the likely importance of positive expectancy, many researchers at the end of the 1980s (e.g., Adams & McNeil, 1991) had decried the lack of attention paid to negative expectancy and it is now unusual for expectancy researchers not to assess *both* constructs in exploring associations between expectancy and consumption: either using discrete positive and negative expectancy questionnaires in combination (e.g., AEQ/NAEQ; McMahon, Jones, & O'Donnell, 1994) or using a single questionnaire developed with both positive and negative expectancy components (e.g., the Comprehensive Effects of

Alcohol Questionnaire [CEOA]; Fromme, Stroot, & Kaplan, 1993; Alcohol Outcome Expectancy Questionnaire [AOEQ]; Leigh & Stacy, 1993).

The Scope of Alcohol Expectancies

A second major issue is where an exhaustive list of positive and negative expectancy items should be sought. Best practice for questionnaire development discussed by Floyd and Widamen (1995) identifies the importance of choosing appropriate samples from which contending items should be collected and through which different data sets can be generated to carry out the exploratory and confirmatory factor analyses essential for questionnaire refinement. Yet, in alcohol expectancy research, items have most frequently been generated from convenience samples of drinkers (e.g., "captive" college students for the AEQ and CEOA, "captive" drinkers in treatment for the NAEQ) and the lack of a standardized expectancy questionnaire is probably most responsible for the difficulty in making the secure generalizations about positive or negative expectancy required of a common explanatory framework.

General Findings for Expectancies and Consumption

Positive Expectancies

These difficulties notwithstanding, there is general evidence that the greater the number of positive expectancy items an individual endorses, the more alcohol they report consuming. The fact that this positive relationship appears to hold along the length of the continuum of consumption delivers one of the principal advantages of seeking a common explanatory framework for drinking. This might have been one of the reasons for the early high confidence in positive expectancy as a drinking explanation.

Negative Expectancies

The considerably fewer results with negative expectancy appeared less consistent and there was not the same confidence in the 1980s that negative expectancy would be as explanatorily useful as positive. These few studies roughly divide into three categories: (1) a small number of studies in the early 1980s that found no relationship with consumption, (2) a small number of studies at the turn of the decade that found a *negative* relationship (individuals who consumed more endorsed fewer negative expectancy items), and (3) a small number of studies in the mid 1990s that found a *positive* relationship (individuals who consumed more endorsed more negative expectancy items). These studies are reviewed by Jones and McMahon (1996a) and Jones, Needham, and McMahon (1998), who offer the following conclusions: (1) the *null* results are due to the use of a severely restricted, unrepresentative, negative expectancy set; (2) the *negative* relationship is also due to the use of a restricted, unrepresentative, but, in addition, particularly "lightweight" negative expectancy set (e.g., "I would expect my handwriting to be affected" and "expect to feel fuzzy") which, compounded by the use of alcohol-illegal adolescents, freshmen, and other young college students as subjects, are less prominent the more a young person becomes familiar with drinking and therefore, under these circumstances, are endorsed less often; and (3) the *positive* relationship derives from studies using a considerably more comprehensive, life-appropriate and life-representative negative expectancy set that includes many "heavyweight" items (e.g., "I would expect to get into a fight," "expect to get into debt," and "expect to lose my job"). This is consistent with increases in consumption bringing increases in negative consequences that would, with repetition, translate through learning to increasing endorsements of negative expectancy items. Initially as epiphenomena, Jones and colleagues conclude, negative expectancies increase as consumption increases with, at first, no effect upon behavior until they pass a certain point and begin to impact alcohol consumption. This view, which the authors propose as the proper role of negative expectancy, is discussed more fully later in the chapter.

POSSIBLE EXPECTANCY-BASED INTERVENTIONS

If the associative link between expectancy and consumption is assumed to be directional, namely levels of expectancy cause levels of consumption, then possible expectancy-based interventions emerge for alcohol misuse and abuse. Simply put, on the one hand, positive expectancy might be a target for *reduction* (reducing the potential for drinking); on the other, negative expectancy might be a target for *enhancement* (increasing the potential for restraint). There is an IndyCar analogy (Jones & McMahon, 1994a). An IndyCar driver wanting to slow his car at a corner (or reduce alcohol consumption) has similar possibilities: ease off the gas (i.e., reduce positive expectancy) or apply the brake (i.e., enhance negative expectancy). Both will have an effect, but one is likely to be more effective. In IndyCar, it will be the brake. The question is, to what extent does the IndyCar analogy translate to alcohol interventions?

ORIGINS AND COURSE OF EXPECTANCIES

It is clear that through *direct* experience of alcohol consumption, social learning theory can readily account for the origins of alcohol expectancies. However, it is also a feature of social learning theory that *indirect* experience of behavior is a salient input and indirect experience of alcohol is such a case (learning through observing the effect of alcohol on parents and relatives). This theoretical position predicts that individuals hold alcohol expectancies prior to their first experiences of drinking alcohol. Discovering whether this is the case and whether there are asymmetries in the development of, for example, positive and negative expectancies, as well as asymmetrical associations with consumption, might have implications for a focus for intervention (as education, prevention, or treatment).

ALCOHOL EXPECTANCIES IN YOUNG CHILDREN

Alcohol expectancies are evident at a surprisingly early age. Zuckner, Kincaid, Fitzgerald, and Bingham (1995), for example, have shown that preschool children (some as young as 3) have developed alcohol schema that are capable of influencing their behavior. Their expectancies appear to become more focused as they age from 3 to 7. Many others have also shown that alcohol expectancies are present in young children before drinking occurs (most recently, Dunn & Goldman, 1996; Kraus, Smith, & Ratner, 1994) and yet others have studied how these expectancies change as young children age. Social expectancies, in particular those relating to peer approval, increase during this time (Johnson & Johnson, 1996). There is also evidence that both positive and negative expectancies increase with age (from 5 to 12; Miller, Smith, & Goldman, 1990) but, at all ages (where it is possible to compare), it is negative expectancies rather than positive that appear to be *spontaneously* attributed to alcohol (e.g., Casswell, Gilmore, Silva, & Brasch, 1988; Johnson & Johnson, 1995).

ALCOHOL EXPECTANCIES IN ADOLESCENTS

By early adolescence, and where comparisons of positive and negative expectancies are possible (e.g., Gustafson, 1992; Miller *et al.,* 1990), positive (not negative) expectancies appear to be more prominent, although the questionnaires used considerably underrepresent the negative expectancies that adolescents might hold. By contrast, however, Grube, Chen, Madden, and Morgan (1995), with what was a more equally balanced questionnaire (though still limited in scope), have shown negative (not positive) expectancies to be more prominent. Of recent studies, Grube and colleagues' is unusual in this category since it relates expectancies held to self-reported alcohol consumption rather than simply measuring expectancies held, as most others have done.

ALCOHOL EXPECTANCIES IN YOUNG AND MATURE ADULTS

Most studies with young adults have addressed positive (not negative) expectancies and demonstrated convincingly (in common with studies of mature adults) that the more positive alcohol expectancies held, the more individuals consume. It is surprising that very few studies have *concurrently* assessed the associations of positive and negative expectancies with alcohol consumption, for if, as was suggested earlier in this chapter, there might be two logical routes for expectancy-based alcohol interventions (i.e., reducing positive or enhancing negative), then discovering the relative status of each of these expectancies with respect to concurrent consumption should be a priority. However, only two small sets of research have explored the relative status of positive and negative expectancy—one using the CEOA (three studies) and the other using an AEQ/NAEQ combination (three studies). They have produced quite contradictory results and the contradiction has proved instructive.

Research Using the CEOA

Fromme, Kivlahan, and Marlatt (1986), have found with young adults a positive relationship between positive expectancy and consumption and negative relationship between negative expectancy and consumption. This has been replicated by Needham, Jones, and Taghavi-Laryani (1998) in young and mature adults and, except for negative expectancy, which replicated descriptively but not

significantly, by Werner, Walker, and Greene (1993) in young adults. These findings appear plausible, first, because the positive expectancy result is consistent
with most other studies in which only positive expectancy has been assessed
(higher expectancy, higher consumption); second, because for negative expectancy, one might reasonably expect that individuals who strongly believe consuming alcohol will bring them negative consequences will restrain their drinking
whereas others with less strong beliefs will have less restraint. However, Jones and
colleagues (1997) have a contrary view and argue the negative relationship is an
artifact of the CEOA design—an artifact that derives from the CEOA's containing
only 18 negative items of a particularly mild and temporally immediate or short-
term nature. With such a "lightweight" CEOA, they argue, even moderate and
moderately experienced drinkers are likely to report and endorse the milder negative consequences of alcohol much less frequently, because of their experience.
Lighter drinkers, however, are likely to have much higher expectations of such
negative outcomes and, through their relative inexperience, have yet to discover
that the negative expectations they hold of some of the milder consequences of
consumption might be inappropriately taught and inappropriately learned "over-
estimates" (Shewan *et al.,* in press).

Research Using the AEQ/NAEQ Combination

Whereas the CEOA contains 18 negative expectancy items of a relatively mild
and temporally immediate or short-term nature, Jones and colleagues (1998) argue
that the NAEQ contains 60 items representing a more comprehensive range of negative consequences, including many more severe items and items drawn from not
just short-term, but medium- and longer-term temporal contexts. Indeed, in cap-
turing a more life-appropriate range of negative consequences, the "heavyweight"
NAEQ comprises three explicit temporal negative expectancy subscales representing same-day consequences (that surround consumption), next-day consequences
(that occur the day after consumption), and continued-drinking consequences (that
occur should consumption continue at the current rate over months or years).
When the AEQ/NAEQ combination was used, McMahon and colleagues (1994,
with mature adults) and Jones and colleagues (1998, with young and mature adults)
found a positive relationship between negative expectancy and consumption (not
a negative relationship, as with the CEOA).

A Model for Integrating the Roles of Positive and Negative Expectancy

Although the results reported in the previous section might at first sight appear
implausible, McMahon and colleagues (1994) have argued otherwise: as individuals begin their normal drinking career "negative expectancy should *rise* [italics
added] with consumption because as consumption rises (presumably under the
control of positive expectancies) so, *inevitably,* will rise the frequency and intensity
of negative consequences and these will normally translate to negative expectancies through learning. Subsequently, at some point, negative expectancy will reach
levels at which it will begin to influence drinking decisions and drinking behavior"
(p. 351). Jones and McMahon's (1992) finding that there can be differences in levels
of negative expectancy between groups of heavy drinkers according to their usual

drinking contexts suggests that the translation is not necessarily even and might account for the generation of unrecognized alcohol problems. The three studies just cited are consistent with the view that the level of negative expectancy rises with consumption *without necessarily impacting behavior* (although the expectancies are still held and can be measured). In further support of this, McMahon and Jones (1994) have shown that rising levels do, indeed, begin to impact alcohol decisions *before* behavior is affected, in the same way that contemplators' cognitions, but not their behavior, are different from precontemplators' in the stages of change framework (Prochaska & DiClemente, 1982).

There is a final source of support for the dynamics that are proposed for negative expectancy (silently rising through a threshold to become cognition- then behavior-effective). Evidence from outside mainstream expectancy research has shown that drinkers who seek help for their alcohol problems by entering treatment or who resolve their problems in a less formal manner do so because of levels of "negative expectancy" they hold as compared with when they were drinking without problems (reviewed by McMahon & Jones, 1993). Moreover, the few studies from mainstream expectancy research that have assessed clients' negative expectancy at treatment confirm this high level (Jones & McMahon, 1994b, 1994c, 1996a, 1996b; McMahon & Jones, 1996; Morgenstern, Kahler, & Labouvie, 1997). It is difficult to see how the three studies revealing a negative association between negative expectancy and consumption in social drinkers can be extrapolated to, or economically predict these high levels. It is more defensible to conclude, as do McMahon and colleagues (1994), that the deceptively plausible negative relationship between negative expectancy and consumption is an artifact.

Expectancy Asymmetries

On the basis of what is known about the etiology of expectancies, both positive expectancy reduction and negative expectancy enhancement remain contending intervention routes for alcohol education, problem prevention, and treatment, and the IndyCar conundrum remains. The foregoing does suggest, however, that when expectancy change and consumption change are addressed, negative expectancy might be the more important construct. The next section examines this more closely for both positive and negative expectancy.

EXPECTANCY AND TREATMENT

Positive Expectancies

Although countless publications have suggested that manipulating positive expectancy might be an effective intervention, few explicitly discuss possible strategies. Brown, Millar, and Passman (1988), Connors, Maisto, and Dermen (1992), and Goldman (1989), however, do. They discuss variations on two principal strategies: (1) reducing the positive expectancies an individual might hold (a route in the IndyCar model) and (2) teaching methods alternative to alcohol consumption that deliver the same benefits consumption was thought to deliver (not a route in the IndyCar model but with no less potential). For the first strategy to have treatment utility, expectancy would have to be modifiable through some process (such as counseling) and the changes in expectancy would have to relate to subsequent changes in consumption. For the second strategy to have treatment utility, the teaching of skills or alternatives designed to deliver the anticipated alcohol benefits (as assessed by an expectancy profile) would have to produce a subsequent reduction in drinking. It is an important point that changes in the evaluations or the impact of positive expectancies (reviewed by Jones & McMahon 1996b; Jones et al., 1998), rather than the expectancies themselves, might be predicted here (Fromme et al., 1986).

Reducing Positive Expectancy

The most frequently cited (albeit indirect) evidence that reducing positive expectancy of drinkers in treatment might result in improved outcome is Brown (1985). In a follow-up of 34 patients she found that those with lower positive expectancy assessments in treatment (AEQ) had better abstinence and problem drinking outcomes twelve months after discharge. Connors, Tarbox, and Faillace (1993) and Jones and McMahon (1994c) have partially replicated this study. Other indirect evidence that reducing positive expectancies might improve outcome (sobriety) is provided by Rather and Sherman (1989), who have shown that AA attenders who have been sober longest have lower positive expectancies. Of course, this could be due to positive expectancies reducing with time since last reinforcement. But another reason could be that those with higher positive expectancies relapse sooner and cease attending, providing further indirect evidence that reducing positive expectancy is of outcome value.

Conclusions about the role of positive expectancy reduction based on indirect evidence such as this are only speculative, however, for associations do not necessarily mean causality. Darkes and Goldman (1993) have recognized this and have preferred a procedure called "expectancy challenge" that seeks to reduce the positive expectancies held by subjects (by challenging their expectations) and relate the changes in expectancies to subsequent changes in consumption. Although Kraus and colleagues (1994) have shown that positive expectancies can be reduced in adolescents using this method, they did not collect consumption data to discover what the subsequent impact might be. Darkes and Goldman (1993), however, did. They randomly allocated male college students (average age 20 years, no problem drinkers) to one of three groups: experimental (expectancy challenge), traditional prevention (alcohol education), and assessment only. Positive expectancy decrease, with a concomitant decrease in consumption 1 month later, was found only in the expectancy challenge group. These results directly show that, at least with nonproblem-drinking students and in the short term, reducing positive expectancy can reduce subsequent consumption. Studies with problem drinkers, though, have yet to be done.

Reducing the Impact of Positive Expectancies

Connors and colleagues (1993) measured the positive expectancies of problem drinkers on admission to treatment, at discharge, and at 18-month follow-up. Subjects participated in a program designed to teach moderation and alternatives to drinking. The findings showed that, although positive expectancies did not change across treatment, there was, nevertheless, a significant reduction in expectancy at follow-up. Significant relationships between expectancy and drinking were found but the strongest relationships were retrospective rather than prospective: that is, changes in drinking appeared to precede changes in expectancy, rather than changes in expectancy preceding changes in drinking (consistent with Rather and Sherman's [1989] findings with AA attenders). Interestingly, Fromme and colleagues (1986), in a similar study but with students with less severe alcohol problems, have also shown a subsequent reduction in consumption without positive expectancy changes. They have suggested that although the expectancies might not change as a direct result of the intervention, subjective evaluations of expectancy items (value of the outcome) might, and this might account for the Connors and colleagues (1993) and Rather and Sherman (1984) results. Thus, in these circumstances, less importance might be placed on alcohol as a route to obtaining benefits if alternative routes are available. Indeed, this interpretation is further supported by Miller, Westerberg, Harris, and Tonigan's (1996) finding that while expectancy predicted relapse in a univariate analysis, it did not contribute any unique predictive variance when coping skills were controlled for.

Conclusion

Except from Darkes and Goldman (1993) there is little evidence to suggest that positive expectancy can be modified by interventions that subsequently impact consumption. There is also some speculation that the relationship between expectancy and consumption might be moderated by the subjective evaluations of the expectancy items and that it might be the subjective evaluations rather than expectancies that are intervention-sensitive and subsequently reduce consumption with changes in positive expectancy following in this wake. Although this is speculation, Grube and colleagues (1995), Werner and colleagues (1993), Jones and colleagues (1998), and Needham and colleagues (1998; which includes a reanalysis of Fromme et al., 1993) have provided strong empirical evidence that this moderating effect is an important feature of alcohol consumption, although the evidence from drinkers in treatment is less clear (Jones & McMahon, 1996b; Jones, McMahon, & Needham, 1995). There is not much evidence that easing off the gas will help the IndyCar negotiate the bend. The next section looks at its braking.

Negative Expectancies

The bulk of evidence shows that individuals entering treatment are relatively ambivalent with regard to changing their behavior (e.g., Miller & Rollnick, 1991) for, although problems may be occurring, they still believe that drinking brings benefits. There is little experimental evidence (reviewed earlier) that suggests that challenging these beliefs (positive expectancies) might be a successful solution and although teaching coping skills and alternative routes to reinforcement undoubtedly has treatment utility, it raises the question whether these methods are worth the effort.

Negative Expectancies as Problem Recognition

The question why individuals in treatment should *bother* to learn coping skills has been largely ignored by expectancy researchers. Yet evidence on help-seeking and natural recovery (reviewed by McMahon & Jones, 1993) is clear on the fact that individuals seek help to (or do themselves) change their drinking in response to the anticipation of continuing or increasing future negative consequences. This points to the probable importance of *negative* expectancies in understanding alcohol problems and interventions.

Evidence reviewed earlier showed that when negative expectancy was appropriately measured, it rose with consumption in social drinkers. It was proposed that it rose "silently" to criterial level, when it would begin to impact alcohol decisions and consumption. The evidence reviewed and the model proposed is consistent with what is known of help-seeking and natural recovery. McMahon and Jones (1991) make explicit three stages in this rise (from nonproblem, through the criterion, to problem levels of consumption). First, there needs to be recognition of the problem (social, financial, health, etc.). Second, there needs to be recognition of the problem source: If, for example, a heavy drinker has marital or work problems and identifies the spouse or employer as the problem source, then little effort will be made to change drinking behavior. Such misattributions of causal direction in problem behaviors, when problems are viewed as antecedents rather than consequences of behavior, are common (Beck, Emery, & Greenberg, 1985; Thom, 1987). Finally, there needs to be a developed expectation that the problem will continue and increase in frequency or severity should the source remain unchanged.

Predictions about Negative Expectancies

If negative alcohol expectancy is tantamount to alcohol-related problem recognition, if as more problems are recognized as alcohol-related, the number of negative expectancies increases, if they aggregate as "negative expectancy," and if "negative expectancy" becomes supracriterial, then (should such an individual enter treatment) relationships between negative expectancy at treatment and posttreatment activities can be predicted.

Negative Expectancy and Treatment Outcome

Studies of the relationship between negative expectancy at treatment and outcome are few. Using a repertory grid technique to assess expectancies in treatment, Eastman and Norris (1982) showed that, of the subjects who held negative expectancies, only one tenth relapsed, whereas three quarters of those who did not relapsed.

Jones and McMahon (1994c), using the AEQ/NAEQ, measured the expectancies of alcohol-dependent drinkers on entry to residential treatment and found those who had high levels on admission were more likely to be abstinent at a 3-month follow-up. Positive expectancy did not predict outcome. In subsequent studies (Jones & McMahon, 1994b; McMahon & Jones, 1996) they used drinkers treated in a day-center and the more discriminating outcome measure of days of abstinence survivorship. They again showed that negative expectancy was a reliable predictor of outcome—the higher the negative expectancy, the longer to the first drink. Positive expectancy was not predictive in this study. In these studies it was the more serious negative expectancies associated with the "Next-day" and "Continued-drinking" subscales that were the best predictors. The "Same-day" subscale that measured the expected negative consequences accompanying or soon following drinking (and the sorts of consequences more usually represented in questionnaires) was not a predictor. This illustrates the importance of ensuring that expectancy questionnaires are comprehensively representative. Morgenstern and colleagues (1997), using a different method to assess expectancy, have replicated these findings with alcohol and extended them to other drugs. On admission, subjects were asked to rate the harm consequent on continued use in seven life domains: standard of living, work, physical health, relations with family, friendships, love relations, and self-regard. In a survival regression analysis, they found that negative expectancy was a predictor of outcome: subjects with higher negative expectancy returns had a significantly reduced risk of relapse.

A limitation of these studies is that they fail to recognize that whatever treatment is delivered might, itself, change the expectancies held and that either expectancy change during treatment or expectancy at discharge might be a more appropriate predictor of outcome. Consequently, Jones and McMahon (1996a) investigated the relationship of both admission and discharge expectancies with outcome and whether expectancies changed. They found that negative expectancy (but not positive) measured at both admission and discharge reliably predicted abstinence survivorship (days to first drink). Moreover, when admission–discharge *changes* were measured and were controlled for the admission assessment, more negative expectancy enhancement predicted better outcome, whereas positive expectancy changes (reductions) did not predict.

Conclusion

The previous sections suggest that within an alcohol context, braking the IndyCar might be more effective than easing off the gas for negotiating bends: negative expectancy (not positive) measured at admission and discharge, as well as expectancy changes, each relate to outcome. Morgenstern and colleagues (1997), employing a different method of representing negative expectancy, replicated this, adding to the robustness of the position.

The question remains whether negative expectancies can be manipulated in treatment (in the same way that positive expectancies have been through expectancy challenge) and whether whatever changes ensue impact subsequent consumption.

Manipulating Negative Expectancies in Treatment

The finding that changes in negative expectancy relate to subsequent changes in consumption suggests that negative expectancy might offer a focus for treatment. The approach the authors have used to explore this possibility is like traditional therapies in that it addresses "denial" or "problem recognition" and seeks some form of cognitive restructuring through reappraisal. However, the technology chosen to accomplish this is like motivational interviewing (Miller & Rollnick, 1991), through which clients discuss their consumption with reference to self-elected problems and future problems as a means of increasing the likelihood of changing their consumption. A feature of this style of therapy is the importance of the clients' own view of their personal circumstances as a source for nonconfrontational interaction. Important aspects of this view can be represented through clients' endorsements of the 60 items of the NAEQ and can be used to structure a 30-minute motivational enhancement session.

McMahon, Jones, and Smith (1996) allocated 120 self-referred problem drinkers who were day attenders at an alcohol treatment clinic to one of three groups on admission: Specific intervention (SI), General intervention (GI), or Assessment only (AO). Their admission assessment included the NAEQ, administered as a computer program within which each negative expectancy item was presented on the screen on its own with screen buttons representing a 5-point endorsement scale (highly unlikely, unlikely, possible, likely, highly likely). The process was monitored by therapists.

On completion of the computer assessment, subjects in both intervention groups were shown on the screen 20 NAEQ items for feedback and discussion. Each of the 20 items was presented on its own, accompanied below by the subject's previous endorsement embedded in an appropriate sentence. Initiated by the subject, the first of three questions was then displayed below. Question 1 was "What makes you believe this?" designed to encourage discussion of past occurrences. When discussion was finished, Question 2 replaced 1 on the screen: "Does this happen if you are not drinking?" designed to encourage discussion of the source of the problem. Then Question 3 replaced 2: "Do you think that this is becoming more of a problem?" designed to encourage discussion of possible future occurrences.

The 20 NAEQ items for this highly structured motivational enhancement session were chosen as follows: The first 10 items presented were drawn from the pool of items subjects endorsed as "highly likely" and the next 10 were drawn from those endorsed as "possible." For group SI, the 20 feedback items were based on the subjects' *own* endorsements—*specific feedback.* For group GI, they were based on the combined (or *mean)* endorsements of approximately 300 previous attenders at the center—*general feedback.* Group AO received no feedback and like groups SI and GI took part in the conventional treatment sessions delivered by the center for the remaining 8 days of their 10-day attendance. Feedback items were presented in the blocked order "highly likely" and "possible" for two reasons. First, the "highly likely" items and the accompanying discussion were, in the traditions of motivational interviewing (Miller & Rollnick, 1991), used as a vehicle for reinforcement. Second, the subjects should then be more open to discussing the endorsements and outcomes in which there was less certainty (items endorsed as "possible") and around which (unlike items endorsed as "unlikely" or "highly unlikely") cognitive restructuring or alcohol-related problem recognition has the greatest chance of occurring.

Consistent with Jones and McMahon (1996a), a survival regression analysis showed that the change in negative expectancy, with admission assessments controlled, predicted outcome (abstinence survivorship). At 3 months the percentage of each group who had relapsed to a first drink was SI = 68%, GI = 80%, AO =

89% (SI significantly different from GI and AO). The same was found when relapse was defined as "first heavy drink" (12 standard units or more, SI = 57%, GI = 75%, AO = 80%).

POSITIVE AND NEGATIVE EXPECTANCY

Just as with positive expectancy (through expectancy challenge), McMahon and colleagues (1996) have shown that negative expectancy can be changed and that the change can impact subsequent consumption. On the basis of this it is tempting to believe that these two constructs are "equal and opposite" and that generalizations from one to the other might be appropriate. However, Stacy, Widaman, and Marlatt (1990) have shown there is no such symmetry and this is consistent with Prochaska, DiClemente, Velicer, and Rossi's (1992) view that processes underlying the *acquisition* of a behavior (positive expectancies in the terms of this chapter) are likely to be quite different from the processes responsible for *changing* it (negative expectancies). This suggests that an understanding of positive expectancy might be directed toward education and prevention and an understanding of negative expectancy toward prevention and treatment. Consistent with this speculation is Fromme and colleagues' (1986) suggestion that attempts to change positive expectancies might have an effect only with young, naive drinkers whose expectancies are less "crystallized" and Amodeo and Kurtz's (1990) and Saunders's (1996) choice of negative expectancy as a focus for intervention with drinkers entering treatment. Indeed, Amodeo and Kurtz (1990) have found that treated problem drinkers who retained high positive expectancies, which often brought "urges" to drink, reported combating these "urges" by recalling the negative outcomes of drinking. This led them to advocate that formally teaching this negative-based coping mechanism in treatment should be an effective relapse prevention strategy. Saunders (1996) has used a similar approach based on both the negative expectancy items and the temporal construction of the NAEQ subscales. He advocates a process of "thinking through" a relapse situation, in which the therapist encourages the clients to discuss what they would expect "to happen if I went for a drink now," then "to happen later . . . next day" and "to happen in the ensuing days."

IndyCar drivers are quite familiar with the asymmetrical properties of gas and brake for slowing. The limited evidence available from expectancy research suggests that this might also extend to the relationship of positive and negative expectancy with drinking restraint. In terms of the treatment of alcohol problems, the evidence suggests that negative rather than positive alcohol expectancies might lead to a better understanding of the sociocognitive processes involved.

ALCOHOL EXPECTANCIES AS ALCOHOL MOTIVATIONS

To what extent do alcohol outcome expectancies represent alcohol motivations? Alcohol motivations have been at the center of contemporary alcohol treatments for two decades. Two parallel frameworks have had impact. First, Miller and Rollnick (1991) view *motivation for restraint* as emerging from an interactional, nonconfrontational style of counseling in which the interactions create contexts through which the clients' alcohol-related problems might be more read-ily recognized. Second, Prochaska and DiClemente (1982), view the client as oc-cupying different states of *motivation for change* depending upon the extent to which they recognize their alcohol-related problems and the extent to which they want to do something about them. In the first case, motivation is the target of in-tervention and the goal is to enhance it (Chapter 9, this volume). In the second case, the state of motivation is sought and the goal is to use this knowledge to point in the direction of an appropriate intervention (Chapter 1, this volume).

One view might be that knowledge of the dynamics of social learning theory's construct, negative expectancy, does no more than provide a theoretical substrata that is lacking in an otherwise well-articulated but somewhat atheoretical de-scription of client motivation for restraint and how to enhance it. If this is defen-sible, then those who explicitly use the negative expectancy construct to intervene in alcohol problems are doing no more than what good motivational interviewers have been doing for decades (and good counselors for much longer). The similar-ity between the assessment procedure prior to a motivational interview and the procedure for assessing an individual's negative expectancies, let alone, ex-pectancy-based intervention as delivered by McMahon and colleagues (1996), tes-tifies to this. This view on the dynamics of negative expectancy might also extend to categorizing an individual's motivational state as in stages of change frame-works. Those who explicitly use the negative expectancy construct to decide how motivated for change an individual is are doing no more than has been accom-plished during the last decade with existing instruments. Indeed, McMahon and Jones (1996) have demonstrated the equivalence of negative expectancy represen-tations of motivation for restraint and stages of change representations in predict-ing posttreatment outcome, when the Readiness to Change Questionnaire was used (Heather, Gold, & Rollnick, 1991). An advantage of using the negative ex-pectancy construct to represent motivation to change is that the assessment pro-vides information that can be used to assist the client from one state to another whereas the assessment of motivational state does not.

If the view held on the dynamics of negative expectancy was that it provides no more than do other approaches that address motivation for change or restraint, then at least it provides a single common framework where there were previously two—the force behind attempts to make any body of knowledge systematic.

To what extent might these observations on negative expectancy generalize beyond alcohol use, misuse, and abuse? One would expect that generalization would be good, for the observations are based on basic sociocognitive process. En-couragingly, Prochaska (1994) has examined studies on 12 problem behaviors other than those related to alcohol; his metanalysis demonstrates that the con-struct negative expectancy (in Prochaska's terms, "cons") consistently represents a strong principle of change across these quite disparate domains. Moreover, in this same analysis, positive expectancy (Prochaska's "pros") was only a weak prin-ciple of change.

Finally, a note on the role of science. The intelligent layperson might be of the opinion that expectancy research does little more than prove common sense. Just so, but half of common sense is probably right and half is probably wrong; the job of science is to discover which half is which. If the conclusions in this chapter can be sustained, the process of science suggests confidence might be put in developing interventions for treatment that are based on an understanding of negative expectancy, not positive. It remains to be seen whether there is substance to the speculation earlier in this chapter that an understanding of positive expectancy might be more appropriately directed elsewhere.

REFERENCES

Adams, S. L., & McNeil, D. W. (1991). Negative alcohol expectancies reconsidered. *Psychology of Addictive Behaviors, 5,* 9–14.

Amodeo, M., & Kurtz, N. (1990). Cognitive processes and abstinence in a treated alcoholic population. *International Journal of the Addictions, 25,* 983–1009.

Beck, A. T., Emery, G., & Greenberg, R. L. (1985). *Anxiety disorder and phobias: A cognitive perspective.* New York: HarperCollins.

Brown, S. A. (1985). Reinforcement expectancies and alcoholism treatment outcome after a one-year follow-up. *Journal of Studies on Alcohol, 46,* 304–308.

Brown, S. A., Goldman, M. S., Inn, A., & Anderson, L. (1980). Expectations of reinforcement from alcohol: Their domain and relation to drinking patterns. *Journal of Consulting and Clinical Psychology, 48,* 419–426.

Brown, S. A., Millar, A., & Passman, L. (1988). Utilizing expectancies in alcohol treatment. *Psychology of Addictive Behavior, 2,* 59–65.

Casswell, S., Gilmore, L. L., Silva, P., & Brasch, P. (1988). What children know about alcohol and how they know it. *British Journal of Addiction, 83,* 223–227.

Connors, G. J., Tarbox, A. R., & Faillace, L. A. (1993) Changes in alcohol expectancies and drinking behavior among treated problem drinkers. *Journal of Studies on Alcohol, 53,* 676–683.

Connors, J., Maisto, S. A., & Dermen, K. H. (1992). Alcohol-related expectancies and their applications to treatment. In R. R. Watson (Ed.), *Drug and Alcohol Abuse Reviews: Vol 3. Alcohol Abuse Treatment* (pp. 203–231). New York: Humana.

Darkes, J., & Goldman, M. S. (1993). Expectancy challenge and drinking reduction: Experimental evidence for a mediational process. *Journal of Consulting and Clinical Psychology, 61,* 344–353.

Dunn, M. E., & Goldman, M. S. (1996). Empirical modeling of an alcohol expectancy memory network in elementary school children as a function of grade. *Experimental and Clinical Psychopharmacology, 4,* 209–217.

Eastman, C., & Norris, H. (1982). Alcohol dependence, relapse, and self-identity. *Journal of Studies on Alcohol, 43,* 1214–1231.

Floyd, F. J., & Widaman, K. F. (1995). Factor analysis in the development and refinement of clinical assessment instruments. *Psychological Assessment, 7,* 286–299.

Fromme, K., Kivlahan, D. R., & Marlatt, G. A. (1986). Alcohol expectancies, risk identification and secondary prevention with problem drinkers. *Advances in Behavior Research and Therapy, 8,* 237–251.

Fromme, K., Stroot, E., & Kaplan, D. (1993). Comprehensive effects of alcohol: Development and psychometric assessment of a new expectancy questionnaire. *Psychological Assessment, 5,* 19–26.

Goldman, M. S. (1989). Alcohol expectancies as cognitive-behavioral psychology: Theory and practice. In T. Loberg, W. R. Miller, P. E. Nathan, & G. A. Marlatt (Eds.), *Addictive behaviors: Prevention and early intervention.* Amsterdam: Swets and Zeitlinger.

Grube, J. W., Chen, M., Madden, P., & Morgan, M. (1995). Predicting adolescent drinking from alcohol expectancy values: A comparison of additive, interactive, and non-linear models. *Journal of Applied Social Psychology, 25,* 839–857.

Gustafson, R. (1992). The development of alcohol-related expectancies from the age of 12 to the age of 15 for two Swedish adolescent samples. *Alcoholism: Clinical and Experimental Research, 16,* 700–704.

Heather, N., Gold, R., & Rollnick, S. (1991). *Readiness to Change Questionnaire: User's manual.* National Drug and Alcohol Centre, University of New South Wales, Australia.

Johnson, H. L., & Johnson, P. B. (1995). Children's alcohol-related cognitions: Positive versus negative alcohol effects. *Journal of Alcohol and Drug Education, 40,* 1–12.

Johnson, P. B., & Johnson, H. L. (1996). Children's beliefs about the social consequences of drinking and refusing to drink alcohol. *Journal of Alcohol and Drug Education, 41,* 34–43.

Jones, B. T., & McMahon, J. (1992). Negative and positive expectancies in lone and group problem drinkers. *British Journal of Addiction, 87,* 929–930.

Jones, B. T., & McMahon, J. (1994a). *Is negative expectancy the same as motivation for recovery from alcohol problems?* Paper presented at the annual symposium of the Society for the Study of Addiction to Alcohol and Other Drugs, London.

Jones, B. T., & McMahon, J. (1994b). Negative alcohol expectancy predicts post-treatment abstinence survivorship: The whether, when and why of relapse to a first drink. *Addiction, 89,* 1654–1665.

Jones, B. T., & McMahon, J. (1994c). Negative and positive alcohol expectancies as predictors of abstinence after discharge from a residential treatment programme: A one- and three-month follow-up study in males. *Journal of Studies on Alcohol, 55,* 543–548.

Jones, B. T., & McMahon, J. (1996a). Alcohol expectancies at admission and discharge and changes in these expectancies relate to post-treatment abstinence survivorship. *British Journal of Clinical Psychology, 35,* 221–233.

Jones, B. T., & McMahon, J. (1996b). A comparison of positive and negative alcohol expectancy and value and their multiplicative composite as predictors of post-treatment abstinence survivorship. *Addiction, 91,* 89–99.

Jones, B. T., McMahon, J., & Needham, C. J. (1995). *Assessing alcohol motivations on treatment entry: Processing value against expectancy by value-slicing the expectancy pool increases percentage variance explained in post-treatment outcome.* Paper presented at the 7th International Conference on Treatment of Addictive Behaviors, Leeuwenhorst, The Netherlands.

Jones, B. T., Needham, C. J., & McMahon, J. (1998). *Subjective evaluations of adult social drinkers' alcohol expectancies moderate the relationship between expectancies and drinking.* Manuscript submitted for publication.

Kraus, D., Smith, G. T., & Ratner, H. H. (1994). Modifying alcohol-related expectancies in grade-school children. *Journal of Studies on Alcohol, 55,* 535–542.

Leigh, B. C., & Stacy, A. W. (1993). Alcohol outcome expectancies: Scale construction and predictive utility in higher order confirmatory models. *Psychological Assessment, 5,* 216–229.

McMahon, J., & Jones, B. T. (1991). The Negative Alcohol Expectancy Questionnaire (NAEQ) as an instrument for measuring motivation to inhibit drinking and evaluating methods of treating problem drinkers. In F. Tongue & E. Martin (Eds.), *Proceedings of the 36th International Congress on Alcohol and Drug Dependence, I,* (pp. 228–241). Lausanne, Switzerland: ICADD.

McMahon, J., & Jones, B. T. (1993). Negative expectancy in motivation. *Addiction Research, 1,* 145–155.

McMahon, J., & Jones, B. T. (1994). Social drinkers' negative alcohol expectancy relates to their satisfaction with current consumption: Measuring motivation for change with the NAEQ. *Alcohol and Alcoholism, 29,* 687–690.

McMahon, J., & Jones, B. T. (1996). Post-treatment abstinence survivorship and motivation for recovery: The predictive validity of the Readiness to Change (RCQ) and the Negative Alcohol Expectancy (NAEQ) questionnaires. *Addiction Research, 4,* 161–176.

McMahon, J., & Jones, B. T., & O'Donnell, P. (1994). Comparing positive and negative expectancies in male and female social drinkers. *Addiction Research, 1,* 349–365.

McMahon, J., Jones, B. T., & Smith, I. (1996). *Negative expectancy based intervention within a motivational interviewing context.* Paper presented at the annual conference of the British Psychological Society (Social Psychology Division), symposium on Alcohol Motivations. Strathclyde University, Glasgow, Scotland.

Miller, P. M., Smith, G. T., & Goldman, M. S. (1990). Emergence of alcohol expectancies in childhood: A possible critical period. *Journal of Studies on Alcohol, 51,* 343–349.

Miller, W. R., & Rollnick, S. (1991). *Motivational interviewing: Preparing people to change addictive behavior.* New York. Guilford.

Miller, W. R., Westerberg, V. S., Harris, R. R. J., & Tonigan, J. S. (1996). What predicts relapse? Prospective testing of antecedent models. *Addiction, 91,* S3–S4.

Morgenstern, J., Kahler, C. W., & Labouvie, E. (1997). *Negative expectancies and other primary appraisals of substance use: Their role as predictors of treatment outcome.* Manuscript submitted for publication.

National Institute on Alcohol Abuse and Alcoholism (NIAAA). (1995). The Negative Alcohol Expectancy Questionnaire (NAEQ). In J. P. Allen & M. Columbus (Eds.), *Assessing alcohol problems: A guide for clinicians and researchers* (pp. 415–418). Rockville, MD: Author.

Needham, C. J., Jones, B. T., & Taghavi-Laryani, T. (1998). *The Comprehensive Effects of Alcohol questionnaire (CEOA) shows subjective evaluations of alcohol expectancies moderate the expectancy–consumption relationship in young and mature Scottish adults.* Manuscript submitted for publication.

Prochaska, J. O. (1994). Strong and weak principles for progressing from precontemplation to action on the basis of twelve problem behaviors. *Health Psychology, 13,* 47–51.

Prochaska, J. O., & DiClemente, C. C. (1982). Transtheoretical therapy: Toward a more integrative model of change. *Psychotherapy: Theory, Research and Practice, 19,* 276–278.

Prochaska, J. O., DiClemente, C. C., Velicer, W. F., & Rossi, J. S. (1992). Criticisms and concerns of the transtheoretical model in light of recent research. *British Journal of Addiction, 87,* 825–828.

Rather, B., & Sherman, M. F. (1989). Relationship between alcohol expectancies and length of abstinence among Alcoholics Anonymous members. *Addictive Behaviors, 14,* 531–536

Rotter, J. B., Chance, J. E., & Phares, E. J. (1972). *Applications of social learning theory to personality.* New York: Holt, Rinehart and Winston.

Saunders, B. (1996). Relapse revisited: A critique of current concepts and clinical practice in the management of alcohol problems. Paper presented to the Addictions '96 conference, Hilton Head Island, South Carolina.

Shewan, D., Dalgarno, P., Marshall, A., Lowe, E., Campbell, L., McLafferty, Z., Nicholson, S., & Thomson, K. (in press). Patterns of heroin use among a non-treatment sample in Glasgow (Scotland). *Addiction Research.*

Stacy, A. W., Widaman, K. F., & Marlatt, G. A. (1990). Expectancy models of alcohol use. *Journal of Personality and Social Psychology, 58,* 918–928.

Thom, B. (1987). Sex differences in help-seeking for alcohol problems: 2. Entry into treatment. *British Journal of Addiction, 82,* 989–997.

Werner, M. J., Walker, L. S., & Greene, J. W. (1993). Alcohol expectancies, problem drinking and adverse health consequences. *Journal of Adolescent Health, 14,* 446–452.

Zuckner, R. A., Kincaid, S. B., Fitgerald, H. E., & Bingham, C. R. (1995). Alcohol schema acquisition in preschoolers: Differences between children of alcoholics and children of nonalcoholics. *Alcoholism: Clinical and Experimental Research, 19,* 1011–1017.

7

Choice, Behavioral Economics, and Addictive Behavior Patterns

RUDY E. VUCHINICH AND JALIE A. TUCKER

INTRODUCTION

Since the "cognitive revolution" in behavior therapy during the 1970s (e.g., Mahoney, 1974), theories of addictive behavior (e.g., Blane & Leonard, 1987) have emphasized the causal importance of cognitive and affective mediational concepts. This revolution was a positive development, but it led many applied psychologists to lose faith in behaviorism and basic behavioral science as useful for understanding volitional psychological problems such as addictive behaviors. Much has happened in behavioral science since the 1970s, however, that diverges significantly from the behaviorism to which the cognitive revolution reacted. In particular, behavioral choice theory has been developed and has made positive contributions to an analysis of complex human behavior patterns, such as addictive (e.g., Vuchinich & Tucker, 1988) and other health (e.g., Bickel & Vuchinich, in press; Epstein, 1992) behaviors. In this chapter, we (1) discuss a conceptual issue that contributed to the emergence of cognitive behavioral theory and behavioral choice theory, (2) sketch the development of behavioral choice theory and behavioral economics, (3) summarize their applications to research on addictive behaviors, and (4) summarize the intervention implications of the choice perspective.

RUDY E. VUCHINICH AND JALIE A. TUCKER • Department of Psychology, Auburn University, Auburn, Alabama 36849.

Treating Addictive Behaviors, 2nd ed., edited by Miller and Heather. Plenum Press, New York, 1998.

THE PROBLEM OF EXPLAINING PARTICULAR ACTS

A crucial motivator of the cognitive revolution was the fact that most behavior apparently is free from control by the immediate environment. That is, a particular act usually cannot be explained by observable features of the environment at the time of the act (see Mahoney, 1974, p. 31, for four prototypic cases). Thus, the causal context provided by the immediate environment alone is insufficient to account for most particular acts. To address this issue, the cognitive revolution incorporated theoretical terms to represent internal psychological entities that connect the past and current environment to a person's particular acts. With this conceptual strategy, the causal context for an act becomes the immediate environment *plus* the person's internal psychological mechanisms at the time of the act, rather than just the immediate environment alone. This approach directs attention to the internal mechanisms and has led to the now familiar emphasis on mediational concepts to bridge temporal gaps between the environment and particular acts.

Contemporaneous with the cognitive revolution was a quieter evolution in basic behavioral science that adopted a different conceptual strategy to address the same issue (e.g., Herrnstein, 1970; Rachlin, 1974). Behavioral theories of choice developed theoretical terms to represent a particular act as a single instance of a more molar, temporally extended behavior–environment relation. With this strategy, the causal context for a particular act becomes the immediate environment *plus* the more molar behavior–environment relation of which the act is a specific instance, rather than the immediate environment alone. This approach directs attention to molar patterns of behavior and seeks regularities between such patterns and temporally extended features of the environment, and does not require that each particular act be contiguously preceded by either external or internal stimuli. Rachlin (1992, 1994) discussed these issues generally, and Vuchinich (1995) and Vuchinich and Tucker (1996b) discussed them as they apply to addictive behaviors.

Cognitive behavioral theory and behavioral choice theory diverge fundamentally in their theoretical approaches to explaining particular acts. This divergence entails different orienting assumptions and different levels of analysis that probably are not amenable to definitive, comparative empirical tests. Thus, one need not attempt to decide to reject either in favor of accepting the other. Both perspectives are legitimate, and their contributions complement rather than compete with one another. Our goal in this chapter is to describe the contributions of behavioral choice theory and behavioral economics to understanding the variables that control the development and change of addictive behavior patterns.

ORIGINS OF BEHAVIORAL CHOICE THEORY
AND BEHAVIORAL ECONOMICS

Traditional reinforcement-based behavior theories focused on the strength of either individual operants (Skinner, 1938) or individual stimulus–response connections (e.g., Hull, 1943). Premack (1965) showed, however, that engagement in a particular activity depends on what other activities are also available and on the environmental constraints that exist on access to all members of the activity set. Herrnstein (1970) further showed that the frequency of a given activity is a function of its reinforcement relative to the reinforcement obtained from other possible activities. This seminal work revealed that behavioral allocation (i.e., choice) is critically affected by the more general context of environmental conditions and activity opportunities that surrounds individual acts, and it spawned a surge of research aimed at describing how those more molar contextual conditions control choice.

It was soon recognized that the task of describing the behavioral allocation of animals in the laboratory shared essential features with the task of describing the resource allocation of human consumers in the economy (e.g., Rachlin, Green, Kagel, & Battalio, 1976). This connection led some behavioral psychologists to use concepts from consumer demand theory in economics and led some economists to use behavioral methods, which resulted in a mutually beneficial merger now known as behavioral economics (Kagel, Battalio, & Green, 1995).

APPLICATIONS TO ADDICTIVE BEHAVIORS

The potential utility of these basic science developments for studying addictive behaviors was recognized soon after their conception (e.g., Allison, 1979; Vuchinich, 1982), and this has since grown into an active research area (e.g., Bickel, DeGrandpre, & Higgins, 1993; Green & Kagel, 1996; Vuchinich, 1997). From the choice perspective, addictive behavior patterns emerge, develop, and change over time within temporally extended environmental contexts that are characterized by stability and change in access to drug and nondrug-related activity opportunities. This molar view is consistent with two general and important features of addictive behaviors. First, the temporally extended nature of such problems is central to virtually all definitional criteria (e.g., American Psychiatric Association, 1994), and the course of addictive behaviors, including development, stability, recovery, and relapse, is apparent only over lengthy time periods (e.g., Vaillant, 1983). Moreover, addictive behaviors typically exhibit variability over time (e.g., Marlatt, Curry, & Gordon, 1988; Moos, Finney, & Cronkite, 1990) that is not well represented by a "snapshot" of behavior at one particular time. Second, the molar context of other activity opportunities that surrounds addictive behavior patterns is likewise conceived from a broad temporal perspective. Such a temporally extended context is necessary to represent the complex life circumstances within which addictive behavior problems are embedded and that strongly influence their development and change (e.g., Moos et al., 1990; Tucker, Vuchinich, & Gladsjo, 1990/91).

Behavioral choice theory directs attention to two broad classes of variables as critical influences on addictive behavior patterns (e.g., Green & Kagel, 1996; Vuchinich & Tucker, 1988): (1) environmental constraints on access to the abused substance, and (2) alternative, nonsubstance-related activity opportunities and the constraints on access to them. Extensive research on the first variable class has repeatedly demonstrated an inverse relation between substance use and abuse and direct constraints on access to the substance (e.g., through changes in price, response requirement, or availability) (Bickel et al., 1993; DeGrandpre & Bickel, 1996; Vuchinich & Tucker, 1988). This relationship has generality across species, substances of abuse, normal and clinical populations, and laboratory and natural environments. Moreover, technical concepts from behavioral economics, including demand, elasticity of demand, and unit price, have proven quite useful in organizing data from studies of substance use and abuse (e.g., DeGrandpre & Bickel, 1996; Vuchinich, 1997). These behavioral economic analyses of demand for abused substances indicate that that demand can be accurately described with the same analytic tools that apply to all commodities. This suggests that consumption of abused substances is but one instance of a "ubiquitous behavioral process" (Bickel *et al.*, 1993, p. 181) and that they are not a special class of commodities that requires unique analytic concepts.

Research on the second class of variables generally has found a direct relation between drug use and constraints on access to nondrug alternative activities (Carroll, 1996; Higgins, 1997; Vuchinich & Tucker, 1988). This class of variables may be more important for understanding drug-taking patterns in natural environments (Vuchinich & Tucker, 1988), because under natural conditions drug availability typically is minimally constrained and constant relative to the considerable variability that exists in access to valued nondrug alternatives. This second variable class also emphasizes concepts of impulsiveness and self-control in an analysis of addictive behaviors, which are critical concepts in virtually all problem definitions (see Chapter 5, this volume). Behavioral choice theory and research frame these concepts within the context of intertemporal choice between smaller sooner rewards (the impulsive choice) and larger later rewards (the self-controlled choice) (e.g., Ainslie, 1992; Rachlin, 1974). As applied to substance abuse, individuals repeatedly choose to engage in drug use, which typically is readily available, or to engage in alternative behavior patterns that, over time, increase access to more valued but delayed nondrug activities.

Figure 1A depicts self-control situations studied in the laboratory (e.g., Rachlin, 1974) that involve an intertemporal choice between a smaller sooner reward (SSR) and a larger later reward (LLR). Choice of the SSR reduces access to the LLR, and obtaining the LLR requires forgoing the SSR. The curves to the left of the rewards represent their value during the times before they are available and are drawn according to a hyperbolic temporal discounting function, which has extensive empirical support (e.g., Ainslie, 1992). A key feature of hyperbolic discounting is that preference between the LLR and SSR will reverse simply with the passage of time, as indicated by the crossing of the reward value curves between time 3 and time 4. Thus, the LLR would be preferred before that time and the SSR would be preferred after that time.

Figure 1B extends this analysis to choices between substance use, conceptualized as the SSR, and engaging in behavior patterns that, over the long run, increase access to valued alternative activities that may be constrained by continued substance use (e.g., LLRs such as satisfying intimate, family, or social relations; academic or vocational success). Although a substance use episode may reasonably be regarded as a punctate event, the more valuable nondrug activities typically consist of complex activity patterns that occur over time. Thus, in Figure 1B, substance use is represented as a punctate reward at time 6, whereas the more valuable but delayed nondrug alternatives are represented as a series of smaller rewards dispersed over a longer time frame (between time 13 and time 19) that are summed for analytic purposes as a single LLR at time 12.

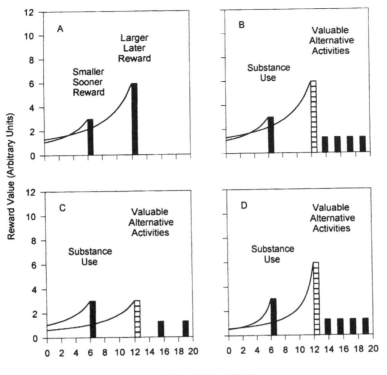

FIGURE 1. Figure illustrates intertemporal choice between smaller sooner and larger later rewards. Rewards are vertical bars; height represents value and abscissa location represents time of availability. The curves represent reward value during times before availability; the reward with the highest value curve at the time of choice will be preferred. Panel A: Basic choice between different amounts of the same reward available at different times. Hyperbolic temporal discounting results in preference reversal with the passage of time. Panel B: Choice between substance use and valuable alternative activities. The latter are shown as a series of smaller rewards distributed over times 13 to 19 that vary together and that sum to the larger reward at time 12. Panel C: Choice between substance use and valuable alternative activities, with fewer of the latter being available than in Panel B. This results in a stronger preference for substance use in Panel C than in Panel B. Panel D: Choice between substance use and valuable alternative activities, with reward structure being the same as in Panel B but with a higher rate of delayed reward discounting than in Panel B. This results in a stronger preference for substance use in Panel D than in Panel B.

The choice dynamics depicted in Figure 1B are consistent with two important aspects of addictive behavior patterns. First, even when the environmental reward structure remains constant, ambivalence about drug use will occur because preference for substance use will vary over time depending on the temporal distance to the availability of the drug and the alternative activity. The LLRs will be preferred before the point where the value curves cross, and drug use will be preferred after that point. But, once the person exits the situation involving drug availability, preference will revert back to the LLRs, and the individual may regret the substance use episode. Second, the LLRs that enter into these intertemporal choice dynamics with substance use will likely differ across individuals and across time for the same individual (Vuchinich & Tucker, 1996a). Such variability is consistent with the diversity of life health problems that are typical of substance abusing populations (e.g., Maisto & McCollum, 1980).

A third choice dynamic that is pertinent to understanding relapse and recovery processes is revealed by comparing Figures 1B and 1C, which depict identical SSR structures but different LLR structures. Figure 1C represents a situation in which access to the LLR is more constrained than in Figure 1B. Even though drug access is constant in both cases, the reward value curves cross much earlier in Figure 1C than in 1B, indicating stronger preference for substance use in the former case. Thus, the risk of relapse increases when the reward structure in an individual's environment goes through a transition from the situation depicted in Figure 1B to that depicted in 1C—i.e., preference for drug use should increase if valued nondrug alternatives become more constrained. Such relationships were found in a prospective study of drinking episodes in problem drinkers during a 6-month interval after treatment (Vuchinich & Tucker, 1996a). Moreover, drinking episodes preceded by life events that signaled increased constraints on valued nondrinking alternatives were found to be more severe than drinking episodes that were not associated with events and that presumably did not involve a change in the overall reward structure. This suggests an environmental basis for distinguishing the controlling variables of lapses and relapses. O'Connell and Martin (1987) found similar relationships with respect to smoking cessation attempts.

Decreasing substance abuse and maintaining the change can be conceptualized as involving the reverse process wherein the environmental reward structure transitions from the situation depicted in Figure 1C to that depicted in Figure 1B. If initial abstinence or reduced drug use increases access to valuable nondrug alternatives, then preference for substance use should decrease and remain low, except in situations where drug availability is imminent, and the LLR reward value curve should supersede that for drug use at most points in time. Such a relation between the maintenance of abstinence or moderation drinking and increased access to valued nondrinking rewards were found in both treated and untreated problem drinkers who had sustained problem resolution for several years (Tucker, Vuchinich, & Gladsjo, 1994; Tucker, Vuchinich, & Pukish, 1995). This choice dynamic also is consistent with a typical behavior change pattern noted by Miller (1996b), in which drinking episodes gradually become less frequent and less severe in problem drinkers who resolve their alcohol abuse. This perspective generally highlights the importance of increasing access to valued nondrug alternatives to motivate and maintain addictive behavior change, and it shows that the amounts and delays of the SSRs and LLRs are critical determinants of preference in intertemporal choice.

Figure 1D depicts another choice dynamic concerning the degree to which the value of delayed rewards are discounted. Higher rates of temporal discounting produce a stronger preference for the SSR (i.e., impulsiveness), which leads to more substance use. This relationship is shown by comparing Figures 1B and 1D. The reward structures are the same in both cases, but the rewards are discounted at a higher rate in 1D than in 1B. The higher discount rate in 1D produces lower reward value curves, which results in an earlier preference shift toward the SSR in 1D compared to 1B. This suggests that substance use should be positively correlated with the rate of discounting. Individuals with a relatively lower discount rate, as in Figure 1B, would spend more time behaving in ways that produce access to the nondrug rewards and less time preferring drug use. Individuals with a higher discount rate, as in Figure 1D, would spend less time behaving in ways that produce access to the nondrug rewards and more time preferring drug use.

Preliminary support has been found for a positive relation between temporal discounting and substance use. In a laboratory study involving choices between different hypothetical amounts of money available after different delays (Vuchinich & Simpson, in press), heavy social drinkers and problem drinkers discounted the value of money at a higher rate than did light social drinkers, with problem drinkers showing the highest discount rate. The same relationship was found in a similar study that compared the discount rates of opioid-dependent and non– drug-using control participants (Madden, Petry, Badger, & Bickel, 1997). Also, in a prospective follow-up of problem drinkers who were attempting to recover without treatment (Tucker & Vuchinich, 1997), successful maintenance for a year or more was predicted by a monetary index of the extent to which individuals organized a portion of their behavior around delayed outcomes when they were drinking heavily. Individuals who maintained abstinence or moderation drinking had saved about 10 times as much money during the year prior to positive behavior change compared to those who resumed abusive drinking, even though the two outcome groups were similar in their total preresolution income and expenditures and in their preresolution drinking practices. This discounting–substance abuse relation suggests that individuals with higher rates of discounting may be more susceptible to developing substance abuse and, once a problem exists, they may be less likely to resolve it.

INTERVENTION IMPLICATIONS

The heterogeneity of addictive behavior problems, coupled with the limited absolute effectiveness of clinical treatments, have made it critical to expand the range of interventions to include clinical, public health, and policy initiatives (e.g., Institute of Medicine, 1990; also see Chapter 8, this volume). Clinical treatments and mutual help groups obviously will remain vital intervention options, but an expanded continuum of care also must include interventions that (1) attract more affected individuals into helping environments, including the underserved majority with less severe problems and those uninterested in stopping drug use but who wish to reduce the harm associated with it; (2) are more accessible and make greater use of social and community resources; and (3) facilitate the natural forces that promote behavior change (Marlatt, Tucker, Donovan, & Vuchinich, 1997). A related priority among harm reduction proponents (e.g., Heather, Wodak, Nadelmann, & O'Hare, 1993; Marlatt & Tapert, 1993) is to expand prevention, treatment, and policy initiatives aimed at reducing the demand for drugs and the harms associated with drug use. In the United States, drug demand reduction efforts have been neglected during the War on Drugs, which emphasizes reducing drug use by restricting the drug supply through interdiction efforts and by criminalizing drug trafficking and drug use.

These complex intervention needs cut across scientific and professional disciplinary boundaries and require pragmatic concepts that direct attention toward key variables and goals. No single perspective on addictive behaviors is clearly best suited to direct these efforts. Nevertheless, the behavioral choice perspective can contribute to the development and coordination of interventions at several levels, ranging from the individual in treatment, to the community and health services system, to public policy. Given the confluence of principles from behavioral choice theory and economics, this perspective is especially well suited for guiding drug demand reduction strategies since its primary dependent variable is consumer behavior patterns.

A simple but easily overlooked implication of the perspective is that, in characterizing the determinants of drug use and in developing interventions to reduce drug-related problems, more attention should be paid to the *molar context of drug use*. This context is defined by the availability of valuable nondrug activities and by the extent to which access to them is contingent on abstinence or reduced drug use. This focus on the molar context of drug use differs from the singular focus of many interventions and the War on Drugs on the drug-taking behavior itself, which presumes that eliminating drug use will eliminate the problems associated with it as well. The behavioral economic literature is clear that reducing drug use depends critically on increasing access to valued nondrug alternatives (Carroll, 1996; Vuchinich & Tucker, 1988) and that simply increasing the constraints on drug access usually will not be sufficient to reduce or eliminate use (Bickel & De-Grandpre, 1995; Hursh, 1991). Indeed, constraining drug access or increasing the price of drugs without also providing alternative activities usually intensifies drug-seeking behavior and any associated criminal activity.

Drug demand interventions aimed at increasing access to nondrug alternatives can be implemented at several levels. At the individual treatment level, interventions should move rapidly to improve clients' access to nondrug alternatives that would reduce demand for drugs, rather than focusing nearly exclusively on reducing or eliminating drug use, as is common practice. This approach also is responsive to the fact that most substance abusers seek help for problems related to substance use rather than because of excessive drug use per se and thus may help promote treatment engagement and retention (Marlatt *et al.*, 1997). The importance of this general intervention principle was stated succinctly by Cox and Klinger (1988): "any treatment technique will be doomed to failure if it enables alcoholics to stop drinking but does not provide them with alternative sources of . . . satisfaction" (p. 176). The conceptually compatible and effective Community Reinforcement Approach (e.g., Higgins, in press; also see Chapter 11, this volume) illustrates this principle and may include increasing access to employment, drug-free housing, and drug-free social interactions. At the community level, introducing customized activity opportunities that can compete with drug use is a prevention strategy suggested by experimental work showing that environmental enrichment with nondrug alternatives reduces both the acquisition of drug taking and levels of drug use once drug taking has been acquired (Carroll, 1996).

Another implication of the choice perspective is that, in developing services for persons with addictive behavior problems, more attention should be paid to the needs and preferences of the consumers of those services. This theme is shared by harm reduction (e.g., Marlatt & Tapert, 1993) and motivational (e.g., Miller & Rollnick, 1991) interventions that emphasize "meeting clients where they are." Research on help-seeking (Marlatt *et al.*, 1997) clearly shows that the abstinence-oriented U.S. service delivery system has not created sufficient demand for services and that coercive elements often are present in the helping environments of the minority who seek assistance (about 20% of persons with problems). Several factors probably contribute to the help-seeking problem, including the stigma associated with substance abuse and its treatment, the lack of a range of effective intervention alternatives that are responsive to the heterogenous needs and concerns of substance abusers, and the typical requirement that they abstain if they are to receive services.

If an important goal of a broadened intervention system is to attract and retain more substance abusers in helping environments, then the behavioral choice and harm reduction perspectives converge in recommending that the traditional abstinence requirement be relaxed in some circumstances. The choice dynamics discussed earlier indicate that, by seeking help when abstinence is required, the substance abuser must forgo a readily available valued commodity (drug use) in order to gain access to higher valued but delayed and probabilistic outcomes (benefits of treatment or abstinence). The help-seeking and treatment motivation literatures strongly suggest that the discounted value of the delayed and probabilistic treatment effects often do not outweigh the value of more immediate and certain substance use. This suggests that the abstinence requirement could be relaxed until the client's access to nondrug alternatives is increased, unless that access is dependent upon abstinence or if there are health reasons for abstaining. This provides a functional basis for initial goal selection and is responsive to the forces that often promote help-seeking. Moreover, harm reduction programs that do not require abstinence for participation (e.g., clean needle exchanges) can function as gateways for referrals to more intensive abstinence-oriented treatment or to medical care (e.g., Carvell & Hart, 1990).

CONCLUSIONS

The mediational psychological concepts of the cognitive revolution have contributed much to individual clinical approaches to intervention, but their utility may be diminished in an expansion of the intervention system beyond conventional clinical settings to levels other than the individual client. In part because of its interdisciplinary foundation, behavioral economics offers guidance about variables and goals that cut across several intervention levels. At all levels, the perspective highlights the molar context dependence of choice and the importance of increasing access to nondrug alternatives in attempts to reduce drug use and drug-related problems.

The behavioral choice perspective and the transtheoretical model (Prochaska, DiClemente, & Norcross, 1992) converge on some points (Vuchinich & Tucker, 1996b) but diverge in complementary ways on others. Both emphasize that addictive behavior change is a temporally extended process, that clinical treatment is only one of several important forces that can influence change, and that extratherapeutic factors play an important role in change. These commonalities run counter to traditional views that tie recovery from addictive behaviors to lengthy participation in mutual help groups or intensive treatment. The divergence occurs in how the two views characterize the key variables that produce behavior change. The transtheoretical model has continued the tradition of the cognitive revolution by characterizing many of its key variables (e.g., the change processes) as psychological mediating mechanisms that operate primarily within the person, although these processes sometimes are triggered by temporally contiguous events in the environment. The choice perspective has continued the tradition of behavioral choice theory by characterizing the key variables as molar behavior patterns in the context of temporally extended environmental constraints on access to valued activities.

The transtheoretical model has promoted consideration of the range of intervention alternatives needed in an expanded approach to addictive behavior change, but the temporally contiguous and interiorized conceptual structure of the model may not provide the most effective guidance for all components of such an expanded initiative. Behavioral economics can make unique contributions to this initiative that go beyond conventional efforts to change behavior by changing the contiguous environment and expectancies, self-efficacy, and other internalized states thought to mediate between human behavior and that environment.

Despite these differences, the two views share an interest in making sense of the fundamental puzzle succinctly framed by Miller (1996a):

> The voluntary road away from the gratification cycles of addiction seems to involve . . . the processes of valuing and choosing and deciding. Models for effective and lasting change may have more to do with processes colloquially described as "making up one's mind" than with counterconditioning or skill training. I do not discount the demonstrated value of behavioral approaches. . . . I do puzzle, however, about what really constitutes motivation for change, and what finally sets in motion the process of altering that which has been so persistent. (p. 841)

Dealing effectively with the phenomena of "valuing and choosing and deciding" and "making up one's mind" is a critical aspect of improving our understanding of development and change in addictive behavior patterns. Although these phenomena were neglected by the behavioral theoretical frameworks that generated interventions such as counterconditioning or skill training, that neglect is no longer the case. As discussed in this chapter, these phenomena are precisely what behavioral choice theory and behavioral economics have been developed to address (cf. Rachlin, 1994).

REFERENCES

Ainslie, G. (1992). *Picoeconomics: The strategic interaction of successive motivational states within the person.* Cambridge, England: Cambridge University Press.

Allison, J. (1979). Demand economics and experimental psychology. *Behavioral Science, 24,* 403–415.

American Psychiatric Association. (1994). *Diagnostic and statistical manual of mental disorders* (4th ed.). Washington, DC: Author.

Bickel, W. K., & DeGrandpre, R. J. (1995). Price and alternatives: Suggestions for drug policy from psychology. *The International Journal of Drug Policy, 6,* 93–105.

Bickel, W. K., & Vuchinich, R. E. (in press). *Reframing health behavior with behavioral economics.* New York: Erlbaum.

Bickel, W. K., DeGrandpre, R. J., & Higgins, S. T. (1993). Behavioral economics: A novel experimental approach to the study of drug dependence. *Drug and Alcohol Dependence, 33,* 173–192.

Blane, H. T., & Leonard, K. E. (Eds.). (1987). *Psychological theories of drinking and alcoholism.* New York: Guilford.

Carroll, M. E. (1996). Reducing drug abuse by enriching the environment with alternative nondrug reinforcers. In L. Green & J. Kagel (Eds.), *Advances in behavioral economics: Vol. 3. Substance use and abuse* (pp. 37–68). Norwood, NJ: Ablex.

Carvell, A. M., & Hart, G. J. (1990). Help-seeking and referrals in a needle exchange: A comprehensive service to injecting drug users. *British Journal of Addiction, 85,* 235–240.

Cox, M., & Klinger, E. (1988). A motivational model of alcohol use. *Journal of Abnormal Psychology, 97,* 168–180.

DeGrandpre, R. J., & Bickel, W. K. (1996). Drug dependence as consumer demand. In L. Green & J. H. Kagel (Eds.), *Advances in behavioral economics: Vol. 3. Substance use and abuse* (pp. 1–36). Norwood, NJ: Ablex.

Epstein, L. H. (1992). The role of behavior theory in behavioral medicine. *Journal of Consulting and Clinical Psychology, 60,* 493–498.

Green, L., & Kagel, J. H. (Eds.). (1996). *Advances in behavioral economics: Vol. 3. Substance use and abuse.* Norwood, NJ: Ablex.

Heather, N., Wodak, A., Nadelmann, E. A., & O'Hare, P. (Eds.). (1993). *Psychoactive drugs and harm reduction: From faith to science.* London: Whurr.

Herrnstein, R. J. (1970). On the law of effect. *Journal of the Experimental Analysis of Behavior, 13,* 243–266.

Higgins, S. T. (in press). Potential contributions of the Community Reinforcement Approach and contingency management to broadening the base of substance abuse treatment. In J. A. Tucker, D. M. Donovan, & G. A. Marlatt (Eds.), *Changing addictive behavior: Moving beyond therapy assisted change.* New York: Guilford.

Higgins, S. T. (1997). The influence of alternative reinforcers on cocaine use and abuse: A brief review. *Pharmacology Biochemistry and Behavior, 57,* 419–427.

Hull, C. L. (1943). *Principles of behavior.* New York: Appleton-Century.

Hursh, S. R. (1991). Behavioral economics of drug self-administration and drug abuse policy. *Journal of the Experimental Analysis of Behavior, 56,* 377–393.

Institute of Medicine. (1990). *Broadening the base of treatment for alcohol problems.* Washington, DC: National Academy Press.

Kagel, J. H., Battalio, R. C., & Green, L. (1995). *Economic choice theory: An experimental analysis of animal behavior.* New York: Cambridge University Press.

Madden, G. J., Petry, N. M., Badger, G. J., & Bickel, W. K. (1997). Impulsive and self-control choices in opioid-dependent patients and non–drug-using control participants. *Experimental and Clinical Psychopharmacology, 5,* 256–263.

Mahoney, M. J. (1974). *Cognition in behavior modification.* Cambridge, MA: Ballinger.

Maisto, S. A., & McCollam, J. B. (1980). The use of multiple measures of life health to assess alcohol treatment outcome: A review and critique. In L. C. Sobell, M. B. Sobell, & E. Ward (Eds.), *Evaluating alcohol and drug abuse treatment effectiveness* (pp. 15–76). New York: Pergamon.

Marlatt, G. A., & Tapert, S. R. (1993). Harm reduction: Reducing the risks of addictive behaviors. In J. S. Baer, G. A. Marlatt, & R. McMahon (Eds.), *Addictive behaviors across the lifespan* (pp. 243–273). Newbury Park, CA: Sage.

Marlatt, G. A., Curry, S., & Gordon, J. R. (1988). A longitudinal analysis of unaided smoking cessation. *Journal of Consulting and Clinical Psychology, 56,* 715–720.

Marlatt, G. A., Tucker, J. A., Donovan, D. M., & Vuchinich, R. E. (1997). Help-seeking by substance abusers: The role of harm reduction and behavioral economic approaches to facilitate treatment entry and retention. In L. S. Onken, J. D. Blaine, & J. J. Boren (Eds.), *Beyond the therapeutic alliance: Keeping the drug dependent individual in treatment* (NIDA Research Monograph No. 165, pp. 44–84). Rockville, MD: National Institute on Drug Abuse.

Miller, W. R. (1996a). Motivational interviewing: Research, practice, puzzles. *Addictive Behaviors, 21,* 835–842.

Miller, W. R. (1996b). What is a relapse? Fifty ways to leave the wagon. *Addiction, 91* (Suppl.), S15–S27.

Miller, W. R., & Rollnick, S. (1991). *Motivational interviewing: Preparing people to change addictive behavior.* New York: Guilford.

Moos, R. H., Finney, J. W., & Cronkite, R. C. (1990). *Alcoholism treatment: Context, process, and outcome.* New York: Oxford University Press.

O'Connell, K. A., & Martin, E. J. (1987). Highly tempting situations associated with abstinence, temporary lapse, and relapse among participants in smoking cessation programs. *Journal of Consulting and Clinical Psychology, 55,* 367–371.

Premack, D. (1965). Reinforcement theory. In D. Levine (Ed.), *Nebraska Symposium on Motivation* (pp. 123–180). Lincoln: University of Nebraska Press.

Prochaska, J. O., DiClemente, C. C., & Norcross, J. C. (1992). In search of how people change: Applications to addictive behaviors. *American Psychologist, 47,* 1102–1114.

Rachlin, H. (1974). Self-control. *Behaviorism, 2,* 94–107.

Rachlin, H. (1992). Teleological behaviorism. *American Psychologist, 47,* 1371–1382.

Rachlin, H. (1994). *Behavior and mind: The roots of modern psychology.* New York: Oxford University Press.

Rachlin, H., Green, L., Kagel, J., & Battalio, R. (1976). Economic demand theory and psychological studies of choice. In G. Bower (Ed.), *The psychology of learning and motivation* (pp. 129–154). New York: Academic Press.

Skinner, B. F. (1938). *The behavior of organisms: An experimental analysis.* Englewood Cliffs, NJ: Prentice-Hall.

Tucker, J. A., & Vuchinich, R. E. (1997). Unpublished data, Auburn University, AL.

Tucker, J. A., Vuchinich, R. E., & Gladsjo, J. A. (1990/91). Environmental influences on relapse in substance abuse disorders. *International Journal of the Addictions, 25,* 1017–1050.

Tucker, J. A., Vuchinich, R. E., & Gladsjo, J. A. (1994). Environmental events surrounding natural recovery from alcohol-related problems. *Journal of Studies on Alcohol, 55,* 401–411.

Tucker, J. A., Vuchinich, R. E., & Pukish, M. A. (1995). Molar environmental contexts surrounding recovery from alcohol problems by treated and untreated problem drinkers. *Experimental and Clinical Psychopharmacology, 3,* 195–204.

Vaillant, G. E. (1983). *The natural history of alcoholism.* Cambridge, MA: Harvard University Press.

Vuchinich, R. E. (1982). Have behavioral theories of alcohol abuse focused too much on alcohol consumption? *Bulletin of the Society of Psychologists in Substance Abuse, 1,* 151–154.

Vuchinich, R. E. (1995). Alcohol abuse as molar choice: An update of a 1982 proposal. *Psychology of Addictive Behaviors, 9,* 223–235.

Vuchinich, R. E. (1997). Behavioral economics of drug consumption. In B. A. Johnson & J. D. Roache (Eds.), *Drug addiction and its treatment: Nexus of neuroscience and behavior* (pp. 73–90). Philadelphia: Lippincott-Raven.

Vuchinich, R. E., & Simpson, C. A. (1997). Hyperbolic temporal discounting in social drinkers and problem drinkers. *Experimental and Clinical Psychopharmacology* (in press).

Vuchinich, R. E., & Tucker, J. A. (1988). Contributions from behavioral theories of choice to an analysis of alcohol abuse. *Journal of Abnormal Psychology, 97,* 181–195.

Vuchinich, R. E., & Tucker, J. A. (1996a). Alcoholic relapse, life events, and behavioral theories of choice: A prospective analysis. *Experimental and Clinical Psychopharmacology, 4,* 19–28.

Vuchinich, R. E., & Tucker, J. A. (1996b). The molar context of alcohol abuse. In L. Green & J. Kagel (Eds.), *Advances in behavioral economics: Vol. 3. Substance use and abuse* (pp. 133–162). Norwood, NJ: Ablex.

8

Policy Change as a Means for Reducing the Prevalence and Impact of Alcoholism, Smoking, and Obesity

KATHERINE BATTLE HORGEN AND KELLY D. BROWNELL

INTRODUCTION

This chapter proposes that policy change is the most immediate, least expensive, and most powerful way to have an impact on alcohol abuse, smoking, and obesity. Although existing approaches to treatment provide some relief from the enormous individual and collective suffering from these problems, the cost is high, and clinical relief reaches relatively few.

We make the distinction at the outset between what the field recognizes as "public health approaches" and policy. In psychology and related disciplines, most authors discussing public health approaches refer to ways of delivering conventional treatment in less costly ways (i.e., with brief treatment, see Chapter 10) and in settings where more people can be reached than in individual treatment (e.g., schools, worksites, entire communities). In fact, the field of public health is much broader than such approaches, and includes what we discuss here—public policy. We believe there is considerable utility in a focus on policy in the addictions field. Current work on treatment and enhanced focus on policy could be mutually reinforcing (Heather, 1996; also see Chapter 10).

KATHERINE BATTLE HORGEN AND KELLY D. BROWNELL   •   Department of Psychology, Yale University, New Haven, Connecticut 06520.

Treating Addictive Behaviors, 2nd ed., edited by Miller and Heather. Plenum Press, New York, 1998.

PREVALENCE AND COSTS OF ADDICTIVE DISORDERS

The addictive behaviors create staggering costs, both to the individuals affected and to public health and well-being. Smoking, alcohol abuse, and obesity are issues of great importance. Collectively, the toll is enormous. Approximately 34% of the American population is overweight (Williamson, 1995), and the prevalence continues to rise. Considering the monetary toll of approximately $40 billion per year in the United States (Colditz, 1992) and the associated psychological and physical health problems including cardiovascular disease, certain cancers, hypertension, stroke, and diabetes mellitus (Pi-Sunyer, 1995), obesity is a major public health concern.

In the context of diet-related diseases, eating disorders (anorexia nervosa, bulimia nervosa, and binge eating disorder) must also be considered. The prevalence of diagnosed eating disorders is approximately 2% of the population, but milder forms of the disorders may be five times as common (Garfinkel, 1995). Medical complications include reproductive, cardiovascular, gastrointestinal, metabolic, neurological, and dermatological problems (Goldbloom & Kennedy, 1995).

Smoking is the single greatest cause of preventable death in the United States (Centers for Disease Control, 1989), accounting for approximately 30% of all cancer deaths (American Cancer Society, 1989), and contributing to heart disease, chronic bronchitis, emphysema, respiratory problems, peptic ulcers, and retardation of fetal development (Centers for Disease Control, 1989). There will be 10 million tobacco-related deaths a year worldwide by the year 2010 (Peto, Lopez, Boreham, Thun, & Heath, 1992). Secondhand smoke places those in the vicinity of the smoker at risk for a variety of health disorders (Marshall, 1986).

Alcohol consumption is associated with cirrhosis of the liver, some cancers, fetal abnormalities, and cognitive impairment (Goldman, 1983; Streissguth, Landesman-Dwyer, Martin, & Smith, 1980). This behavior affects not only the drinker but those with whom the drinker has contact. Drunk driving crashes claimed 16,589 lives in 1994 and caused 297,000 injuries (Hingson, McGovern, Heeren, Winter, & Zakocs, 1996). Economists estimate that alcohol abuse costs the United States $42 billion yearly in absenteeism and decreased job performance, while approximately 15% of the national health budget is expended on treatment for alcoholism and related disorders (Holden, 1987; Saxe, Dougherty, & Esty, 1983). The indirect costs of alcohol use in the United States, estimated at approximately $120 billion annually, are even more disturbing (Schifrin, Hartzog, & Brand, 1980).

With the high prevalence of these costly problems, it is important to understand the efficacy and effectiveness of available treatments. To the extent the impact of current treatments is limited, approaches derived from alternative models must be considered.

EFFICACY AND EFFECTIVENESS OF CURRENT TREATMENTS

Efforts to address obesity have been equivocal. Although behavioral interventions have produced significant weight loss in mildly to moderately obese patients, with some research indicating good maintenance of weight loss at 2 years, 5-year follow-up data show that maintenance is difficult to achieve (Wilson,

1995). Few long-term studies have been done, and weight regain varies over studies, but the general trend indicates a return to baseline (Wilson, 1995). This erodes faith in tertiary care efforts for the problem and has even led to an antidieting movement in which some claim that weight loss cannot be sustained and should not be attempted (Garner & Wooley, 1991). This stance is extreme (Brownell & Rodin, 1994), but it reflects considerable frustration with current treatments.

Obesity is viewed by the culture, and still by many professionals, as a moral deficit of the individual; this attitude disregards the culpability of environment, which produces excessive pressure to be thin coupled with pervasive inducements to eat (Brownell, 1994). Although individuals have some control over weight, both biology and culture play important roles. Treatments focused solely on the behavior of the individual have provided little relief from the epidemic. A promising alternative is to shift the focus from demand (focus on the behavior of the obese individual) to supply (focus on the environmental problems perpetuating the problem).

Treatment of eating disorders is also a challenge. Treatment of anorexia nervosa with behavioral, family, psychoanalytic, and even pharmacological treatment is only partially successful (Johnson, 1995; Russell, Szmukler, Dare, & Eisler, 1987; Vitousek, 1995). When the disorder is life-threatening, medical or psychiatric hospitalization, or both, is warranted, but this is very expensive. Treatment of bulimia nervosa has been more successful, but only models involving intensive and expensive psychotherapy have been tested (Fairburn, 1995; Fairburn, Agras, & Wilson, 1992)

Smoking cessation interventions have also produced mixed results. Cognitive-behavioral treatments, emphasizing skills for managing cravings and smoking triggers, have shown modest but clinically significant success (Lichtenstein & Glasgow, 1992; Tiffany & Baker, 1988). However, many people drop out of such programs, and for those who remain, the chance of relapse is high. Nicotine replacement strategies are the only pharmacological agents that have been related to long-term abstinence, and the combination of such strategies with cognitive and behavioral methods has been endorsed by the American Psychological Association (see Chapter 18, this volume). Lichtenstein and Glasgow (1992) have argued that the necessarily intensive nature of treatment makes it available to few and not cost-effective. Intensive clinical interventions, though not in and of themselves practical, are valuable research tools for examining strategies that may then be extended to public health programs (Lichtenstein & Glasgow, 1992).

Research on treatment for alcoholism has shown promise, although a gap still exists between research and treatment in the community. A review by Miller, Andrews, Wilbourne, and Bennett (Chapter 15, this volume) notes that brief interventions are superior to wait-list or no treatment. While treatment results are promising, an important issue is determining which combination of treatment components is best for which client. Research programs such as Project MATCH (Project MATCH Research Group, 1997) have begun to explore matching patients with the most appropriate form of treatment (see Chapter 12, this volume).

Aversion therapies and nausea-inducing drugs such as antabuse and emetine can decrease consumption, although side effects preclude them from being prescribed in many cases, and less motivated alcoholics may simply discontinue use (Cannon, Baker, Gino, & Nathan, 1988; Goldstein, 1994; Porterfield, 1992). The opiate antagonist naltrexone has shown promising results, not by precluding a single drink, but by preventing a drink from triggering a binge and by decreasing cravings. However, relapse rates are high following discontinuation of the drug (Goldstein, 1994). McClellan and colleagues (1994) found that substance abuse services such as alcohol and drug education, group therapy for denial, and 12-step meetings may change alcohol use but do not affect the psychosocial problems of the alcohol abuser. Social skills training offers promise as a treatment component, as does behavioral skills training (see Chapter 15, this volume). Psychotherapy, family counseling, and employment counseling improve post-treatment psychosocial functioning but do not appear to reduce posttreatment substance use.

When one looks at the overall picture across the addictions, there is considerable promise in clinical treatment. Another innovative variant to traditional approaches is matching treatment combinations to the patient. As noted by Miller and colleagues (1995), "the best hope lies in assembling a menu of effective alternatives, and then seeking a system for finding the right combination of elements for each individual" (p. 33). Furthermore, those treatments with the highest cost do not necessarily produce the best results (Finney & Monahan, 1996), and treatment that proves efficacious in clinical trials may not be as effective in natural settings.

Even when the gap between research and practice is successfully bridged, one must consider that only a few have access to these services. Efficacy of treatments across the addictions ranges from poor to promising, but in no case has effectiveness been documented or has a sizable fraction of the affected population been reached. A logical addition to clinical treatment programs may be public policy changes, which reach large numbers of people at lower cost.

RATIONALE FOR POLICY

Treatment effectiveness has been limited by the high cost of treatment, lack of trained professionals to deliver treatment, and the fact that only a small fraction of those with the problems are treated and helped. The lack of access will only worsen with managed care. Even those who can afford treatment may not receive it, due to lack of information, misgivings about therapy, or the associated stigma of the addictive behaviors.

Intervening at the structural or environmental level is an appealing complement or even alternative to prevailing approaches. If the environment is responsible for these problems to a significant extent, the environment is a natural place to look for solutions.

APPLICATION OF POLICY TO ADDICTIVE BEHAVIORS

Policy interventions and environmental change have taken many forms across the addictive behaviors. Legislation has altered the price of cigarettes and alcohol through taxes, has imposed penalties for some forms of abuse (e.g., drunk driving), has defined the age at which substances can be purchased legally, has regulated the sale of the substances, and has imposed some limits on advertising. Regulation requires warning labels on cigarettes, food labels, and prohibition of smoking in public places. National initiatives such as Mothers Against Drunk Driving aim to influence policy, attitudes, and behavior.

It is beyond the scope of this chapter to review each such area in detail. The purpose of this chapter is to draw attention to the potential influence of policy and to underscore the importance of the process of policy making as an area of inquiry. We will, therefore, cover two areas of policy change: taxes imposed on cigarettes, alcohol, and food, and regulation of the media. These serve as examples of the potential of policy as a means of changing behavior.

ALTERING PRICE STRUCTURE

Changing the cost of cigarettes, alcohol, and food may affect use. Should this be the case, legislation increasing the price of tobacco, alcohol, and poor food through taxes, or subsidies for the sale of more healthy food, could influence millions of people with a single act.

Taxes on Alcohol

Economic studies have demonstrated that higher taxes decrease alcohol consumption, even in heavy drinkers (Hacker, 1987). Godfrey and Maynard (1995) assert, however, that sensitivity to price varies across countries and that the most popular beverage in a country is generally the least price-sensitive. Such was the case with wine in France between 1954 and 1971 and with beer in Ireland between 1953 and 1967 (Osterberg, 1995). Osterberg notes, however, that despite variety in price elasticity due to social circumstances, the data support the conclusion that alcohol consumption is affected by its price. Swedish taxes between 1976 and 1983 were associated with a 21% decline in per capita alcohol consumption ("Alcohol and drug abuse in Sweden," 1984). A 16-year American study examining the effects of a one dollar per proof gallon increase in the liquor excise tax indicated that the tax was related to a sharp decrease in per capita liquor consumption and a decline in the mortality from cirrhosis of the liver (Cook & Tauchen, 1982). Although alcohol sales have been shown to be highly price-sensitive, one must consider the amount of taxation in relation to income. Godfrey and Maynard (1992) estimate that a 5% annual increase in alcohol price in the United Kingdom would reduce alcohol consumption by 31% by the year 2000, but that any growth in income would offset this decline in consumption.

Taxes on Cigarettes

Cigarette taxes have decreased smoking, with similar price elasticities in different countries (Godfrey & Maynard, 1995). A study evaluating the effects of state tax increases in all 50 states from 1955 to 1988 linked tax increases to a 2.4% per capita consumption decline, with larger taxes related to larger reductions (Peterson, Zeger, Remington, & Anderson, 1992). The 1989 cigarette excise tax of 25 cents per pack in California resulted in a 5% to 7% decline in consumption attributable to the tax and the generation of over $600 million in revenue during the first year (Flewelling *et al.*, 1992). Price has been cited as the single most important determinant of consumption in Finland (Meier & Licari, 1997). The World Health Organization (1987) estimated an approximate inverse linear relationship between price per pack of cigarettes and consumption in 22 European countries.

A 12-cent increase in the New York State cigarette tax from 21 to 33 cents reduced smoking by about 3%. This 3% is impressive when one considers that more than 3 million people were influenced, not including those newly protected from secondhand smoke. It was estimated that 115,967 New Yorkers would either quit or not start smoking as a result of the tax, and that 28,992 smoking-induced premature deaths would be prevented in the subsequent generation. Almost $200 million in revenue was generated in the first year (Cummings & Sciandra, 1990). The U.S. Department of Agriculture reported that domestic consumption of cigarettes decreased by 14 billion cigarettes, or 4%, attributable to the doubling of the federal excise tax (Warner, 1984). Similarly, a British study predicted that approximately 100,000 additional people would live to age 65 as a result of the government's doubling the federal cigarette tax in 1983 (Lewit, 1989). Even a relatively small percentage decrease in behavior can have an impressive public health impact.

Snack Food Tax

In July of 1991, California enacted a short-lived 8.25% "Twinkie Tax" on "nonessential" foods in an attempt to close a $14.3 billion budget gap (Zuck, 1992). A list of approximately 5,000 taxable and nontaxable food items was sent to retailers. The distinctions were arbitrary, with donuts being taxed but not donut holes, slices of cake taxed, but not whole cakes (Molpus, 1995). The law taxed cheaper foods (e.g., potato chips) while leaving luxury items such as brie and caviar untouched (McCraw, 1993). Only 5,000 of California's 18,000 stores used electronic scanners, leaving most to have personnel memorize what was and was not taxable (Motamedi, 1991). Organizations providing food for the needy reported more people relying on their services, an increase one opponent attributed to the regressive nature of the tax that penalized those without access to fresh foods (Lozano, 1991). However, purchases made with food stamps were not taxable. The 1992 *Consumer Snacking Behavior Report* (Snack Food Association, 1992) indicated that from 1989 to 1990, the heaviest buyers of snack foods were those classified as "white collar families," with almost 70% of heavy buyers reporting average household incomes of over $27,500.

First year revenues were $200 million from the California tax. Estimates were that snack sales decreased about 10% during that period (Boroughs & Collins, 1992). Californians repealed the tax in December of 1992 with a 60% rejection rate through Proposition 163. Following the repeal, store owners reported a 16.7% increase in snack food sales over the previous year ("California," 1993).

Maryland imposed a 5% snack food tax in 1992. Following the legislation, a Frito-Lay spokesperson noted that "demand in Maryland has been off" (Harrison, 1993). The legislation received severe opposition from the Snack Food Association, an international trade association of about 850 members that represents snack manufacturers and suppliers to the snack industry (Harrison, 1993). The director of government affairs for Frito-Lay, Inc., reported a loss of $500,000 in sales attributable to the decline in consumer demand (Harrison, 1993). Currently, Maryland is moving toward repeal of the tax (Abramowitz, 1995). Maine is the only other state to have experimented with snack taxes; it implemented a 7% tax in 1991 on "nonnutritious" foods (Zuck, 1992).

According to critics, these taxes were arbitrary in their classification system (Garry, 1992) and difficult for retailers to enact (Gasparello, 1991). Future taxes might be imposed at the wholesale level before they reach retail stores to bypass such problems. Consumer discontent with taxes in general has increased, coupled with resentment toward government interference (Molpus, 1995). Finally, vested economic interests including candy, snack food, and soft drink manufacturers have lobbied heavily against the tax. It appears, however, that the taxes decreased consumption and generated revenue. Furthermore, information from the Snack Food Association (1992) indicates that those classified as "snackers" in the 1992 *Consumer Snacking Behavior Report* based their purchases on price, used coupons, shopped for bargains, and bought sale items more than did their nonsnacking counterparts.

Conclusions on Price Modification with Taxes

Research with cigarette and alcohol taxes is clear and consistent: As price rises with increasing taxes, consumption declines. Because these taxes have been levied more to raise revenue for states than to decrease consumption, the optimal level of taxation that would decrease consumption while being acceptable to voters has not been determined. Should voters be told that the purpose is to decrease consumption (given the large toll on public health) and that the revenue will be put to good use (e.g., stemming the rise in health care costs), greater taxation than is currently in use might be viable.

The case is less clear with food. The only attempts at taxation on unhealthy foods have been aimed at revenue generation. Practical implementation problems have made these taxes unpopular, and only anecdotal data are available on changes in consumption. This area needs attention in research. An alternative and probably more publicly popular approach might be to decrease the prices of healthful foods with subsidies. No data are available to address the potential impact of such an approach.

MEDIA REGULATION

Over the past two decades, alcohol and cigarettes have been among the world's most heavily advertised products (Clark, 1988; Viscusi, 1992). Advertising is intended to differentiate brands in order to either promote brand loyalty, induce brand switching, or recruit new smokers to a brand (Edwards *et al.*, 1994; Viscusi, 1992). This has led to competitive advertising among brands, to the point of promoting some cigarettes as "more healthful" than others, as was the case in early Camel cigarette ads touting the brand as a "milder" cigarette and others promoting the ability of filters to remove tar. This concession involving mentioning the health risks denotes an implicit recognition of the consumer's awareness of the product dangers (Viscusi, 1992).

Studies have suggested short-term increases in the amount of alcohol consumed following alcohol advertisements (Edwards *et al.,* 1994). Studies examining the effects of advertisements embedded in television shows indicate an increase in consumption relative to those not viewing the commercials (Kohn & Smart, 1984, 1987). A study on repeated exposure to ads indicated immediate increased consumption, but the effect tapered off; exposure to 12 advertisements instead of the 6 did not significantly increase consumption (Wilks, Vardanega, & Callan, 1992).

Even more alarming are studies on younger individuals. A study on drinking in young adults indicated that those who reported high exposure to alcohol advertisements in the previous month had consumed an average of 30 beers, compared to those reporting low exposure, who drank around 15 beers (Atkin & Block, 1984). An examination of the attitudes and intentions of "pre-drinkers" suggested that children who could identify more beer advertisements held more positive attitudes toward drinking and expressed greater intention to drink as adults (Grube & Wallack, 1994). Edwards and colleagus (1994) noted that the positive correlations between advertisement exposure, attitudes, and consumption remain when demographic factors, social influences, and other media exposure are controlled.

One must consider that the techniques used to assess the impact of advertising are often unlike realistic drinking situations, tend to rely on self-report measures, and measure only short-term effects. Still, measurable impacts of advertising have been reported and should be taken as cause for concern. One means by which ads may influence behavior is through alcohol expectancies, in that more positive expectancies about the benefits of drinking would encourage drinking behavior. As advertising depicts alcohol as normal and desirable and associates it with wealth, social approval, and success, regulating these ads might influence expectancies and thus affect alcohol consumption (Edwards *et al.,* 1994).

Studies examining the effects of advertising bans on alcohol have yielded equivocal results. Two studies in single provinces in Canada indicated no effects (Ogborne & Smart, 1980; Smart & Cutler, 1976), which Edwards and colleagues (1994) speculate may have been due to a failure to control for ads from other provinces. However, a cross-national study of 20 countries during the 1970s showed significant reductions in both alcohol consumption and alcohol-related problems, measured by the vehicle fatality rate.

A ban on television and radio cigarette advertising, signaling the end of the Fairness Doctrine (equal time for antismoking ads), and the mandate of hazard-warning labels were only two of the social changes occurring as cigarette consumption began decreasing around 1970, but it is evident that various government efforts to influence cigarette consumption have been successful. Not only have half of all American adults who once smoked quit, but fewer people have started to smoke (Viscusi, 1992). Norway has banned smoking advertising since 1975; this led to a sharp decrease in the percentage of adolescents who smoke (British Medical Association, 1986; Chapman, 1985; White, 1988).

One can speculate how advertising bans on unhealthy foods might affect obesity (Brownell, 1994). Jeffery (1995) noted that controlling advertising is a method of limiting promotion of products to population groups for which the products would constitute a significant hazard. The average American child, an easily influenced target, sees 10,000 food commercials per year, 95% of which are for candy, fast food, soft drinks, and sugared cereal (Battle & Brownell, 1996). Brownell (1994) and Jeffery (1995) suggest restricting the promotion of low-nutrition items as one strategy, and one could focus on those television programs and viewing hours targeted at children.

While the notion of banning advertisements raises cries of violation of the First Amendment, commercial free speech has long been considered different from any other form of speech, and until 1976 did not enjoy any First Amendment privileges. The courts remain undecided on this issue (Cox, 1980; Miller, 1985). The Supreme Court has stated that "false, deceptive, and misleading advertising can be prohibited, and even non-deceptive advertising can be banned where necessary to accomplish a substantial government purpose" (Blasi & Monaghan, 1986, p. 503, summarizing *Central Hudson Gas & Electric Corp. v. Public Service Commission*, 447 U.S. 557, 566 [1980]).

The tobacco companies have also asserted that a product legally for sale can be advertised (Goodin, 1989). Opponents argue that states permit various practices between consenting adults in private while prohibiting them in public, hence it is acceptable to relegate dangerous behaviors to the private sphere in the realm of consenting adults (Lundberg & Knoll, 1986). A second argument is that tobacco companies have generally been unable or unwilling to target their advertising at adults without appealing to minors (Goodin, 1989; P. Taylor, 1985). Advertising to attract new consumers to a product that might improve their lives is permissible, but for a product to "service an addiction" (Goodin, 1989, p. 106) could be challenged on the ground of damage to the public health. Recently, negotiations between federal and state officials and tobacco companies have made advertising a key issue. We see this as a sign of progress.

Public opinion is important to policy decisions. An analysis of Gallup Poll surveys from 1962 to 1988 indicates that support for a complete ban on cigarette ads rose from 36% in 1977 to 55% in 1988 (Viscusi, 1992). One might expect an even higher percentage today. Edwards and colleagues (1994) note that restrictions on advertising may have an effect on the social attitudes toward substance use rather than a direct effect on behavior. This impact may then translate into a social and political context fertile for future legislation in which policy is used to decrease addictive behaviors.

Although the scope of this chapter does not allow a comprehensive review of public health media campaigns, it should be noted that advertising can have a positive impact on health, as seen when a National Cancer Institute (NCI) initiative collaborated with Kellogg's cereal company to publicize the benefits of a high-fiber, low-fat diet. The 2-year campaign included messages on cereal boxes and television advertisements, along with a telephone number to call for information. More than 20,000 telephone calls and 30,000 written inquiries were received by the NCI. Sales of all types of high-fiber cereal increased in the Washington, DC area, indicating that consumers were able to generalize the message to other brands (Freimuth, Hammond, & Stein, 1988). One might consider such an intervention in the realm of alcohol, where the promotion of one type of nonalcoholic beverage could extend to many other nonalcoholic beverages, especially if the campaigns focused on the drinks as healthful alternatives to alcohol (Holder & Howard, 1992).

CONCLUSIONS: THE UNREALIZED POTENTIAL OF POLICY

Perhaps the greatest unrealized potential for reversing the massive public health costs and personal toll of the addictions is to intervene with policy. There are cases where policy mandates, leading to changes in legislation and regulation, have had rapid and powerful effects on behavior, with effects that dwarf the results of treatments delivered in clinical settings.

Policy changes have been considered much more in the tobacco and alcohol fields than has been the case with obesity and eating disorders. With tobacco and alcohol, legislators and regulators have long considered it the purview of government to protect its citizens from exposure to potentially deadly substances. Professionals in the addictions fields have worked with those in the government to consider issues such as taxes on the substances, ages at which substances may be purchased, and advertising practices.

The general conclusions that can be drawn from such interventions are that substance problems are strongly related to per capita consumption, that a reduction in consumption, regardless of its impetus, leads to a decline in problems related to the substance, and that both cigarette and alcohol sales are highly price-sensitive. These conclusions support the promise of policy interventions as a supplement to clinical treatment of the addictive behaviors.

The results of policy changes have been evaluated frequently in some cases but little in others. In too many cases, there is no evaluation at all. The fact that policy implementation is far ahead of policy evaluation is probably due to several factors. First, policy changes have sometimes occurred for purposes other than to affect substance use. Sin taxes on tobacco and alcohol, and snack taxes on food, have been used by states and federal legislators to generate revenue, so judgments of their utility would not be based on behavior and health. Second, the effect of policy is not easy to evaluate, and obstacles to research funding complicate the matter further. The grant review process may delay the collection of baseline data so that the new policy may be in place before the funding to evaluate it has even been obtained. Finally, and perhaps most important, there is not a sufficient pool of addiction researchers who evaluate policy.

We chose several examples of policy that have had positive impact. We could have chosen others where policy has had no effects or even has had paradoxical effects. An example of the latter was the voluntary removal of cigarette advertisements from television by the tobacco industry. This occurred after legislation required equal time for antismoking messages for every cigarette advertisement. The tobacco companies, seeing the negative impact on sales of the antismoking messages, and fearing broad-based restriction on advertising, withdrew from television. It was later reported that the advertising of cigarettes in other media (e.g., billboards, magazines) was more cost-effective than was television advertising. This shows a need for evaluation of policy changes to ensure a positive impact.

An example of a policy victory is the use of taxes on cigarettes and alcohol. The literature shows an orderly relationship of price with per capita consumption. As price increases, consumption declines. Should legislators wish to decrease smoking and drinking, increasing taxes may be the most rapid, effective, and least costly method. An internal memo from the Philip Morris Tobacco Company written in the 1980s but made public in the *New York Times* ("Why the Tobacco Industry Found Taxes Hazardous to Its Health") only in 1997 shows the key role such policies can play. The memo estimated that "a 10% increase in the price of cigarettes would lead to a decline of 12 percent in the number of teenagers who would otherwise begin to smoke," and that "if future reductions in youth smoking are desired, an increase in the Federal excise tax is a potent policy" (p. A1). A 1997 review of taxes on cigarettes concluded, "Excise tax increases are clearly one policy weapon that is effective in reducing the consumption of tobacco" (Meier & Licari, 1997).

It is unfortunate that so little attention has been paid to policy in the area of diet. Brownell (1994) proposed that Americans and people in many other countries are exposed to a "toxic environment" in which they are surrounded by low-cost, widely available, high-fat, and high-calorie foods. The expected result has occurred—high levels of diet-related diseases, especially obesity. We (Battle & Brownell, 1996; Brownell, 1994) and others (Jeffery, 1995; L. B. Taylor & Stunkard, 1993) have proposed intervention at the structural level through policy. Specifically, we have proposed that taxes be used to decrease the consumption of unhealthy foods, subsidies be used to enhance intake of healthful foods, advertising practices be regulated, and efforts be made to increase physical activity. There is only anecdotal evidence that any of these would be effective.

Advertising is a natural target for policy change. Limits have been placed on advertising cigarettes and alcohol to children. School health education programs routinely teach children skills to buffer them against messages that encourage substance use. There is no similar effort aimed at inducements to eat unhealthful foods. Policy dealing with advertising clearly needs more attention.

It is our belief that the lack of attention to policy is the most glaring gap in the addictions field. Policy is not a regular part of training in any field other than public health. Given the potential power of policy change, the difficulty in treating these problems, and the desperate need to take action, the gap between how much attention policy is given and how much it deserves needs to be closed. For those who study human behavior, policy making may be the most important behavior of all to study.

REFERENCES

Abramowitz, M. (1995, May 8). Snack tax crunched. *The Washington Post*, p. BO3.

Alcohol and drug abuse in Sweden. (1984, July). *Fact Sheets in Sweden. FS77 j Ohi*. Stockholm: The Swedish Institute.

American Cancer Society. (1989). *Cancer facts and figures—1989*. Atlanta, GA: Author.

Atkin, C. K., & Block, M. (1984). The effects of alcohol advertising. In T. C. Kinnear (Ed.), *Advances in consumer research* (pp. 688–693). Provo, UT: Association for Consumer Research.

Battle, E. K., & Brownell, K. D. (1996). Confronting a rising tide of eating disorders and obesity: Treatment vs. prevention and policy. *Addictive Behaviors, 21,* 755–765.

Blasi, V., & Monaghan, H. P. (1986). The First Amendment and cigarette advertising. *Journal of the American Medical Association, 256,* 502–509.

Boroughs, D. L., & Collins, S. (1992, January 27). The 10 worst economic moves. *U.S. News and World Report*, 54.

British Medical Association (BMA) Public Affairs Division. (1986). *Smoking out the barons: The campaign against the tobacco industry*. Chichester, England: Wiley, for the BMA.

Brownell, K. D. (1994, December 15). Get slim with higher taxes [Editorial]. *New York Times*, p. A29.

Brownell, K. D., & Rodin, J. (1994). The dieting maelstrom: Is it possible and advisable to lose weight? *American Psychologist, 49,* 781–791.

California. (1993, January 8). *Daily Report for Executives,* p. 5.

Cannon, D. S., Baker, T. B., Gino, A., & Nathan, P. E. (1988). Alcohol aversion therapy: Relationship between strength of aversion and abstinence. In T. B. Baker & D. S. Cannon (Eds.), *Assessment and treatment of addictive disorders* (pp. 205–237). New York: Praeger.

Centers for Disease Control. (1989). *Reducing the health consequences of smoking: 25 years of progress—A report of the Surgeon General* (DHHS publication CDC 89-8411). Rockville, MD: U.S. Public Health Service.

Chapman, S. (1985). *Cigarette advertising and smoking: A review of the evidence.* London: British Medical Association. Reprinted in BMA 1986, pp. 79–98.

Clark, E. (1988). *The want makers: Lifting the lid off the world advertising industry: How they make you buy.* London: Hodder & Stoughton.

Colditz, G. A. (1992). Economic costs of obesity. *American Journal of Clinical Nutrition, 55,* 503s–507s.

Cook, P. J., & Tauchen, G. (1982) The effect of liquor taxes on heavy drinking. *Bell Journal of Economics, 13,* 379–390.

Cox, A. (1980). Foreword: Freedom of expression in the Burger Court. *Harvard Law Review, 94,* 1–73.

Cummings, K. M., & Sciandra, R. (1990, April). The public health benefit of increasing tobacco taxes in New York State. *New York State Journal of Medicine,* 174–175.

Edwards, G., Anderson, R., Babor, T. F., Casswell, S., Ferrence, R., Giesbrecht, N., Godfrey, C., Holder, H. D., Lemmens, P., Makela, K., Midanik, L. T., Norstrom, T., Osterberg, E., Romelsjo, A., Room, R., Simpura, J., & Skog, O. (1994). *Alcohol policy and the public good.* Oxford, England: World Health Organization.

Fairburn, C. G. (1995). Short-term psychological treatments for bulimia nervosa. In K. D. Brownell & C. G. Fairburn (Eds.), *Eating disorders and obesity: A comprehensive handbook* (pp. 344–348). New York: Guilford.

Fairburn, C. G., Agras, W. S., & Wilson, G. T. (1992). The research on the treatment of bulimia nervosa: Practical and theoretical implications. In G. H. Anderson & S. H. Kennedy (Eds.), *The biology of feast and famine: Relevance to eating disorders* (pp. 317–340). San Diego, CA: Academic Press.

Finney, J. W., & Monahan, S. C. (1996). The cost-effectiveness of treatment for alcoholism: A second approximation. *Journal of Studies on Alcohol, 57,* 229–243.

Flewelling, R. L., Kenney, E., Elder, J. P., Pierce, J., Johnson, M., & Bal, D. G. (1992). First-year impact of the 1989 California cigarette tax increase on cigarette consumption. *American Journal of Public Health, 82,* 867–869.

Freimuth, V., Hammond, S., & Stein, J. (1988). Health advertisement: Prevention for profit. *American Journal of Public Health, 78,* 557–561.

Garfinkel, P. E. (1995). Foreword. In K. D. Brownell & C. G. Fairburn (Eds.), *Eating disorders and obesity: A comprehensive handbook* (pp. 336–343). New York: Guilford.

Garner, D. M., & Wooley, S. C. (1991). Confronting the failure of behavioral and dietary treatments for obesity. *Clinical Psychology Review, 11,* 729–780.

Garry, M. (1992). To tax or not to tax? California's Proposition 163 would repeal the snack tax. *Progressive Grocer, 71,* 10.

Gasparello, L. (1991, November 15). Repeal of snack tax effort begins in California. *Food & Drink Daily, 1*(175).

Godfrey, C., & Maynard, A. (1992). *A health strategy for alcohol: Setting targets and choosing policies* (YARTIC Occasional Paper 1). York and Leeds, England: Centre for Health Economics, University of York and Leeds Addiction Unit.

Godfrey, C. & Maynard, A. (1995). The economic evaluation of alcohol policies. In H. D. Holder & G. Edwards (Eds.), *Alcohol and public policy: Evidence and issues* (pp. 238–259). Oxford, England: Oxford University Press.

Goldbloom, D. S., & Kennedy, S. H. (1995). Medical complications of anorexia nervosa. In K. D. Brownell & C. G. Fairburn (Eds.), *Eating disorders and obesity: A comprehensive handbook* (pp. 266–270). New York: Guilford.

Goldman, M. S. (1983). Cognitive impairment in chronic alcoholics: Some cause for optimism. *American Psychologist, 38,* 1045–1054.

Goldstein, A. (1994). *Addiction: From biology to drug policy.* New York: Freeman.

Goodin, R. E. (1989). Note: The First Amendment and legislative bans of liquor and cigarette advertisements. *Columbia Law Review, 85,* 632–658.

Grube, J. W., & Wallack, L. (1994). The effects of television beer advertising on children. *American Journal of Public Health, 84,* 254–259.

Hacker, G. A. (1987). Taxing booze for health and wealth. *Journal of Policy Analysis and Management, 6*(4), 701–716.

Harrison, D. J. (1993). Empty Frito-Lay plant awaits change in political tastes. *Baltimore Business Journal, 10,* 11.

Heather, N. (1996). The public health and brief interventions for excessive alcohol consumption: The British experience. *Addictive Behaviors, 21*(6), 857–868.

Hingson, R., McGovern, J. H., Heeren, T., Winter, M., & Zakocs, R., (1996). Reducing alcohol-impaired driving in Massachusetts: The Saving Lives Program. *American Journal of Public Health, 86,* 791–797.

Holden, C. (1987). Is alcoholism treatment effective? *Science, 236,* 20–22.

Holder, H. D., & Howard, J. M. (1992). *Community prevention trials for alcohol problems: Methodological issues.* London: Praeger.

Jeffery, R. W. (1995). Public health approaches to the management of obesity. In K. D. Brownell & C. G. Fairburn (Eds.), *Eating disorders and obesity: A comprehensive handbook* (pp. 558–563). New York: Guilford.

Johnson, D. (1995). Psychodynamic treatment of bulimia nervosa. In K. D. Brownell & C. G. Fairburn (Eds.), *Eating disorders and obesity: A comprehensive handbook* (pp. 349–353). New York: Guilford.

Kohn, P. M., & Smart, R. G. (1984). The impact of television advertising on alcohol consumption: An experiment. *Journal of Studies on Alcohol, 45,* 295–301.

Kohn, P. M., & Smart, R. G. (1987). Wine, women, suspiciousness, and advertising. *Journal of Studies on Alcohol, 48,* 161–166.

Lewit, E. M. (1989). U.S. tobacco taxes: Behavioral effects and policy implications. *British Journal of Addiction, 84,* 1217–1235.

Lichtenstein, E., & Glasgow, R. E. (1992). Smoking cessation: What have we learned over the past decade? *Journal of Consulting and Clinical Psychology, 60,* 518–527.

Lozano, C. V. (1991, July 23). Tax bite's sour aftertaste. *The Los Angeles Times,* p. B1.

Lundberg, G. D., & Knoll, E. (1986) Tobacco for consenting adults in private only [Editorial]. *Journal of the American Medical Association, 255,* 1051–1053.

Marshall, E. (1986). Involuntary smokers face health risks. *Science, 234,* 1066–1067.

McClellan, A. T., Alterman, A. I., Metzger, D. S., Grissom, C. R., Woody, G. E., Luborsky, L., & O'Brien, C. P. (1994). Similarity of outcome predictors across opiate, cocaine, and alcohol treatments: Role of treatment services. *Journal of Consulting and Clinical Psychology, 62,* 1141–1158.

McCraw, V. (1993, March 5). Kelly budget is too taxing, council says. *The Washington Times,* p. B1.

Meier, K. J., & Licari, M. J. (1997). The effect of cigarette taxes on cigarette consumption, 1955 through 1994. *American Journal of Public Health, 87,* 1126–1130.

Miller, M. L. (1985). Note: The First Amendment and legislative bans of liquor and cigarette advertisements. *Columbia Law Review, 85,* 632–655.

Miller, W. R., Brown, J. M., Simpson, T. L., Handmaker, N. S., Bien, T. H., Luckie, L. F., Montgomery, H. A., Hester, R. K., & Tonigan, J. S. (1995). What works? A methodological analysis of the alcohol treatment outcome literature. In R. K Hester & W. R. Miller (Eds.), *Handbook of alcoholism treatment approaches: Effective alternatives* (pp. 12–44). Boston: Allyn & Bacon.

Molpus, M. (1995, May 17). Prepared testimony of Manly Molpus, President and Chief Executive Officer of the Grocery Manufacturers of America, Inc., before the House Agriculture Committee, Subcommittee of Department Operations and Nutrition. *Federal News Service.*

Motamedi, B. (1991, July 13). Confusing new law: Snack tax drives grocers crackers. *The San Francisco Chronicle,* p. A1.

Ogborne, A., & Smart, R. (1980). Will restrictions on alcohol advertising reduce alcohol consumption? *British Journal of Addiction, 75,* 293–296.

Osterberg, E. (1995). Do alcohol prices affect consumption and related problems? In H. D. Holder & G. Edwards (Eds.), *Alcohol and public policy: evidence and issues* (pp. 145–163). Oxford, England: Oxford University Press.

Peterson, D. E., Zeger, S. L., Remington, P. L., & Anderson, H. A. (1992). The effect of state cigarette tax increases on cigarette sales, 1955 to 1988. *American Journal of Public Health, 82,* 94–96.

Peto, R., Lopez, A. D., Boreham, J. Thun, M., & Heath C., Jr. (1992). Mortality from tobacco in developed countries: Indirect estimation from national vital statistics. *Lancet, 339*, 1268–1278.

Pi-Sunyer, F. X. (1995). Medical complications of obesity. In K. D. Brownell & C. G. Fairburn (Eds.), *Eating disorders and obesity: A comprehensive handbook* (pp. 401–405). New York: Guilford.

Porterfield, K. M. (1992). *Teenage perspectives: Focus on addiction.* Oxford, England: ABC-CLIO.

Project MATCH Research Group. (1997). Matching alcoholism treatments to client heterogeneity: Project MATCH posttreatment drinking outcomes. *Journal of Studies on Alcohol, 58*, 7–29.

Russell, G., Szmukler, G. I., Dare, C., & Eisler, I. (1987). An evaluation of family therapy in anorexia nervosa and bulimia nervosa. *Archives of General Psychiatry, 44*, 1047–1056.

Saxe, L., Dougherty, D., & Esty, J. (1983). *The effectiveness and costs of alcohol treatment* (Congressional Office of Technology Assessment Case Study, Publication No. 052-003-00902-1). Washington, DC: U.S. Government Printing Office.

Schifrin, L. G., Hartzog, C. E., & Brand, D. H. (1980). Costs of alcoholism and alcohol abuse and their relationship to alcohol research. In *Alcoholism and related problems: Opportunities for research* (pp. 165–186). Washington, DC: National Academy of Sciences.

Smart, R. G., & Cutler, R. (1976). The alcohol advertising ban in British Columbia: Problems and effects on beverage consumption. *British Journal of Addiction, 71*, 13–21.

Snack Food Association. (1992). *Consumer snacking behavior report.* Alexandria, VA: Author.

Streissguth, A. P., Landesman-Dwyer, S., Martin, J. S., & Smith, D. W. (1980). Teratogenic effects of alcohol in humans and laboratory animals. *Science, 209*, 353–361.

Taylor, C. B., & Stunkard, A. J. (1993). Public health approaches to weight control. In A. J. Stunkard & T. A. Wadden (Eds.), *Obesity: Theory and treatment* (pp. 335–353). New York: Raven.

Taylor, P. (1985). *The smoke ring.* London: Sphere Books.

Tiffany, S. T., & Baker, T. B. (1988). The role of aversion and counseling strategies in treatments for cigarette smoking. In T. B. Baker & D. S. Cannon (Eds.), *Assessment and treatment of addictive disorders* (pp. 238–289). New York: Praeger.

Viscusi, W. K. (1992). *Smoking.* Oxford, England: Oxford University Press.

Vitousek, K. B. (1995). Cognitive-behavioral treatment for anorexia nervosa. In K. D. Brownell & C. G. Fairburn (Eds.), *Eating disorders and obesity: A comprehensive handbook* (pp. 324–329). New York: Guilford.

Warner, K. E. (1984). Cigarette taxation: Doing good by doing well. *Journal of Public Health Policy, 5*, 312–319.

White, L. C. (1988). *Merchants of death: The American tobacco industry.* New York: Beach Tree Books, Morrow.

Why the tobacco industry found taxes hazardous to its health. (1997, April 6). *New York Times*, p. A1.

Wilks, J., Vardanega, A. T., & Callan, V. J. (1992). Effects of television advertising of alcohol on alcohol consumption and intentions to drive. *Drug and Alcohol Review, 11*, 15–21.

Williamson, D. F. (1995). Prevalence and demographics of obesity. In K. D. Brownell & C. G. Fairburn (Eds.), *Eating disorders and obesity: A comprehensive handbook* (pp. 391–395). New York: Guilford.

Wilson, G. T. (1995). Behavioral approaches to the treatment of obesity. In K. D. Brownell & C. G. Fairburn (Eds.), *Eating disorders and obesity: A comprehensive handbook* (pp. 479–483). New York: Guilford.

World Health Organization. (1987). *Tobacco price and the smoking epidemic: Smoke-free Europe—9.* Copenhagen, Denmark.

Zuck, R. A. (1992). What balancing acts follow tax on snacks? *Paper, Film, & Foil Converter, 66*, 4.

III

Preparing for Change

There is a broad consensus that motivation is a key obstacle in addressing addictive behaviors. It could be argued, in fact, that it lies at the very heart of the problem, that fundamentally, addictions are human motivation gone wrong. The idea that some clients need help with motivation (rather than a focus on behavior change) seems to be part of the clinical appeal of the stages of change. Our first edition contained a series of chapters that focused on processes for moving clients from precontemplation and contemplation to preparation (then called "determination") and on to action. That remains the organizing theme of Part III.

The vast majority of individuals with currently problematic addictive behavior, perhaps 80%, are in precontemplation or contemplation stages, and not ready for change. Rather than waiting for the person to "hit bottom," clinicians emphasize enhancing readiness to change. These chapters address practical clinical issues related to motivation for change. Chapter 9 provides an overview of therapeutic strategies for increasing motivation for change in specialist settings, and an updated review of pertinent outcome research. Many other opportunities for identification and brief intervention are found in health care settings; Chapter 10 explores issues and research in this area.

A different motivational challenge involves the calls for help that are inevitably received from significant others concerned about addictive behavior in a loved one. Here the caller is often highly motivated, but the loved one is not. Robert Meyers and his colleagues briefly review in Chapter 11 the several methods used in common practice, and document an effective new unilateral family therapy method based on the community reinforcement approach.

The preparation stage has been included in Part III as a motivational challenge, in that clients in this stage are still in the process of gearing up for action. Two chapters are focused on processes involved in helping clients identify optimal change strategies, which might be thought of as a health services issue. The "matching hypothesis" was quite popular at the time of our first edition, positing that the effectiveness of services would be improved by assigning clients to the right treatment alternative the first time. Since then a number of new studies have appeared, including the results of Project MATCH, now the field's largest randomized psychotherapy trial. In Chapter 12, Margaret Mattson takes up this complicated issue in light of these new findings. James McKay and Thomas McLellan offer a different slant on client–treatment matching in the final chapter of this section, focusing on the challenges of polyproblem clients. When your client has multiple problems, where do you start? An issue here is the prioritizing of goals and problems in order to arrive at a reasonable opening treatment plan.

It is plain that the scope of these chapters is broad, spanning the rather different challenges of the precontemplation, contemplation, and preparation stages. What binds them together is the work of enhancing motivation for change.

9

Enhancing Motivation
for Change

WILLIAM R. MILLER

THINKING ABOUT MOTIVATION

Every therapist knows that motivation is a vital element of change. Nowhere is this clearer than in the treatment of addictive behaviors, which are, if one thinks about it, fundamentally motivational problems. Addictive behaviors are by definition highly motivated, in that they persist against an accumulating tide of aversive consequences. When one continues to act despite great personal risk and cost, something is overriding common sense. In the context of war, we call it bravery or heroism. In the context of pleasure, we call it addiction.

How does one change a motivated pattern of behavior that seems relatively impervious to deterrence by fear and pain? All manner of bizarre measures have been tried over the centuries. Some have bet on intensifying the deterrent pain by dunking, flogging, imprisonment, public humiliation, hot-seat attack therapy, fines, even the threat of execution. Oddly enough, the effectiveness of punishment seems extremely limited, and may even increase adamant defiance to persist. "If punishment worked," one client sagely observed, "there would be no alcoholics." Addiction is not for insufficient suffering.

Other reformers have put their faith in knowledge and education. Yet, as evidenced in Chapter 15, it would be difficult to find a strategy that has proved less successful in changing established substance use disorders. Those who are in trouble with alcohol and other drugs, or with gambling or other self-destructive behavior patterns, are often rationally aware of the risk and harm they face. What

WILLIAM R. MILLER • Department of Psychology, University of New Mexico, Albuquerque, New Mexico 87131.

Treating Addictive Behaviors, 2nd ed., edited by Miller and Heather. Plenum Press, New York, 1998.

smoker does not know that his or her habit causes chronic heart disease, deforming and disabling cancers, and suffocating emphysema, some of the cruelest ways to die? Even prevention strategies based on educating about drugs have been ineffective at best (Moskowitz, 1989). Addiction is not for lack of knowledge.

The psychodynamic era left us with insight-focused concepts of the dynamics of addiction: What addicts need is a "breaking through" or "breaking down of defenses" or an understanding of the unconscious motives beneath their self-defeating and perplexing behavior. Systems theory took this a step further to view the motivated pathology as resident not in an individual, but in a family or social system. Through a strange concatenation of Synanon, ego defenses, and correctional systems, the American addiction field for two or three decades placed its faith in confrontation. Confrontational counseling, groups, communities, and boot camps arose. Videotape self-confrontation was tried. People were allegedly "scared straight." Again the outcomes were poor, sometimes worse than no treatment at all. LSD was tried to evoke breakthrough insights in alcoholics, to no avail. Supposedly universal defense mechanisms in alcoholism eluded attempts to measure and document them. Insight-focused group and individual psychotherapy likewise proved dramatically unsuccessful in controlled trials (see Chapter 15, this volume). Addiction does not seem to be for lack of insight.

Still others have appealed to innately irresistible motivations hardwired into victims. Early disease models of alcoholism postulated an abnormal constitution rendering the person permanently incapable of controlling alcohol use. In the current era of fascination with genetic and biochemical mechanisms, this takes the form of hereditary or toxic brain disease that predisposes neurotransmitter systems to light up when presented with particular drugs, overriding normal self-control mechanisms (e.g., Milam & Ketcham, 1981). Psychoactive drugs do, of course, work their magic primarily through neurochemistry. Yet effective pharmacologic solutions remain elusive. (A notable exception here is methadone maintenance, which in essence is a continuation of opioid addiction in a more manageable form.) In the end, even in more biologically oriented treatment programs, clients in effect are left to use their rational capacities of deciding, accepting, choosing, and controlling themselves. And so they do, by the millions, with or more often without treatment. Ask people who have successfully quit an addiction how they did it (see Chapter 14, this volume). Motivation does not seem to be a matter of insurmountable biology.

What, then? If the motivational problem of addiction is not remedied by enhancing suffering, knowledge, insight, or neurochemistry, then what is motivation? I propose a simple and pragmatic approach: *Motivation is doing something to get better.*

Note I am not saying that motivation *leads to* doing something. Much time has been spent focusing on mental mechanisms believed to trigger change, and this may yet prove to be a useful pursuit. For practical purposes, however, think of motivation as the *probability of a behavior* (Miller, 1985). How, in fact, do we know that a client is motivated? It might be from what the person says about wanting to change or admitting a problem, but these are relatively weak predictors of change. In general, we know that our clients are motivated when they get moving—take their medication as prescribed, go to AA meetings, show up for sessions on time, complete their homework assignments, or find a job. Motivation *is* getting moving.

This emphasis, if a bit narrow, is not misguided. It turns out that doing something—almost anything—to get better is one of the stronger predictors of success in overcoming alcohol problems. Those who attend AA more regularly, or who finish the recommended number of sessions, or who faithfully take their medication (even if it is a placebo) are more likely to show successful change (Miller, 1998). If this is so, then the question becomes: What can I do to help my clients do *something,* to take action on their own behalf?

Happily, research has already provided many answers to this question. The purpose of the rest of this chapter is to pull together what research has revealed that is of use to the practicing clinician in enhancing motivation for change. The summary is organized around three general topics: therapeutic *style,* motivational *techniques,* and the broader context of behavior.

MOTIVATIONAL STYLE

The reader of a chapter like this often scans for the techniques, the practical tips or tricks for inducing change. There are indeed some strategies to share, but to focus first on techniques is to miss the essential fundamental *style* of motivational interviewing and the spirit that underlies it (Rollnick & Miller, 1995). It is particularly important to consider this in the addiction field, where a very different zeitgeist has haunted us.

Understanding Ambivalence

A working assumption in motivational interviewing is that the change process often gets stalled in *ambivalence,* the resolution of which is a key in facilitating change. Ambivalence involves simultaneously held and conflicting motivations, or in everyday language, feeling two ways about something. Ambivalence can be immobilizing. One thinks of the not-so-good things about a present situation, then about the good things, then again about the reasons for a change, then again about the reasons not to change, finally moving on to think of something else less stifling. Ambivalence is a normal phase in the process of change.

The Confrontation–Denial Trap

An important clinical aspect here is that if you take one side of the inner argument of an ambivalent person, he or she is quite likely to argue the opposite side. If you then, for whatever reason, further press your side of the argument more ardently, you find that the ambivalent person normally defends the opposite more vehemently. It is as though the person's inner conflict were being acted out on a stage.

In the American addiction field, pathological meaning has been attributed to this normal scenario. Assume that most people who walk through the door for alcohol or drug counseling are ambivalent about doing so; they see both good things and not-so-good things about their substance use. A counselor trained to confront this problem directly may take up one side of the inner conflict, arguing that there is a problem (you are an alcoholic) in need of change (and you have to quit drinking). The predictable client response would be, "No I'm not, and no I don't." Addiction counselors, if trained to identify this as denial, may respond by intensifying their confrontation in order to break through the perceived wall of defenses. The client, in turn, resists more defensively, thereby confirming the diagnosis. They are complementary roles, confrontation and denial. One elicits the other, creating a predictable two-step that is frustrating for both dancers.

The counselor, of course, does not intend or perceive that he or she is doing harm. The dance has the feel of a life or death struggle, and the counselor is on the good side. The client's resistance, from the counselor's perspective, seems to be emanating from a nearly bottomless well of denial. Yet it is clear that a client's "resistance" or "denial" is strongly influenced by how the therapist responds (Miller, Benefield, & Tonigan, 1993). A therapist can drive denial up and down with the same client within the same session simply by alternating between directive confronting and empathic listening (Patterson & Forgatch, 1985). A high level of resistance or denial is not a client problem, but a therapist skill problem. Said another way, resistant or defensive behavior from a client should be a signal to the therapist to change what he or she is doing.

First, Do No Harm

The dance might be harmless enough, were it not for another principle of normal social psychology: that when we defend a position aloud, we become more committed to it. One would predict, therefore, that if a therapist elicits defensive statements, the client would become more committed to the status quo and less committed to change. This is precisely what we found in a study of problem drinkers, where the level of client resistance in a single session was a strong predictor of drinking one year later. "Of course!" one might say. "Resistant clients are harder to change." We were able, however, to show that the client's level of resistance was driven by intentional control of the therapist's level of confrontation. The more the therapist confronted, the more the client resisted during the session, and the more the client drank a year later (Miller et al., 1993). This is consistent with the larger outcome literature on confrontational approaches (see Chapter 15). Whether in the form of individual sessions, videotape feedback, or group therapy, confrontational approaches have a poor track record. Confrontationally directive therapist styles tend to be associated with lower success rates in treating clients with alcohol problems (Miller, Taylor, & West, 1980; Miller et al., 1993; Valle, 1981).

BASIC ASSUMPTIONS

This suggests a needed departure from an authoritarian approach in counseling, from a stance that implies, "I have the answers, and I am going to give them to you." An authoritarian counseling stance places the client one-down, in a passive-receptive and disempowered role. Although this may serve a therapist's needs, it does not tend to inspire change.

The Process of Change

In motivational interviewing, change is understood as a normal life process that can be facilitated by but does not arise from the counselor. Rather, the therapist can be thought of as removing obstacles so that the client can move forward in a normal process of growth. This view is akin to that of Carl Rogers (1957, 1959), who regarded human beings as inherently health-seeking, as drawn to an innately positive identity unless their path is somehow diverted. Such diversions frequently occur, of course, and Rogers placed strong emphasis on creating a therapeutic atmosphere of acceptance, warmth, and understanding. Discontented to leave these as vague ideals, Rogers and his students carefully defined them and developed methods for training therapists in how to manifest them (Truax & Carkhuff, 1967). Given the proper therapeutic conditions such as acceptance, Rogers maintained, people will grow and change in a positive direction *on their own,* much as a seed becomes a flower if given soil, water, and sunshine.

A now large body of research on brief interventions lends some support to this view (Bien, Miller, & Tonigan, 1993). With surprising consistency, brief counseling of one to three sessions has been found in dozens of studies to trigger change in people with alcohol problems (see Chapters 10 and 15). It is as though the counseling freed or set in motion a natural process of change within the person, that is continued and maintained for years afterward. Interestingly, the magnitude of change observed with such briefer counseling is often similar to that associated with longer and more intensive forms of treatment (Bien *et al.*, 1993; Project MATCH Research Group, 1997).

The Locus of Change

This suggests that the locus of and responsibility for change lie within the client. Emphasizing this responsibility is one common element of effective brief intervention (Bien *et al.*, 1993; Miller & Sanchez, 1994). "No one can change your drinking for you," the client is told. "Even if I wanted to make the decision for you, I could not. You are free to continue drinking and using just as you have been, or to make a change. It's really up to you." A moment's reflection might suggest that it could be no other way, and yet there has often been a strong paternalistic undertone in addiction counseling: "Addicts can't make good decisions for themselves," and, "You can't let an alcoholic drink." In the end, no one but the client *can* make those choices. Being honest about that with yourself and your clients doesn't endanger change; rather, it seems to facilitate it.

The Possibility of Change

Expectancies have a way of coming true. This applies to clients' own expectancies, of course. Ask someone what their chances are of staying clean and sober, and they are likely to give you a reasonably accurate prediction. This might be because people know themselves well, but it could also be because what we expect to happen has an influence on what actually occurs (cf. Chapters 4 and 6, this volume).

This is true of therapists' expectancies as well. In one study, alcoholics in a treatment program were tested for certain personality characteristics. The researcher then privately shared with program staff the names of a few clients who were particularly ready and likely to succeed in treatment. During treatment those clients did indeed prove to be more responsive, and over the course of a year's follow-up they had particularly positive outcomes. The researcher's secret was that the "good prognosis" clients had been chosen *at random.* The therapists' expectations that they would succeed had become self-fulfilling prophecies (Leake &

King, 1977). Another important element of motivational style, then, is belief in the possibility of change. Imparted to clients, this becomes enhanced *self-efficacy,* the belief that one can achieve a particular goal or task (Bandura, 1982; see Chapter 4, this volume).

EMPATHY

The therapeutic quality of *empathy* represents a conceptual opposite of aggressive confrontation. Empathy here does not mean the ability to identify with clients based on personal history. Studies consistently show that counselors who are in recovery themselves are neither more nor less likely to help their clients overcome substance use disorders. Rather, empathy is defined here as Rogers (1957) meant it: the ability to develop an accurate understanding of the client's meaning through reflective listening. It is not so much an attribute as a skill that is observable and learnable. High levels of skillful empathy have been shown to be associated with high success rates in treatment (Miller *et al.,* 1980; Valle, 1981).

SUPPORT

More generally, a supportive and client-centered approach in counseling tends to yield more positive outcomes (see Chapter 15). Again, this is more a style of counseling than a particular technique. For this reason, it may be combined effectively with a wide range of treatment methods or pharmacotherapies (e.g., O'Malley *et al.,* 1992). In a study cited above, we found the effectiveness of behavior therapy to be strongly influenced by the extent to which the therapist practiced empathy during self-control training sessions (Miller *et al.,* 1980). Clients are heartened by the sense that their therapist is very actively and personally interested in their welfare.

MOTIVATIONAL TECHNIQUES

PRACTICAL MATTERS

Like social support more generally, a therapist's support can be quite practical, expressed in simple but important ways. Suppose a client comes for a first evaluation visit, and a second appointment is scheduled. Should you get in touch again before the second session, or leave it to the client to return? A simple handwritten note sent after the first session, to express concern and caring, can nearly double the chances that the client will come back (Koumans & Muller, 1965). The same is true of a simple telephone call to show interest and caring (Koumans, Muller, & Miller, 1967). After a client misses a scheduled appointment, such a letter or phone call can significantly reduce the likelihood of treatment dropout (Panepinto & Higgins, 1969; Wedel, 1965).

Suppose you want to make a referral. Is it better to give your client the telephone number and make him or her take the responsibility for calling, or to make the call yourself while the client is still in your office? The latter can more than double the chances that your client will actually make it to the referral (Kogan, 1957). Similarly, suppose you want a client to go to a 12-step meeting. A common approach is to give clients a list of the times and locations of local meetings, and recommend that they pick one. A more active approach is to pick up the telephone while the person is in your office, and call a member with whom you have a prior arrangement for "twelve-stepping." The client gets on the phone with the member, who offers to transport and accompany the client to this first meeting, and they agree on a mutually convenient time. In a comparison of these two approaches, 100% of clients in the active support condition got to a meeting, whereas none of those in the list-only condition did so (Sisson & Mallams, 1981)—a fairly large difference in "motivation"!

Attendance at aftercare meetings can be increased substantially by measures as simple as reminder telephone calls (Intagliata, 1976). In another study, planning together on a calendar the aftercare meetings to be attended was effective in doubling the number of sessions kept (Ahles, Schlundt, Prue, & Rychtarik, 1983). Even a practical factor such as the distance one has to travel can have a substantial effect on attendance (Prue, Keane, Cornell, & Foy, 1979).

Practical support in essence involves making it easier to take the next step, removing obstacles, and showing active interest and caring. It can make quite a difference in whether or not clients will do something toward their own recovery, and *doing something* is one of the antecedents of successful change.

DEVELOPING DISCREPANCY

If it is countertherapeutic to elicit a client's arguments against change (resistance), then it may be therapeutic (change-promoting) to engage the client in talking about reasons for change. In motivational interviewing (Miller & Rollnick, 1991), these have been termed *self-motivational statements,* which tend to fall into four classes: (1) statements recognizing problems or negative consequences of current behavior, (2) expressions of concern about one's current state; (3) statements of a desire for change, and (4) expressions of optimism about the possibility of change. The goal, remember, is to have the *client* voice these statements. When the therapist is arguing for change and the client is resisting it, they are caught in the confrontation–denial dance.

There are many ways to elicit self-motivational statements from clients. Perhaps the simplest of all is to ask for them. For example, corresponding to the four types above:

1. What are the not-so-good things about cocaine for you? (This might follow from a discussion of what the client likes about cocaine.)
2. What do you think might happen if you keep on drinking as you have been?
3. What are the most important reasons for you to quit smoking?
4. What makes you think you could give up marijuana if you decided to? What successful changes have you made in your life in the past?

In a motivational interviewing style, it is best to follow a question with reflective listening. There is a strong temptation to continue asking questions, but this can quickly put the client into a passive or defensive mode and the therapist in a directive expert role. Imagine a visit to your general practitioner. A series of questions (particularly short-answer questions) implies that at the end of the questioning the practitioner will have an answer. This, then, leads back into the authoritarian asymmetry. A simple rule of thumb is, never ask three questions in a row. Self-motivational statements may also follow from asking the client about how things were in the past, before problems developed, or about what the client would like for life to be like in 5 years. Then listen. As the client describes personal hopes, goals, and dreams, the therapist eventually can ask, "And how does (drinking) fit into all this?"

The underlying goal here is to help the client see the discrepancy between a risky or harmful behavior pattern and important personal goals. There seems to be something about *simultaneously* experiencing the good and the not-so-good that helps the person become unstuck from ambivalence. Another approach for creating discrepancy is to give the client direct, objective feedback about risk and harm. We have developed and tested a *drinker's check-up* that provides feedback about personal alcohol use and related problems, based on a structured assessment (Miller, Zweben, DiClemente, & Rychtarik, 1992). The feedback is given in a supportive, empathic style, and the client is asked to reflect and respond (rather than being told what he or she must do about it). This motivational enhancement approach has been found in controlled trials to trigger reductions in alcohol use among problem drinkers (Handmaker, 1993; Miller, Sovereign, & Krege, 1988; Miller et al., 1993), and to increase the effectiveness of outpatient (Bien, Miller, & Boroughs, 1993), methadone (Saunders, Wilkinson, & Phillips, 1995), and inpatient (Brown & Miller, 1993) treatment for substance dependence. In Project MATCH (1997), clients treated by motivational enhancement therapy showed outcomes similar to those for clients receiving longer cognitive-behavioral and 12-step treatment programs.

A MENU OF OPTIONS

One gains nothing by bringing a client to the point of readiness, only to offer a change method that is unacceptable, unattainable, or otherwise inappropriate. The good news here is that the addiction field is blessed with a wide range of effective change strategies (see Chapters 15 to 21). This means that clients can be offered an informed choice among various options, each of which has a good likelihood of being helpful (e.g., Project MATCH Research Group, 1997).

From this perspective, it makes good clinical sense to involve the client in selecting and designing his or her own treatment program. First of all, clients are likely to have some wisdom about what may be most helpful to them, and no one knows them better. Among options of roughly equal potential benefit, clients know which they would find most acceptable—an important factor, because adherence is a good predictor of success. Then there is the fact that when a person has freely chosen a course of action, he or she is more likely to be committed to it than if it had been assigned without a perceived choice. These factors all point toward the utility of helping clients choose their own change plan from among effective alternatives.

THE BROADER CONTEXT FOR CHANGE

If enhancing motivation means increasing the probability that a behavior (doing something) will happen, one needs to look beyond the counseling room. Many of the reinforcers that influence moment-to-moment and day-to-day behavior are found in the client's ongoing social environment.

Carrots, Honey, and Vinegar

One of the most often misrepresented analogies regarding motivation has to do with a carrot and a stick. The common misunderstanding has to do not with the carrot—almost everyone knows what that is for—but with the stick. For some reason, people have thought of the carrot as positive reinforcement, and the stick as punishment (for whipping or prodding). In fact, the original image is that of suspending a carrot on a string tied to the end of a stick, which thus dangles in front of the donkey just out of reach. Trying to reach it, the donkey moves forward and pulls the cart. The carrot and stick, then, represents an effective alternative to punishment. In the words of another bit of ancestral wisdom, "You catch more bees with honey than with vinegar."

The point, of course, is that positive reinforcement is what motivates much behavior. People do what feels good and right to them, what brings about a pleasing result. Drugs of abuse are reinforcing. Many of them elicit pleasant experiences, at least at first. Many of them also directly stimulate the brain's reinforcement systems, artificially activating the natural channels that tell us "do that again." In this way, drugs can be reinforcing even without bringing euphoria; the person keeps on using them even after the thrill and pleasure are gone.

People give up something good for something better. In order for being clean and sober to stick, then, it has to be better than the reinforcement that comes from using. In commonsense language, "If you're sober but not enjoying it, you're probably not going to stay that way." Motivation, then, involves much more than talking a person into changing their drinking and drug habits. It also means considering the client's other sources of positive reinforcement, the broader family and social environment (Meyers & Smith, 1995; Moos, Finney, & Cronkite, 1990).

Working with Significant Others

The most significant sources of reinforcement and influence are often (though not always) those who live with the client, or with whom he or she spends the most time. It is helpful, therefore, to know who the people are in the client's social support system, and how they are currently responding to the client's alcohol or drug use. Knowingly or not, they may be supporting substance use in a variety of ways. When a behavior leads to rewarding consequences, the behavior is more likely to be repeated (positive reinforcement), as, for example, when drinking increases the likelihood of having sex. A behavior may also turn off unpleasant consequences (negative reinforcement), again with result that the behavior is more likely to continue or increase. The popping of a beer can may be the family's fearful cue to stop nagging, making noise, or making requests, and to leave the drinker "in peace." Still another form of support for continued use is when others protect the user from the natural punishing consequences of alcohol or drug use (sometimes called "enabling").

The more support there is for drinking, the less likely it is to change (Project MATCH Research Group, 1997). In contrast, the more a person's family and friends do not support drinking and instead support (reinforce) sobriety, the more likely it is that drinking will decrease (Sisson & Azrin, 1986). The same appears to be true with illicit drug use. When positive reinforcement is tied to being drug-free, drug use decreases (Higgins *et al.,* 1993; Higgins *et al.,* 1995).

One practical problem is that it is harder to notice and reward the *absence* of a behavior. Smokers experience this when they quit. They receive some positive comments, but mostly people don't notice what they are *not* doing. Sometimes loved ones are even disinclined to reward the new desirable behavior ("She's just doing what she's *supposed* to do!"). Here is a place, then, where working with significant others can be very helpful in motivating the maintenance of change. The task is to remove as many of the supports for alcohol or drug use as possible, and to increase the supports for a drug-free lifestyle. The former involves identifying and removing positive reinforcement and attention when the person is using. The latter involves reinforcing drug-free alternative behaviors, so that the individual's life literally becomes more rewarding without than with drugs (Meyers & Smith, 1995).

It is possible to do this even if the drinker or drug user is not yet physically involved in treatment. Research on "unilateral family therapy" has provided encouraging evidence that even a single family member can be taught effective skills for discouraging alcohol or drug use and for reinforcing drug-free alternatives, ultimately engaging the user in treatment (Sisson & Azrin, 1986, 1993; Thomas & Ager, 1993). Whether or not the identified patient is in treatment, then, do not neglect the family and larger social support system as significant sources of motivating reinforcement.

FINAL NOTE: THE CONTEXT OF VALUES

Our work more recently has turned to the study of human values as a context for motivating change. In essence, the question is, "What does this person care more about than drinking or using drugs?" There are some cases where the answer seems to be "nothing," but with exploration one can usually find people or values that are more dear to the client than the drug(s) of choice. The motivational style and techniques described here are not tricks for duping people into doing what they do not want to do. Rather, they are ways of bringing them face to face with the reality that their drinking or drug use is jeopardizing that which they hold most dear. I believe that unless one taps into this dimension of values, and accesses what the person cares about more than their drug habit, no amount of motivational wizardry will change their behavior. It may happen through the introspective process of motivational interviewing, or through feedback of risk and harm. It may occur by helping the family to change contingencies so that using comes to cost more than it is worth. People move forward toward their happiness, whether a carrot or a star or a few moments of drug-induced respite. Motivation has to do with helping people find what makes it worth their while to change, to leave artificial paradise for the real thing.

REFERENCES

Ahles, T. A., Schlundt, D. G., Prue, D. M., & Rychtarik, R. G. (1983). Impact of aftercare arrangements on the maintenance of treatment success in abusive drinkers. *Addictive Behaviors, 8,* 53–58.

Bandura, A. (1982). Self-efficacy mechanism in human agency. *American Psychologist, 37,* 122–147.

Bien, T. H., Miller, W. R., & Boroughs, J. M. (1993). Motivational interviewing with alcohol outpatients. *Behavioural and Cognitive Psychotherapy, 21,* 347–356.

Bien, T. H., Miller, W. R., & Tonigan, J. S. (1993). Brief interventions for alcohol problems: A review. *Addiction, 88*, 315–336.

Brown, J. M., & Miller, W. R. (1993). Impact of motivational interviewing on participation and outcome in residential alcoholism treatment. *Psychology of Addictive Behaviors, 7*, 211–218.

Handmaker, N. S. (1993). *Motivating pregnant drinkers to abstain: Prevention in prenatal care clinics.* Unpublished doctoral dissertation, University of New Mexico, Albuquerque.

Higgins, S. T., Budney, A. J., Bickel, W. K., Hughes, J. R., Foerg, F. E., & Badger, G. J. (1993). Achieving cocaine abstinence with a behavioral approach. *American Journal of Psychiatry, 150*, 763–769.

Higgins, S. T., Budney, A. J., Bickel, W. K., Badger, G. J., Foerg, F. E., & Ogden, D. (1995). Outpatient behavioral treatment for cocaine dependence: One-year outcome. *Experimental and Clinical Psychopharmacology, 3*, 205–212.

Intagliata, J. (1976). A telephone follow-up procedure for increasing the effectiveness of a treatment program for alcoholics. *Journal of Studies on Alcohol, 37*, 1330–1335.

Kogan, L. S. (1957). The short-term case in a family agency: Part II. Results of a study. *Social Casework, 38*, 296–302.

Koumans, A. J. R., & Muller, J. J. (1965). Use of letters to increase motivation in alcoholics. *Psychological Reports, 16*, 1152.

Koumans, A. J. R., Muller, J. J., & Miller, C. F. (1967). Use of telephone calls to increase motivation for treatment in alcoholics. *Psychological Reports, 21*, 327–328.

Leake, G. J., & King, A. S. (1977). Effect of counselor expectations on alcoholic recovery. *Alcohol Health and Research World, 1*(3), 16–22.

Meyers, R. J., & Smith, J. E. (1995). *Clinical guide to alcohol treatment: The community reinforcement approach.* New York: Guilford.

Milam, J. R., & Ketcham, K. (1981). *Under the influence: A guide to the myths and realities of alcoholism.* Seattle, WA: Madrona.

Miller, W. R. (1985). Motivation for treatment: A review with special emphasis on alcoholism. *Psychological Bulletin, 98*, 84–107.

Miller, W. R. (in press). Why do people change addictive behavior? The 1996 H. David Archibald Lecture. *Addiction.*

Miller, W. R., & Rollnick, S. (1991). *Motivational interviewing: Preparing people to change addictive behavior.* New York: Guilford.

Miller, W. R., & Sanchez, V. C. (1994). Motivating young adults for treatment and lifestyle change. In G. Howard (Ed.), *Issues in alcohol use and misuse by young adults* (pp. 55–82). Notre Dame, IN: University of Notre Dame Press.

Miller, W. R., Taylor, C.A., & West, J. C. (1980). Focused versus broad-spectrum behavior therapy for problem drinkers. *Journal of Consulting and Clinical Psychology, 48*, 590–601.

Miller, W. R., Sovereign, R. G., & Krege, B. (1988). Motivational interviewing with problem drinkers: II. The Drinker's Check-up as a preventive intervention. *Behavioral Psychotherapy, 16*, 251–268.

Miller, W. R., Zweben, A., DiClemente, C. C., & Rychtarik, R. G. (1992). *Motivational Enhancement Therapy manual: A clinical research guide for therapists treating individuals with alcohol abuse and dependence.* Rockville, MD: National Institute on Alcohol Abuse and Alcoholism. (Single copies available free of charge from the National Clearinghouse for Alcohol and Drug Information, P.O. Box 2345, Rockville, MD, 20847–2345.)

Miller, W. R., Benefield, R. G., & Tonigan, J. S. (1993). Enhancing motivation for change in problem drinking: A controlled comparison of two therapist styles. *Journal of Consulting and Clinical Psychology, 61*, 455–461.

Moos, R. H., Finney, J. W., & Cronkite, R. C. (1990). *Alcoholism treatment: Context, process, and outcome.* New York: Oxford University Press.

Moskowitz, J. M. (1989). The primary prevention of alcohol problems: A critical review of the research literature. *Journal of Studies on Alcohol, 50*, 54–88.

O'Malley, S., Jaffe, A. J., Chang, C., Schottenfeld, R. S., Meyer, R. E., & Rounsaville, B. (1992). Naltrexone and coping skills therapy for alcohol dependence. *Archives of General Psychiatry, 49*, 881–887.

Panepinto, W. C., & Higgins, M. J. (1969). Keeping alcoholics in treatment: Effective follow-through procedures. *Quarterly Journal of Studies on Alcohol, 30*, 414–419.

Patterson, G. A., & Forgatch, M. S. (1985). Therapist behavior as a determinant for client noncompliance: A paradox for the behavior modifier. *Journal of Consulting and Clinical Psychology, 53*, 846–851.

Project MATCH Research Group. (1997). Matching alcoholism treatments to client heterogeneity: Project MATCH posttreatment drinking outcomes. *Journal of Studies on Alcohol, 58,* 7–29.

Prue, D. M., Keane, T. M., Cornell, J. E., & Foy, D., W. (1979). An analysis of distance variables that affect aftercare attendance. *Community Mental Health Journal, 15,* 149–154.

Rogers, C. R. (1957). The necessary and sufficient conditions for therapeutic personality change. *Journal of Consulting Psychology, 21,* 95–103.

Rogers, C. R. (1959). A theory of therapy, personality, and interpersonal relationships as developed in the client-centered framework. In S. Koch (Ed.), *Psychology: The study of a science: Vol. 3. Formulations of the person and the social context* (pp. 184–256). New York: McGraw-Hill.

Rollnick, S., & Miller, W. R. (1995). What is motivational interviewing? *Behavioural and Cognitive Psychotherapy, 23,* 325–334.

Saunders, B., Wilkinson, C., & Phillips, M. (1995). The impact of a brief motivational intervention with opiate users attending a methadone programme. *Addiction, 90,* 415–424.

Sisson, R. W., & Azrin, N. H. (1986). Family-member involvement to initiate and promote treatment of problem drinkers. *Journal of Behavior Therapy and Experimental Psychiatry, 17,* 15–21.

Sisson, R. W., & Azrin, N. H. (1993). Community reinforcement training for families: A method to get alcoholics into treatment. In T. J. O'Farrell (Ed.), *Treating alcohol problems: Marital and family interventions* (pp. 34–53). New York: Guilford.

Sisson, R. W., & Mallams, J. H. (1981). The use of systematic encouragement and community access procedures to increase attendance at Alcoholics Anonymous and Al-Anon meetings. *Behavior Therapy and Experimental Psychiatry, 17,* 15–21.

Thomas E. J., & Ager, R. D. (1993). Unilateral family therapy with spouses of uncooperative alcohol abusers. In T. J. O'Farrell (Ed.), *Treating alcohol problems: Marital and family interventions* (pp. 3–33). New York: Guilford.

Truax, C. B., & Carkhuff, R. R. (1967). *Toward effective counseling and psychotherapy.* Chicago: Aldine.

Valle, S. K. (1981). Interpersonal functioning of alcoholism counselors and treatment outcome. *Journal of Studies on Alcohol, 42,* 783–790.

Wedel, H. L. (1965). Involving alcoholics in treatment. *Quarterly Journal of Studies on Alcohol, 26,* 468–479.

10

Using Brief Opportunities for Change in Medical Settings

NICK HEATHER

INTRODUCTION

This chapter is concerned with the use of opportunistic brief interventions in medical settings as a means of initiating change in the addictive behaviors. In other words, it is concerned with short and inexpensive interventions among individuals who are not complaining or seeking help for an addictive disorder. Advantage is taken of settings where people present for some other kind of problem to screen for hazardous or harmful substance use and to offer a brief intervention delivered by nonspecialist health professionals to those screening positive. Although there may well be direct benefits to the individual, especially if behavior can be changed before seriously adverse consequences arise, opportunistic interventions are often justified on public health grounds, as a way of reducing the aggregate harm to a society from the addictive behavior in question (Heather, 1996).

In terms of the stages of change model, the assumption is that the majority of the targets of brief intervention are in earlier stages of change with respect to substance use problems, since they are identified in situations where they are not complaining about or seeking help for such problems. There is some empirical support for this assumption. In a study concerned with the development of a measure of the stages of change among excessive drinkers (the Readiness to Change Questionnaire) found on general hospital wards (Rollnick, Heather, Gold, & Hall, 1992), we classified 73% of such patients as being in the precontemplation or contemplation stages, with the remainder in the action stage. In contrast to this, in a

NICK HEATHER • Centre for Alcohol and Drug Studies, Newcastle City Health NHS Trust, Newcastle upon Tyne NE1 6UR, England.

Treating Addictive Behaviors, 2nd ed., edited by Miller and Heather. Plenum Press, New York, 1998.

later study designed to develop a treatment version of the same instrument, in which we studied clients attending specialist treatment centers for alcohol problems, 74% were deemed to be in the action stage and 26% in contemplation, with none being classified as being in precontemplation (Heather, Luce, Peck, Dunbar, & James, 1997). Thus, although the teaching of skills to those already seeking to change their substance using behavior may sometimes be appropriate, the primary objective in delivering opportunistic brief interventions is motivational—to move people from precontemplation to contemplation and from contemplation to preparation and action.

The chapter reviews research evidence on the effects and applications of opportunistic brief interventions in a range of medical settings and for three types of addictive behavior: tobacco smoking, long-term use of benzodiazepines, and excessive alcohol consumption. There have been applications of brief interventions in social service, criminal justice, and occupational settings, with interesting possibilities, but research on the effectiveness of these interventions is not sufficiently mature to arrive at meaningful conclusions. There have also been attempts to apply the concept of brief interventions to the illicit drugs field and to other addictive behaviors but, again, this has not been sufficiently developed as yet to warrant inclusion here. This chapter makes no attempt to provide an exhaustive coverage of the evidence; rather, selected research reports and reviews will be described in order to illustrate dominant themes in the literature and important conclusions that may be derived from it. The chapter shows that the evidence strongly justifies the implementation of brief interventions in medical settings but that the major obstacle to progress is the difficulty in ensuring that this implementation takes place.

SMOKING CESSATION INTERVENTIONS

A pioneering study of the effects of general practitioners' (i.e., family physicians') advice against smoking was carried out by Russell, Wilson, Taylor, and Baker (1979). They allocated 2,138 smokers attending their general practitioners (GPs) in five health centers in London to one of four groups: (1) a nonintervention control; (2) a questionnaire-only group; (3) a group given simple advice by the GP to stop smoking; and (4) a group advised to stop smoking, given a leaflet to assist them, and warned that they would be followed up. The proportions in these groups who had stopped smoking during the first month and still were not smoking one year later were 0.3%, 1.6%, 3.3%, and 5.1%, a linear trend that was highly statistically significant.

It must immediately be conceded that many clinicians would find these success rates unacceptably low. However, given that in most Western industrialized societies up to 80% of the population visit a healthcare professional, usually in primary care, at least once a year (e.g., Freer, Boyle, & Ryan, 1986; Silagy et al., 1992), these rates could translate into substantial achievements in smoking cessation if interventions were consistently applied by all family doctors in a country. Russell and colleagues (1979) were themselves able to show that, if all GPs in the United Kingdom adopted the simple routine described in their highest level of intervention (group 4 in the preceding paragraph), the yield would exceed half a million ex-smokers per year, a figure that could not be matched by increasing the number of specialist withdrawal clinics in the country from about 50 to 10,000.

Another important issue Russell and colleagues were able to comment on was the relative contributions to the success of the brief intervention of motivational and skills components. Changes in motivation and intention to stop smoking were measured immediately after advice had been given and this enabled the authors to conclude that the beneficial effect of brief intervention was achieved by motivating more smokers to try to quit, rather than by increasing the success rate among those who did try. However, in a later study in which nicotine gum was added to brief advice in one condition, Russell, Merriman, Stapleton, and Taylor (1983) found that the beneficial effects were more prolonged; this intervention motivated more smokers to try to give up but also increased the success rate among those who tried and reduced relapse among those who stopped. The inference was that the latter benefits were the result of the nicotine gum rather than the brief advice.

EFFECTIVENESS OF BRIEF SMOKING CESSATION INTERVENTIONS

Since Russell and colleagues' (1979) original report, there have been many studies of brief interventions in medical practice aimed at smoking cessation. In an influential review, Kottke, Battista, DeFriese, and Brekke (1988) estimated that brief advice and support in primary care settings achieved long-term abstinence rates of between 5% and 10%, while more intensive interventions produced rates between 15% and 30%.

The latest review in this area was conducted on behalf of the Cochrane Collaboration by Silagy and Ketteridge (1996) but conclusions were less favorable regarding the beneficial effects of brief smoking cessation interventions than those of Kottke and colleagues (1988). Nevertheless, a small benefit of minimal advice to smokers by a medical practitioner was found and this was said to justify the routine use of minimal interventions by primary care physicians. "Minimal interventions" here were defined as advice provided during a single consultation of less than 20 minutes duration plus up to one follow-up visit. Compared with no advice, the effect of advice equated to a success rate of 2% or one quitter for every 50 smokers receiving the intervention. From studies in which minimal and more intensive interventions had been directly compared, there was also evidence that the latter showed an incremental advantage but this was not sufficiently large to justify a recommendation for routine use among unselected smokers. Relatively more intensive brief interventions, however, could be of benefit to more motivated individuals, such as those already suffering from smoking-related diseases.

NICOTINE REPLACEMENT THERAPY

As noted previously, the addition of nicotine gum appeared to prolong the beneficial effects of brief advice given to smokers (Russell *et al.*, 1983). The effectiveness of nicotine replacement therapy (NRT) in general has recently been reviewed by Silagy, Mant, Fowler, and Lancaster (1997). This review embraced 47 trials of nicotine gum, 22 of transdermal patches, three of intranasal nicotine spray, and two of nicotine inhaler devices. The majority of trials were carried out in primary care settings but others were conduced in specialized smoking cessation clinics and hospital wards or with community volunteers recruited by media advertisements.

The main conclusion of the review was that all commercially available forms of NRT are effective as part of smoking cessation strategies and produce a two- to threefold increase in quit rates. NRT is especially useful for smokers with high levels of nicotine dependence, as defined by a score of 7 or more on Fagerström's (1978) Tolerance Questionnaire. Of particular interest for present purposes was the finding that nicotine gum and transdermal patches were more effective when offered to smokers recruited in the community or attending specialized cessation clinics than to those identified opportunistically in primary health care settings. However, this is likely to be explained, at least in part, by the higher level of motivation to quit among the volunteers and clinic attenders. It certainly does not mean that the opportunistic use of NRT in primary care is ineffective and should be abandoned; as already implied, primary care allows much greater access to smokers and probably therefore much greater impact on cessation rates in the general population.

How is the effectiveness of NRT influenced by the addition of brief advice, counseling, or support? Silagy, Mant, and colleagues (1997) conclude that the effectiveness of NRT appears to be largely independent of the intensity of additional support given to the smoker. Although a higher intensity of support, with or without NRT, increases the likelihood of quitting, it is not essential to the success of NRT. On the other hand, all the trials of NRT included in the review contained at least some form of brief advice to the smoker, so that brief advice represents a minimum that should be offered to enable NRT to be effective. The authors warn, "In the light of recent advertising campaigns to promote use of NRT, it is important that smokers do not misinterpret these results by believing that NRT offers an easy option 'medical cure' for the far more complex problem of addictive behavior" (Silagy, Mant, et al., 1997, p. 9).

IMPLEMENTING BRIEF INTERVENTIONS FOR SMOKING CESSATION

Given the large number of studies investigating the effects of physicians' and other health professionals' advice against smoking delivered in routine clinical care, it is reasonable to conclude that further research in this area would follow the law of diminishing returns. This is not to say that no issues remain that could be clarified by research; for example, the incremental effectiveness of relatively more intensive intervention in the form of follow-up telephone counseling has been doubted (e.g. Ockene et al., 1991) and this general issue needs clarification in further research. Nevertheless, brief advice alone, with or without the addition of some form of NRT, has been clearly shown to be effective as a minimum level of intervention. What is now needed is more research on how best to increase the use of brief interventions by family physicians, other medical practitioners, and other healthcare professionals.

The starting point for such research should be the discovery of ways to increase the frequency with which smokers are identified. Present evidence suggests that many smokers are completely missed by general practitioners. For example, a study by Dickinson, Wiggers, Leeder, and Sanson-Fisher (1989) using videotaped consultations found that only 56% of smokers were correctly identified by GPs.

Further, the number of patients who receive advice from health professionals on how to stop smoking and other risky substance use is disappointingly low (Richmond, Kehoe, Heather, Wodak, & Webster, 1996; Silagy *et al.*, 1992; Wallace, Brennan, & Haines, 1987).

Clearly, providing relevant training to health professionals is one way of increasing their involvement in smoking cessation interventions. A review of the results of 12 studies aiming to assess the effectiveness of such training, all carried out in primary care medical and dental practices in the United States and Canada, has been reported by Silagy, Lancaster, Fowler, and Spiers (1997). The conclusion was that healthcare professionals who had received training were more likely to carry out elements of smoking cessation interventions (i.e., offering counseling, setting dates to quit, making follow-up appointments, giving out self-help materials, or recommending nicotine chewing gum) than those who had not been trained. Moreover, there was a modest increase in rates of stopping smoking among patients of trained health professionals compared with those who had attended practitioners with no training, but this was not a robust effect. The authors concluded, therefore, that training alone was unlikely to be an effective strategy for improving the quality of healthcare unless organizational and other factors were also considered. What these other factors might be is considered at the end of this chapter.

INTERVENTIONS FOR LONG-TERM BENZODIAZEPINE USE

For practical purposes, long-term benzodiazepine (BZD) use means dependence on prescribed tranquilizers, sedatives, or hypnotics in the BZD class of drugs. Long-term use is usually defined as taking tablets for over 1 year; it can be assumed that most people in this category are taking BZDs for reasons unconnected with the original complaint for which they were prescribed and have become dependent on them. Although there has been a steady fall in the United Kingdom since the late 1970s (Wells, 1993), the number of prescriptions for BZDs continues to cause concern in health circles (Department of Health, 1992), particularly in view of an apparent increase in long-term users (Williams & Bellantuono, 1991).

Two recent studies have shown that brief and inexpensive interventions by family physicians can lead to a cessation or reduction in intake of BZDs by long-term users. Cormack, Sweeney, Hugh-Jones, and Foot (1994) divided 219 mostly elderly, long-term users identified from medical records into two intervention groups and a control group. One intervention group received a letter from their GP asking them gradually to reduce the use of BZDs and perhaps in time stop; the second intervention group received the same letter plus four information sheets at monthly intervals. Results showed that, after 6 months, both intervention groups had reduced their intake to roughly two thirds of their original BZD consumption, with a statistically greater reduction than in the control (usual care) group. Eighteen percent of patients in the intervention groups had received no prescriptions at all during the 6-month monitoring period. There was no added effect of the information sheets. The authors conservatively estimated that the use of their letter throughout general practice in England would save the National Health Service at least £4 million (in 1989 prices).

Bashir, King, and Ashworth (1994) undertook a study to assess the effects of a brief intervention given by GPs in helping chronic BZD users to withdraw from their medication. On this occasion, the intervention took the form of a short consultation with the doctor which the patients were invited to attend, plus a self-help booklet. This was compared to a control group receiving routine care. Results were that 18% of 50 patients in the intervention group showed a reduction in BZD prescriptions in their medical records over the following 6 months, compared with 5% of 55 patients in the control group, a difference that was statistically significant. It is important to note that this result was obtained in a population with high rates of past depression, anxiety, and attempted suicide. Yet asking patients to withdraw from their medication did not lead to any observable psychological harm or distress or to increased consultation rates with the family doctor. This applied whether or not patients were successful in cutting down or stopping, suggesting that asking patients to withdraw from BZDs by means of a brief intervention of this kind is a relatively safe procedure.

In a study just started in Newcastle, we aim to compare the effectiveness and cost-effectiveness of these two forms of brief intervention for long-term BZD users—the letter from the GP and the short consultation. We also aim to discover the characteristics of patients who respond best to each of these two interventions and to brief interventions in general, with particular attention to the possibility that some types of patient may need more intensive intervention to benefit. On this basis, we hope to be able to develop guidelines for the rational and coordinated deployment of brief and more intensive interventions for the patient population in question. These guidelines will need to take account of difficulties that have been described in attempting to implement nonpharmaceutical strategies among benzodiazepine users in general practice (Simpson, 1993).

INTERVENTIONS AGAINST EXCESSIVE ALCOHOL CONSUMPTION

Excessive alcohol consumption is a term that is meant to embrace both hazardous drinking at levels that increase the risk of medical or other harm from alcohol and harmful drinking where some form of alcohol-related damage is already evident. Opportunistic brief interventions in this area have usually been targeted at drinkers with only low levels of dependence on alcohol and are typically aimed at a goal of moderate (i.e., low-risk) drinking rather than total abstinence. They are carried out in the interests of early detection and secondary prevention of alcohol problems, although previous comments in this chapter on the contribution of brief interventions to the wider public health agenda should also be borne in mind (see Heather, 1996; Chapter 8, this volume).

Research on the general effectiveness of brief interventions against excessive drinking has been reviewed several times (e.g., Bien, Miller, & Tonigan, 1993; Fremantle et al., 1993; Heather, 1995; Kahan, Wilson, & Becker, 1995) and need not be repeated here in any detail. The major conclusion is that brief intervention results in a net reduction in alcohol consumption of between 20% and 30% among excessive drinkers receiving it. Perhaps the most influential study in this area was the WHO clinical trial of brief intervention in primary health care (Babor & Grant, 1992), an international collaboration involving 10 countries and 1,655 heavy drinkers recruited from a combination of various, mostly medical, settings. This clearly established that, among male excessive drinkers at least, a brief intervention delivered at the primary care level and consisting of 5 minutes of simple advice based on 15 minutes of structured assessment is effective in reducing alcohol consumption, with concomitant improvements in health. No additional benefit of more extended counseling was observed. Opportunistic brief interventions are discussed here in more detail for three kinds of medical setting.

PRIMARY HEALTH CARE

Studies by Wallace, Cutler, and Haines (1988) and by Anderson and Scott (1992) in the United Kingdom established the effectiveness of brief intervention delivered by GPs in reducing the proportion of patients drinking above medically recommended guidelines, although the Anderson and Scott report was confined to men. Among women, Scott and Anderson (1990) found no difference in reductions between an intervention and a control group. The public health potential of GP-based brief interventions was highlighted by Wallace and colleagues (1988) when they estimated, on the basis of their findings, that consistent implementation of their program by GPs throughout the United Kingdom would result in a reduction from excessive to low-risk levels of the drinking of 250,00 men and 67,500 women each year.

Wallace and colleagues' (1988) key findings have recently been replicated in the United States by Fleming, Barry, Manwell, Johnson, and London (1997) in a randomized controlled trial (Project TrEAT) based closely on the design of the British study. A total of 64 family physicians from 17 community-based primary care practices in Wisconsin took part in the trial. The main result was that excessive drinking patients randomized to an intervention group offered two 10 to 15 minute-structured counseling sessions by the physician showed significantly greater reductions in alcohol consumption, including binge drinking and frequency of drinking, at 12-month follow-up than a control group receiving usual care. On this occasion, women in the intervention group showed a greater average drop in consumption (31%) than men (14%). A novel finding of the study was that men in the intervention group reported less than half the total number of hospital days in the 12 months following intervention than men in the control group, a finding with obvious implications for the economics of the health care system. The importance of Fleming and colleagues' study is that it provides the first direct evidence that intervention by primary care physicians reduces hazardous and harmful alcohol consumption and health care utilization in the U.S. health care system. The authors conclude that their findings are applicable throughout the United States and could have an enormous impact on the heath care system of that country (see also Parish, 1997).

It must be pointed out, however, that the trials of brief intervention considered so far in this section were, in terms of Flay's (1986) distinction, *efficacy* rather than *effectiveness* trials; i.e., they provided a test of brief interventions under optimum conditions rather than under real-world conditions of routine primary health care. For example, patients entering the study were identified and recruited by the research team rather than by the busy physician in the normal course of his or her practice and this may have resulted in more motivated patients being selected for study (Kahan *et al.,* 1995). In a project in which brief interventions were evaluated in naturalistic general practice settings in Australia (Richmond, Heather, Wodak, Kehoe, & Webster, 1995), far fewer patients returned for consultation following assessment and the beneficial effects of brief intervention were less obvious. Accepting that the beneficial effects of brief interventions among excessive drinkers found in primary health care settings has been demonstrated in efficacy trials, we need now to focus research on effectiveness trials concerning the real-world circumstances under which excessive drinkers are recognized and brief interventions offered to them.

A recent report by Israel and colleagues (1996) is helpful in this regard. These authors persuaded 81% of all primary care physicians in the city of Cambridge, Ontario, to agree to their excessive drinking patients being randomly allocated to an intervention group that received a maximum of 3 hours of cognitive-behavioral counseling by a nurse spread over 1 year or to a control group in which patients were simply advised by the nurse to reduce their intake. At 1-year follow-up, patients who had received counseling showed significantly greater reductions in reported alcohol consumption, psychosocial problems, and serum gamma-glutamyl transferase levels than controls. Intervention group patients also showed significantly reduced physician visits following counseling, another finding with important economic implications for the health care system.

Equally interesting, however, was the method of screening employed in this study. Rather than asking directly about alcohol consumption and related problems, medical receptionists handed out a "trauma questionnaire" developed by Skinner, Holt, Schuller, Roy, and Israel (1984). Only patients giving a positive response to this questionnaire were subsequently asked about drinking by the doctor. It is known that heavy drinkers have a much higher prevalence of trauma than the normal population and the authors estimated that they were able to detect approximately 70% of the excessive drinkers attending primary care. The advantages of this nonobtrusive and nonthreatening screening system were (1) the proportion of patients screened was restricted to about one in seven, thus avoiding the possibility of offending the majority of patients with a low chance of screening positive and cutting down the time needed to carry out screening; (2) it was much more acceptable to receptionists than asking patients about their alcohol consumption; (3) physicians were given a legitimate clinical rationale for inquiring about drinking, i.e., as a possible factor leading to trauma. This study illustrates an innovative and context-sensitive approach to research and service development regarding the use of brief interventions in the real-world primary care setting.

THE GENERAL HOSPITAL

In some ways, the general hospital ward offers a setting more conducive to brief alcohol interventions than does primary health care, mainly because patients have more time available for screening and counseling. There is abundant evidence that many types of hospital wards contain high numbers of excessive drinkers, especially for men; depending on the definitions used, estimates range up to 40% excessive drinkers among male patients (McIntosh, 1982).

Two studies (Chick, Lloyd, & Crombie, 1985; Elvy, Wells, & Baird, 1988) have provided suggestive evidence that counseling by a nurse or a psychologist lasting up to 1 hour could be an effective brief intervention in this setting. However, neither of these studies demonstrated a reduction in alcohol consumption among counseled patients after discharge from the hospital. This has now been shown in a study reported by Heather, Rollnick, Bell, and Richmond (1996). Compared with an assessment-only control condition, counseling on the ward (either brief motivational interviewing or skills-based counseling for 30 to 40 minutes) resulted in an average reduction in consumption of roughly 10 drinks per week 6 months after discharge. An interesting matching effect involving the stages of change model was also shown in this study. Patients' stage of change was assessed before counseling by the Readiness to Change Questionnaire (Rollnick, Heather, Gold, & Hall, 1992). Those deemed to be in early stages of change (precontemplation or contemplation) showed greater reductions in drinking if they had received brief motivational interviewing than if they had received skills-based counseling, as the stages of change model would predict. However, for those in the action stage there was no difference between the two forms of counseling in their effect on consumption and most patients did well. This latter finding might be interpreted as showing that, given the low level of alcohol dependence among these patients, those who have reached the action stage do not need counseling to help them cut down drinking; very brief advice and encouragement may suffice. Resources could perhaps be more efficiently used by reserving motivational-type counseling for those patients assessed as being not ready to change. This interesting possibility deserves research attention.

ACCIDENT AND EMERGENCY SERVICES

It is well established that excessive drinkers are overrepresented among attenders of accident and emergency (A&E) departments (Holt *et al.*, 1980; Lockhart *et al.*, 1986; Weisner & Schmidt, 1993). In the last study cited, patients attending emergency rooms in four hospitals in California were found to have almost twice the risk of showing alcohol-related harm as individuals in the general population. Despite the inherent difficulties in carrying out opportunistic screening in this setting, it seems that it is possible to detect excessive drinkers in A&E departments (Lockhart *et al.*, 1986). Green and colleagues (1993) found that almost half the patients they identified as having an alcohol problem accepted an invitation to return to the department for advice on drinking the following day, suggesting that A&E departments can be appropriate settings in which to offer help to reduce consumption.

Antti-Poika (1988) randomized to an intervention or control (usual care) group 120 heavy drinking men attending an emergency service because of injuries. The intervention group received up to three sessions of counseling from a trained assistant nurse. Results were encouraging: At 6-month follow-up, 45% of patients in the intervention group had either moderated their drinking or abstained compared with 20% in the control group, a statistically significant difference supported by changes in GGT values. This study suggests that brief intervention can be effective in the A&E setting but more research on this possibility is needed.

Phase III of the WHO International Collaborative Project on the Identification and Management of Alcohol-related Problems in Primary Health Care (Monteiro & Gomel, 1998) is concerned specifically with investigating ways in primary care to improve the implementation of brief interventions against excessive drinking. The first strand of this research program was a questionnaire study of primary care physicians' attitudes to preventive medicine in general and secondary prevention of alcohol problems in particular.

In the U.K. arm of the study (Kaner, McAvoy, Heather, Haighton, & Gilvarry, 1997), there emerged some encouraging signs that GPs are receiving more education about alcohol than previously, that they are more prepared than before to counsel patients about reducing consumption, and that a current perception about their lack of effectiveness in helping patients cut down could be improved by more information, training, and support. Nevertheless, in terms of current practice, there was little evidence that GPs had increased their levels of inquiry, identification, and intervention regarding excessive drinking since the start of efforts to involve GPs in this area of work over 20 years ago (see Heather, 1996). Some specific obstacles to progress were identified, including an undue focus on physical rather than social or psychological consequences of excessive drinking, the perception that illicit drug use is more important to health than drinking level, a lack of awareness of positive results from research on brief interventions, and a feeling of lack of support, from both alcohol specialists and government policy, for practice in this area. However, the overriding barrier to implementation of brief interventions identified in the survey was perhaps the most obvious—*lack of time;* busy GPs felt that they simply had insufficient available time for screening and brief intervention against excessive drinking.

The third strand of the WHO project just mentioned is a randomized controlled trial of ways to encourage the uptake and utilization of a brief intervention package by GPs (Kaner, Haighton, McAvoy, Heather, & Gilvarry, 1996). Results from the Australian arm of this study are now available (Gomel, Saunders, Wutzke, Hardcastle, & Carnegie, 1996). A total of 632 primary care physicians were randomly allocated to one of three marketing strategies: direct mail, telemarketing, or "academic detailing" (i.e., a personal marketing interview). Outcome measures were the percentage of physicians who accepted the brief intervention package (uptake) and the percentage who were recruited to take part in the research trial. Uptake rates were significantly higher for the telemarketing (80%) and academic detailing (79%) strategies than for direct mail (48%). A similar order of response was obtained for the recruitment rate. There were no significant differences between the telemarketing and academic detailing strategies but, because the former is cheaper, it appears to be a more cost-effective approach to disseminating brief interventions, in Australia at least (Gomel *et al.,* 1996).

A second phase of this study randomized 127 physicians who had agreed to take part in the trial to one of four groups: (1) training and maximal support, (2) training and minimal support, (3) training and no support, and (4) a control group receiving no training or support. Rates of screening and counseling for excessive drinking were measured at a 3-month follow-up. Both screening and counseling rates were significantly higher in the maximal support condition but a further analysis suggested that the critical factor determining the counseling rate was the number of patients screened. The overall conclusion of this study was that initial training and support facilitate the implementation of brief interventions in primary health care (Gomel *et al.,* 1996). Results from other countries participating in the WHO research project are awaited.

IMPLICATIONS FOR RESEARCH AND PRACTICE

A first conclusion from the evidence reviewed in this chapter is that in the three areas of problem substance use covered—tobacco smoking, long-term benzodiazepine use, and excessive drinking—the use of minimal interventions in a range of medical settings has been justified by research. To achieve their beneficial effects, these interventions need consist of no more than basic advice and support for behavior change delivered in a sympathetic and nonjudgmental fashion and need last no longer than 5 or 10 minutes. (In the smoking cessation field, the addition of nicotine replacement therapy to brief advice is also well justified by research.) Only a relatively small proportion of the recipients of this advice will change their behavior but, given the wide accessibility and potentially high recruitment rates for brief interventions in primary health care, general hospital, and other medical settings, the impact on public health if brief interventions were systematically incorporated into routine medical practice would be enormous.

There are a number of important issues requiring further clarification in research, including the following: (1) There is conflicting evidence on the added benefits of more intensive (but still brief) interventions, consisting perhaps of condensed forms of cognitive-behavioral therapy (Sanchez-Craig, Wilkinson, & Walker, 1987) or motivational interviewing (Rollnick, Heather, & Bell, 1992). We need to know to whom these more intensive interventions should be offered, under what conditions they are most effective, and whether or not they are an efficient and cost-effective use of resources compared with basic advice. (2) The role of health professions other than medicine needs further work. For example, if family doctors are too busy to deliver brief interventions, it is likely that practice or community nurses could make a vital contribution, but we need research specifically relevant to this possibility. (3) In the alcohol field, there is conflicting evidence on the effectiveness of brief interventions in primary health care among female excessive drinkers. This should be clarified because a high proportion of women present to primary care and this represents an ideal opportunity to modify excessive drinking in this population (Kaner, Haighton, McAvoy, Heather, & Gilvarry, 1997). (4) Despite positive evidence for the effectiveness of brief interventions against single problem behaviors, it is still possible that combined interventions directed at changing lifestyle behavior in general should be the preferred strategy. Although one recent review found little evidence for the effectiveness of such a strategy in primary care (Ashenden, Silagy, & Weller, 1997), more extensive and rigorous evaluation is needed here. (5) A particular line of research that needs further development is the possible additional benefits to be gained from matching types of brief intervention to the stage of change of the patient (see Heather *et al.,* 1996).

A more general issue for brief intervention research is the need for movement from, in Flay's (1986) use of these terms, efficacy research to effectiveness research and beyond. It seems that the smoking cessation field is further advanced in this particular respect than is the alcohol field (Richmond, 1996). Having established the efficacy of brief interventions in medical settings, researchers in alcohol and other fields should move on to investigate their effectiveness in real-world situations. As in the smoking cessation field, this should lead to research on optimal conditions for facilitating the implementation of brief interventions and to studies of how they may be widely disseminated in communities.

An objection to brief interventions that is sometimes encountered is that their effects are likely to be modest compared with whole population preventive strategies, such as higher taxation on cigarettes and alcohol, increased environmental restrictions on substance use, and advertising restrictions (Chapman, 1993). But this misses the point; there is no competition between brief intervention strategies and preventive control measures and no reason why both should not contribute synergistically to public health (see Chapter 8, this volume). Indeed, brief interventions could facilitate the introduction of effective control measures by helping to create a climate of opinion in which such measures become politically viable. Conversely, an environment that does not support and encourage smoking or hazardous drinking is likely to render individual brief interventions more effective. On the other hand, if control measures continue to be resisted by governments, widespread implementation of brief interventions is probably the next best alternative for impacting public health.

Accepting then that such a widespread implementation of brief interventions would have a major impact on the health and quality of life of the population, and accepting also that the evidence to support this conclusion has been available for some time, why has it not occurred? Much has been written on this topic and it is a vexed and difficult area of debate. There is little doubt that the situation would be helped by better training of health professionals on the rationale and methods of brief intervention. There is a need, too, to make screening and intervention methods more acceptable to doctors and their patients (Israel et al., 1996; Rollnick, Butler, & Stott, 1997). The disjunction in aims between the public health approach, which regards even very low success rates as beneficial, and the clinical perspective of most practitioners, in which the welfare of the individual patient is paramount, is one problem clearly in need of resolution.

Beyond this, however, it is likely that significant progress will be made only by paying attention at national policy level to the *structural* factors preventing the implementation of brief interventions. These mostly concern two obvious and related factors—time and money. Those interested in encouraging the implementation of brief interventions in general practice and other medical settings must attempt to persuade governments to create the financial incentives and other structural conditions that will allow it to occur.

ACKNOWLEDGMENTS

I am very grateful to the following for insightful comments on earlier drafts of this chapter: Professor Heather Ashton, Alison Bowie, Dr. Chris Butler, Dr. Eileen Kaner.

REFERENCES

Anderson, P., & Scott, E. (1992). The effect of general practitioners' advice to heavy drinking men. *British Journal of Addiction, 87,* 891–900.

Antti-Poika, I. (1988). *Alcohol intoxication and abuse in injured patients* (Dissertationes #19, Commentationes Physico-Mathematicae). Helsinki, Finland: Finnish Society of Sciences & Letters.

Ashenden, R., Silagy, C., & Weller, D. (1997). A systematic review of the effectiveness of promoting lifestyle change in general practice. *Family Practice, 14,* 160–175.

Babor, T. F., & Grant, M. (Eds.). (1992). *Project on Identification and Management of Alcohol-related Problems. Report on Phase II: A Randomized Clinical Trial of Brief Interventions in Primary Health Care.* Geneva: World Health Organization.

Bashir, K., King, M., & Ashworth, M. (1994). Controlled evaluation of brief intervention by general practitioners to reduce chronic use of benzodiazepines. *British Journal of General Practice, 44,* 408–412.

Bien, T. H., Miller, W. R., & Tonigan, J. (1993). Brief interventions for alcohol problems: A review. *Addiction, 88,* 315–336.

Chapman, S. (1993). The role of doctors in promoting smoking cessation. *British Medical Journal, 307,* 518–519.

Chick, J., Lloyd, G., & Crombie, E. (1985). Counselling problem drinkers in medical wards: A controlled study. *British Medical Journal, 83,* 159–170.

Cormack, M. A., Sweeney, K. G., Hugh-Jones, H., & Foot, G. A. (1994). Evaluation of an easy, cost-effective strategy for cutting benzodiazepine use in general practice. *British Journal of General Practice, 44,* 5–8.

Department of Health. (1992). *The health of the nation.* London: Her Majesty's Stationery Office.

Dickinson, J., Wiggers, J., Leeder, S., & Sanson-Fisher, R. (1989). General practitioners' detection of patients' smoking status. *Medical Journal of Australia, 150,* 420–426.

Elvy, G. A., Wells, J. E., & Baird, K. A. (1988). Attempted referral as intervention for problem drinking in the general hospital. *British Journal of Addiction, 83,* 83–89.

Fagerström, K. O. (1978). Measuring degree of physical dependence to tobacco smoking with reference to individualization of treatment. *Addictive Behaviors, 3,* 235–241.

Flay, B. R. (1986). Efficacy and effectiveness trials (and other phases of research) in the development of health promotion programs. *Preventive Medicine, 15,* 451–474.

Fleming, M. F., Barry, K. L., Manwell, L. B., Johnson, K., & London, R. (1997). Brief physician advice for problem alcohol drinkers: A randomized controlled trial in community-based primary care practices. *Journal of the American Medical Association, 277,* 1039–1045.

Freer, C. B., Boyle, P., & Ryan, M. P. (1986). A study of attendance patterns in general practice over three years. *Health Bulletin, 44,* 75–80.

Fremantle, N., Gill, P., Godfrey, C., Long, A., Richards, C., Sheldon, T., Song, F., & Webb, J. (1993). *Brief interventions and alcohol use* (Effective Health Care Bulletin #7). Leeds, England: Nuffield Institute for Health.

Gomel, M. K., Saunders, J. B., Wutzke, S., Hardcastle, D. M, & Carnegie M. A. (1996). *Implementation of early intervention for hazardous and harmful alcohol consumption in general practice.* Final Report prepared for the Research Into Drug Abuse Program. Canberra, Australia: Department of Human Services and Health.

Green, M., Setchell, J., Hames, P., Stiff, G., Touquet, R., & Priest, R. (1993). Management of alcohol abusing patients in accident and emergency departments. *Journal of the Royal Society of Medicine, 86,* 393–395.

Heather, N. (1995). Brief intervention strategies. In R. K. Hester & W. R. Miller (Eds.), *Handbook of alcoholism treatment approaches: Effective alternatives* (2nd ed, pp. 105–122). Needham Heights, MA: Allyn & Bacon.

Heather, N. (1996). The public health and brief interventions for excessive alcohol consumption: The British experience. *Addictive Behaviors, 21,* 857–868.

Heather, N., Rollnick, S., Bell, A., & Richmond, R. (1996). Effects of brief counselling among male heavy drinkers identified on general hospital wards. *Drug & Alcohol Review, 15,* 29–38.

Heather, N., Luce, A., Peck, D., Dunbar, B., & James, I. (1997). *Development of the Readiness to Change Questionnaire (treatment version).* Report to the Northern & Yorkshire R&D Directorate (Ref. NYRO ACJ July 96). Newcastle upon Tyne, England: Centre for Alcohol & Drug Studies.

Holt, S., Stewart, I. C., Dixon, J. M. J., Elton, R. A., Taylor, T. V., & Little, K. (1980). Alcohol and the emergency service patient. *British Medical Journal, 281,* 638–640.

Israel, Y., Hollander, O., Sanchez-Craig, M., Booker, S., Miller, V., Gingrich, R., & Rankin, J. G. (1996). Screening for problem drinking and counseling by the primary care physician–nurse team. *Alcoholism: Clinical & Experimental Research, 20,* 1443–1450.

Kahan, M., Wilson, L., & Becker, L. (1995). Effectiveness of physician-based interventions with problem drinkers: A review. *Canadian Medical Association Journal, 152,* 851–859.

Kaner, E., McAvoy, B., Heather, N., Haighton, K., & Gilvarry, E. (1997). United Kingdom. In J. B. Saunders & S. Wutzke (Eds.), *WHO Collaborative Study on Implementing and Supporting Early Intervention in Primary Health Care: Report on Strand 1, The views and current practices of general practitioners regarding preventive medicine and early intervention for hazardous alcohol use.* Copenhagen, Denmark: WHO Regional Office for Europe.

Kaner, E. F. S., Haighton, C. A., McAvoy, B. R., Heather, N., & Gilvarry, E. (1996). Controlled trial of methods to encourage uptake and utilization by GPs of early intervention against excessive alcohol consumption. *Family Practice, 13,* 347.

Kaner, E. F. S., Haighton, C. A., McAvoy, B. R., Heather, N., & Gilvarry, E. (1997). More women drink at hazardous levels in England than Italy [Letter]. *British Medical Journal, 314,* 1413.

Kottke, T. E., Battista, R. N., DeFriese, G. H., & Brekke, M. L. (1988). Attributes of successful smoking cessation interventions in medical practice: A meta-analysis of 39 controlled trials. *Journal of the American Medical Association, 259,* 2883–2889.

Lockhart, S. P., Carter, Y. H., Straffen, A. M., Pang, K. K., McLoughlin, J., & Baron, J. H. (1986). Detecting alcohol consumption as a cause of emergency general medical admissions. *Journal of the Royal Society of Medicine, 79,* 132–136.

McIntosh, I. D. (1982). Alcohol-related disabilities in general hospital patients: A critical review of the evidence. *International Journal of the Addictions, 17,* 609–639.

Monteiro, M. G., & Gomel, M. (1998). World Health Organization project on brief interventions for alcohol-related problems in primary health care settings. *Journal of Substance Abuse, 3,* 5–9.

Ockene, J. K., Kristeller, J., Goldberg, R., Amick, T. L., Pekow, P. S., Hosmer, D., Quirk, M., & Kalan, K. (1991). Increasing the efficacy of physician-delivered smoking interventions: A randomized clinical trial. *Journal of General Internal Medicine, 6,* 1–8.

Parish, D. C. (1997). Another indication for screening and early intervention: Problem drinking [Editorial]. *Journal of the American Medical Association, 277,* 1079–1080.

Richmond, R., Heather, N., Wodak, A., Kehoe, L., & Webster, I. (1995). Controlled evaluation of a general practice-based brief intervention for excessive drinking. *Addiction, 90,* 119–132.

Richmond, R. L. (1996). Retracing the steps of Marco Polo: From clinical trials to diffusion of interventions for smokers. *Addictive Behaviors, 21,* 683–697.

Richmond, R. L., Kehoe, L., Heather, N., Wodak, A., & Webster, I. (1996). General practitioners' promotion of healthy lifestyles: What patients think. *Australian & New Zealand Journal of Public Health, 20,* 195–200.

Rollnick, S., Heather, N., & Bell, A. (1992). Negotiating behavior change in medical settings: The development of brief motivational interviewing. *Journal of Mental Health, 1,* 25–37.

Rollnick, S., Heather, N., Gold, R., & Hall, W. (1992). Development of a short Readiness to Change Questionnaire for use in brief, opportunistic interventions among excessive drinkers. *British Journal of Addiction, 87,* 743–754.

Rollnick, S., Butler, C. C., & Stott, N. (1997). Helping smokers make decisions: The enhancement of brief interventions for general medical practice. *Patient Education & Counselling, 31,* 191–203.

Russell, M. A. H., Wilson, C., Taylor, C., & Baker, C. D. (1979). Effect of general practitioners' advice against smoking. *British Medical Journal, 283,* 231–235.

Russell, M. A. H., Merriman, R., Stapleton, J., & Taylor, W. (1983). Effect of nicotine chewing gum as an adjunct to general practitioners' advice against smoking. *British Medical Journal, 287,* 1782–1785.

Sanchez-Craig, M., Wilkinson, D. A., & Walker, K. (1987). Theory and methods for secondary prevention of alcohol problems: A cognitively-based approach. In W. Cox (Ed.), *Treatment and prevention of alcohol problems: A resource manual.* New York: Academic Press.

Scott, E., & Anderson, P. (1990). Randomized controlled trial of general practitioner intervention in women with excessive alcohol consumption. *Drug & Alcohol Review, 10,* 313–321.

Silagy, C., & Ketteridge, S. (1996). The effectiveness of physician advice to aid smoking cessation. In T. Lancaster & C. Silagy (Eds.), Tobacco Addiction Module of *The Cochrane Database of Systematic Reviews* (updated September 6, 1996). London: British Medical Journal.

Silagy, C., Muir, J., Coulter, A., Thorogood, M., Yudkin, P., & Roe, L. (1992). Lifestyle advice in general practice: Rates recalled by patients. *British Medical Journal, 305*, 871–874.

Silagy, C., Lancaster, T., Fowler, G., & Spiers, I. (1997). Effectiveness of training health professionals to provide smoking cessation interventions: Systematic review of randomized controlled trials. In T. Lancaster, C. Silagy, & D. Fullerton (Eds.), Tobacco Addiction Module of *The Cochrane Database of Systematic Reviews* (updated March 3, 1997). London: British Medical Journal.

Silagy, C., Mant, D., Fowler, G., & Lancaster, T. (1997). The effect of nicotine replacement therapy on smoking cessation. In T. Lancaster, C. Silagy, & D. Fullerton (Eds.), Tobacco Addiction Module of *The Cochrane Database of Systematic Reviews* (updated March 3, 1997). London: British Medical Journal.

Simpson, R. J. (1993). Benzodiazepines in general practice. In C. Hallström (Ed.), *Benzodiazepine dependence* (pp. 252–266). Oxford, England: Oxford Medical Publications.

Skinner, H. A., Holt, S., Schuller, R., Roy, J., & Israel, Y. (1984). Identification of alcohol abuse using laboratory tests and a history of trauma. *Annals of Internal Medicine, 101*, 847–851.

Wallace, P., Cutler, S., & Haines, A. (1988). Randomized controlled trial of general practitioner intervention in patients with excessive alcohol consumption. *British Medical Journal, 297*, 663–668.

Wallace, P. G., Brennan, P. J., & Haines, A. P. (1987). Are general practitioners doing enough to promote healthy lifestyles? *British Medical Journal, 294*, 940–942.

Weisner, C., & Schmidt, L. (1993). Alcohol and drug problems among diverse health and social service populations. *American Journal of Public Health, 83*, 824–829.

Wells, F. (1993). Benzodiazepines and the pharmaceutical industry. In C. Hallström (Ed.), *Benzodiazepine dependence* (pp. 337–349). Oxford, England: Oxford Medical Publications.

Williams, P., & Bellantuono, C. (1991). Long-term tranquillizer use: The contribution of epidemiology. In J. Gabe (Ed.), *Understanding tranquillizer use* (pp. 69–91). London: Routledge.

11

Working through the Concerned Significant Other

ROBERT J. MEYERS, JANE ELLEN SMITH, AND ERICA J. MILLER

INTRODUCTION

It is estimated that for every individual with an alcohol problem, there are five others who suffer directly (Paolino & McCrady, 1977). The loved ones of a substance-abusing individual often are faced with a variety of stressors, such as experiences of physical violence and verbal aggression, unpredictable and embarrassing behavior of the user, and stealing from family members (Velleman *et al.,* 1993). Reports show that many of these concerned significant others (CSOs) exhibit depressed mood, physical complaints, and lowered self-confidence (Brown, Kokin, Seraganian, & Shields, 1995). Unfortunately, problem alcohol or drug users rarely recognize the full negative impact of their use on themselves or others, and consequently the notion of seeking treatment is incongruous. For these "resistant" users, lack of motivation for change can be a significant obstacle in addressing these problems (Miller & Rollnick, 1991).

Individuals with substance abuse problems often report that the decision to pursue treatment was prompted by the direct influence of CSOs, or CSOs acting in concert with courts, employee assistance programs, or informal social networks (Cunningham, Sobell, Sobell, & Kapur, 1995). In reports of CSOs who were directed by trained clinicians, success rates in persuading unmotivated problem drinkers to enter treatment ranged from 24% for a programmed social-network intervention (Liepman, Nirenberg, & Begin, 1989) to 86% for a cognitive-behavioral procedure (Sisson & Azrin, 1986). It is important that posttreatment

ROBERT J. MEYERS, JANE ELLEN SMITH, AND ERICA J. MILLER • Center on Alcoholism, Substance Abuse, and Addictions, University of New Mexico, Albuquerque, New Mexico 87106.

Treating Addictive Behaviors, 2nd ed., edited by Miller and Heather. Plenum Press, New York, 1998.

improvement in several areas of functioning for the CSOs of drinkers also has been reported (Brennan, Moos, & Kelly, 1994). Furthermore, in the case of problem users who enter treatment, evidence suggests that outcomes are enhanced if CSOs actively participate in the therapy process (Atkinson, Tolson, & Turner, 1993; Edwards & Steinglass, 1995; Galanter, 1993; Humphreys, Moos, & Finney, 1996; Liddle & Dakof, 1995).

Substance abuse facilities regularly receive calls from desperate friends and family members who are concerned about loved ones who are abusing alcohol or drugs. However, although it is widely acknowledged that problems related to alcohol and drug misuse can seriously affect the lives of close associates of the user (Collins, Leonard, & Searles, 1990; Orford & Harwin, 1982), historically there have been few options for individuals seeking help for treatment-resistant loved ones. This is regrettable, given that many significant others have proven to be influential in prompting drinkers and drug users into treatment (Hingson, Mangione, Meyers, & Scotch, 1982; Room, 1987).

ENGAGEMENT APPROACHES

TRADITIONAL STRATEGIES

Facilities' traditional responses to the significant other have been offers of Al-Anon (Al-Anon Family Groups, 1965; Carolyn W., 1984) or the Johnson Institute intervention (Johnson, 1986). The Al-Anon approach, which arises from the fundamentally spiritual 12-step program, advocates loving detachment, acceptance of the CSO's helplessness to control the problem drinker, and group support for the CSO. Despite the wide availability of this program, few studies have tested its efficacy. Some success in improving CSO functioning and engaging resistant drinkers in treatment was reported when Al-Anon was compared with a delayed-treatment control (Dittrich & Trapold, 1984).

The Johnson Institute intervention is a technique in which members of the substance user's social network are assisted in outlining the negative impact the abusive drinking has had on them over the years, and the consequences that they are prepared to carry out should the substance user decide not to enter treatment. This information is presented to the drinker in a confrontational family meeting. A demonstration project utilizing this intervention (Liepman et al., 1989) showed that among those networks who actually confronted the drinker, the rate of treatment engagement was high (86%) in comparison with those who did not confront the drinker (17%). The confronted drinkers also had longer periods of abstinence on average than did those not confronted. However, considering that only 29% actually completed the confrontation, the overall success rate was 24% (Liepman et al., 1989). A recent retrospective case file review provided support for the Johnson intervention in terms of treatment engagement when compared with either unrehearsed or unsupervised variations of the program (Loneck, Garrett, & Banks, 1996). However, the nonexperimental nature of the design makes the findings subject to cautious interpretation.

UNILATERAL FAMILY THERAPY

Among the first treatments specifically designed for working with CSOs of unmotivated, treatment-resistant drinkers was unilateral family therapy (Thomas &
Santa, 1982). Its goals are to improve CSO coping and family functioning and to facilitate sobriety for the drinker. Therapy sessions with the CSO include instruction
in monitoring the loved one's alcohol use, education about the effects of excessive
drinking, relationship enhancement training, encouragement for discontinuing ineffective coping strategies, and planning for sobriety. The idea of treatment is presented to the drinker either through a "programmed confrontation" that is quite
similar to the Johnson Institute intervention, or through a carefully timed and
staged "programmed request."

An early trial of unilateral family therapy showed higher rates of treatment
engagement and decreased alcohol consumption for drinkers whose CSOs were
treated with unilateral family therapy compared with those not treated (Thomas,
Santa, Bronson, & Oyserman, 1987). Despite several methodological limitations of
the study, such as small group sizes and a nonrandomized control group, the results were promising. A later study found similar effects initially, but significant
treatment retention differences were lost at the time of the 18-month follow-up
(Thomas, Yoshioka, Ager, & Adams, 1993). Nevertheless, alcohol consumption remained significantly lower for the substance-abusing spouses of the treated CSOs.
Improvements in the nondrinking spouses' functioning, including reductions in
psychopathology and life distress, and an increase in marital satisfaction also were
reported. This study was again limited by lack of random group assignment.

COMMUNITY REINFORCEMENT AND FAMILY TRAINING

Community Reinforcement and Family Training (CRAFT) is an outgrowth of
the Community Reinforcement Approach (Azrin, 1976; Azrin, Sisson, Meyers, &
Godley, 1982; Hunt & Azrin, 1973; Meyers & Smith, 1995) for problem drinkers.
In the Community Reinforcement Approach problem users' CSOs have always
been viewed as crucial collaborators in the treatment of substance abuse, and
have been included successfully as disulfiram monitors, partners in marital
counseling, active agents in resocialization and reinforcement programs, and relapse or problem detectors. The related CRAFT approach is built on the belief
that since concerned family members or friends tend to be emotionally invested
in and have extensive contact with the user, these CSOs can play a powerful role
in effecting change in the user's behavior. It does *not* assume that the CSOs somehow are *responsible* for the drinking or drug problem of the loved one. A second
belief of CRAFT is that most CSOs can benefit from assistance in learning to take
better care of themselves.

Although there are some similarities between CRAFT and unilateral family
therapy (Thomas & Santa, 1982), there are several important differences. CRAFT
does not utilize "programmed confrontation," nor does it focus on educating CSOs
about excessive alcohol use. Some of CRAFT's unique components include an emphasis on safety issues, a reliance on functional analyses of behavior, a focus on

identifying and utilizing positive reinforcers for both the drinker and the CSO, and an emphasis on personal lifestyle changes for the CSO. CRAFT also relies heavily upon the skills-training strategies found in the Community Reinforcement Approach (Meyers & Smith, 1995).

Sisson and Azrin (1986) conducted the first randomized study examining the viability of community-based reinforcement procedures for working with a problem drinker's CSO. Seven CSOs were assigned to Community Reinforcement Training, and five other CSOs received a traditional program based on the disease concept of alcoholism. For the former group, six of the seven drinkers whose CSOs were involved in the program entered treatment. In contrast, none of the traditional group's drinkers sought treatment. In addition, drinkers associated with CSOs in the Community Reinforcement Training group decreased their average number of drinking days by more than half during the time that only the non-drinker was in treatment.

Three federally funded CRAFT research projects are ongoing at the University of New Mexico's Center on Alcoholism, Substance Abuse, and Addictions (CASAA). In two projects for which recruitment has been completed, 832 telephone calls were received from individuals requesting assistance with a treatment-resistant substance-abusing loved one. From among these callers, 392 CSOs were interviewed, 130 CSOs were accepted into the alcohol project, and 62 were admitted to the drug trial. CSOs for the alcohol study were randomized into one of three treatment modalities: CRAFT, 12-step facilitation, or the Johnson Institute intervention. The CSOs who received CRAFT were successful at engaging 67% of the resistant drinkers in treatment. This outweighed the engagement rates of both the 12-step facilitation (13%) and Johnson Institute (23%) approaches. In the drug trial, wherein all CSOs received CRAFT procedures, the success rate for engaging resistant drug users in treatment was 76%. In addition, findings from both projects indicate that CSOs who were parents were significantly more successful at engaging their sons and daughters in treatment when compared to nonparent CSOs. It is noteworthy that these populations were not only treatment-resistant by definition, but overall were more severe in their alcohol and drug use than participants in several other CASAA-based clinical trials, including Project MATCH (Project MATCH Research Group, 1997).

Although one primary goal of CRAFT was to engage resistant individuals in treatment, another was to improve the emotional, relationship, and physical functioning of the CSOs themselves. Preliminary results for changes in CSO functioning from baseline to the 3-month follow-up show that CRAFT-trained CSOs reported significant overall decreases in state anger, state anxiety, and depression, regardless of whether the loved one had entered treatment.

CRAFT PROCEDURES

Overview

What are the specific treatment procedures that led to such high success rates in treatment engagement? The basic components of CRAFT procedures will be introduced next. (For a more detailed description see Meyers & Smith, 1997; Meyers, Dominguez, & Smith, 1996). CRAFT involves

1. preparing the CSO to recognize and safely respond to any potential for domestic violence as behavioral changes are introduced at home;
2. completing two functional analyses with the CSO, the first to identify the substance user's triggers for using alcohol or drugs, as well as the consequences, and the second to profile the user's triggers for nonusing or prosocial behavior and its consequences;
3. working with the CSO to improve communication with the substance user;
4. showing the CSO how to effectively use and withdraw positive reinforcement such that it discourages a loved one's harmful using behavior;
5. teaching the CSO methods for decreasing stress in general, and emphasizing the importance of having sufficient positive reinforcement in his or her own life;
6. instructing the CSO in the most effective ways to suggest treatment to the substance user, and helping to identify optimal times;
7. laying the groundwork for having outpatient treatment available immediately for the user in the event that the decision is made to begin therapy, and discussing the need for the CSO to support the drinker or drug user during treatment.

DOMESTIC VIOLENCE PRECAUTIONS

It is important to proceed carefully when supporting a CSO's efforts to introduce behavioral changes with a substance user, given the significant association between substance abuse and domestic violence (Coleman & Straus, 1983; Gondolf & Foster, 1991; Leonard & Jacob, 1988; Stith, Crossman, & Bischof, 1991). CRAFT's initial procedures include an assessment of the potential for violence, usually with an instrument such as the Conflict Tactics Scale (Straus, 1979). If a history of violence is discovered, it is useful to conduct a functional analysis of the behaviors that typically precede and follow the violent behavior. For example, assume a CSO describes the following situation: "Some days when my husband gets home he is extremely quiet and distant. I ask him what's wrong and he tells me he's fine. I can tell that he *isn't* fine, because he keeps rubbing his hands together, and acting very nervous. When I approach him a few minutes later to ask if there is anything I can do to help, he usually screams for me to get off his back. I know from past experience that once his voice gets that loud, I'm in for trouble. Next he goes into the den and starts with the 'silent treatment.' It's only a matter of time before he starts to drink. Then if I approach him and ask again how I can help, he gets in my face, yells, and sometimes even shoves me across the room."

Once the domestic violence episode is outlined, CRAFT works with the CSO to identify new responses that may be utilized during the precursors to the aggressive behavior. With proper training this CSO would learn that the precursors to violence (rubbing his hands together, acting distant, screaming, the "silent treatment," drinking) should not be addressed with any conversation at all, because it serves as a trigger for abusive behavior. Instead, these precursors can serve as signals to respond in a safer way. The CSO can simply end the conversation by stating that she will be available when he wants to talk, or she can tell her husband that since he wants to be left alone she will be spending the night at her mother's house. CRAFT devotes time to role-playing these new behaviors that have the potential for decreasing violent outbursts. But given that altering the CSO's behavior in any way could elicit a further negative reaction from the drinker, a safety plan must be built in if there is any threat of violence.

FUNCTIONAL ANALYSIS

CRAFT relies heavily on a functional analysis of substance abuse episodes regardless of whether domestic violence is involved. This approach introduces the idea that although the drinking or drug problem is not the CSO's fault, the CSO's behavior toward the user is worth examining due to sheer frequency of contact. The CSO should be invited to try new strategies that may be instrumental in changing the drinking or using behavior and in getting the individual to seek treatment.

When the CSO is first asked to outline the loved one's pattern of substance use, the emphasis is on the triggers for the drinking or drug use. It is important for the CSO to be cognizant of the *antecedents* to alcohol or drug use, so that strategies can be taught to alter the CSO's behavior at these times. The *consequences* that the user experiences for drug use are also reviewed. In particular, the CSO's responses to the drinking or drug use should be highlighted in the event that more adaptive coping responses need to be taught. The functional analysis is sometimes supplemented with an instrument specifically designed to identify spouses' ineffectual coping strategies, such as the Spouse Enabling Inventory or the Spouse Sobriety Influence Inventory (Thomas, Yoshioka, & Ager, 1994).

CRAFT therapists complete a separate functional analysis to help the CSO find antecedents for several of the loved one's pleasurable *non*substance-abusing behaviors. This forms the basis for later interventions that will be introduced to increase the frequency of enjoyable nonusing activities. The CSO has a wealth of knowledge about the functioning and habits of the substance user, yet knowing how and when to apply this information is the key to positive behavior change. If the CSO can explore which activities elicit prosocial behaviors, he or she will be in a position to use this in a more helpful manner.

COMMUNICATION TRAINING

CRAFT is for family members and friends who hope to maintain their relationship with the substance user, but who want it to change in a positive direction. Typically it is useful to start by examining the manner in which the CSO currently communicates with the loved one. CRAFT relies on the positive communication skills training outlined in the Community Reinforcement Approach (see Meyers & Smith, 1995). The basic communication rules are (1) be brief, (2) be positive, (3) be specific and clear, (4) label your feelings, (5) offer an understanding statement once the issue has been viewed from the user's perspective, (6) accept partial responsibility when appropriate, and (7) offer to help.

Consider a mother who is concerned about her substance-abusing teenage son's habit of staying out all night. The therapist (T) will utilize the behavioral principles of modeling, behavioral rehearsal, and shaping while teaching the CSO (C) how to apply the communication rules to a real-life situation. The dialogue begins after the CSO has made her first attempt at the conversation:

T: You say that one of your major concerns is you don't want your son to spend the night at a friend's house without calling you. Actually, you've been telling me a number of things that you *don't* want. Could you change this into a positive statement and talk about what you *would* like him to do?

C: I'm not sure what you mean.

T: Instead of saying to your son, "You never call me when you're spending the night at a friend's. You know how upset I get," you could say, "I don't mind you staying overnight at a friend's. I would just feel a lot better if I knew you were safe. Would you be willing to call me if you think you may not be coming home?" Do you see how it states briefly and clearly what you want, and does so in a positive tone? And it states how you feel. That covers four of the rules of a good conversation that we discussed. Would you like to give it a try? Let's practice it again.

C: OK. I'll give it a try. "Davey, I know you couldn't care less, but I worry and I'd like you to call me if you're not coming home."

T: Great start. You told him how you felt and you clearly stated what you would like him to do. But the part about him not caring has a negative edge. Could we just change that a little to keep it positive? Maybe you could say, "I know you don't want me to be overly concerned, but I do worry and I'd like you to call me if you know you're not coming home." How does that sound?

C: I see what you mean. That should be easy enough.

T: Great. Now let's add something a little fancy. Let's use an understanding statement, accept partial responsibility, and offer to help. For instance you might say, "Davey, I know you get busy and are having fun, and that makes it hard to stop and call. And I'm probably a little overprotective. But still, I worry. What can I do to make it easy for you to let me know you're OK?" Did you see how I was understanding, accepted some of the responsibility for the problem, and came up with an offer to help?

C: That sounds like a lot to remember. But I get the overall idea. He may be more likely to call if he hears that I'm concerned and not just checking up on him. I might say, "Davey, I know you are able to take care of yourself, but I *am* a worrier, so please call me if you plan on not coming home. You could just leave a message on the machine."

T: Great job. You're doing very well. I'm sure with some practice you'll get even better.

All seven communication guidelines have been incorporated. It would be important to have the CSO continue practicing the same basic conversation (behavioral rehearsal), and for the therapist to illustrate improvements with examples (modeling). The therapist should also reinforce the CSO's efforts and offer feedback so that the CSO's conversation gradually approximates the therapist's model (shaping).

USE OF POSITIVE REINFORCEMENT

Frequently the CSO is in a position to support or discourage the loved one's substance abuse even through a modest change in the CSO's own behavior. But the customary attempts at managing the behavior tend to be ineffective and unsystematic.

Some examples include constantly nagging the user to stop, discarding the substance-abusing alcohol or drugs to "show them what it's like," or even threatening the user. CRAFT presents additional alternatives, since the CSO is taught to arrange positive consequences for nonusing behaviors and to avoid contact with the substance user whenever he or she is using.

The therapist should first explain the concept of a positive reinforcer, or a reward, to the CSO: it is any object or behavior whose presentation increases the rate of the behavior that it follows. The CSO is then asked to identify several small reinforcers that could be introduced when the loved one is not using, such as preparing the individual's favorite meal, discussing the user's favorite topic, offering verbal praise or support for sobriety, suggesting a romantic encounter, or just spending time with the individual. Regardless of the reinforcer selected, it is necessary to discuss whether it is powerful enough to compete with substance-abusing behavior. The therapist next explains the importance of introducing the rewards at a time when the user is clean, sober, and not hungover. The CSO is queried about being able to recognize when the loved one is under the influence of even a small amount of alcohol or drugs (see Meyers et al., 1996). Finally, the therapist might train the CSO to verbally link the reward with nonusing behavior. For example, the CSO could practice saying, "You know, sometimes I absolutely love being with you, Sarah. I can't seem to get enough of you. And I've noticed that I feel this way toward you when you're not high. So that's when I want to spend my time with you. If you begin using, I'll just excuse myself and leave. I thought it was important for you to know how I feel."

Sometimes the anger that has built up over time in a CSO toward the substance user temporarily blocks the CSO's willingness to use positive reinforcement of nonusing activities. Other CSOs believe that it would not be appropriate to do anything special for the user, since this could be considered enabling or rescuing behavior. The therapist needs to clarify that positive reinforcement is not an enabling behavior when it is introduced only when the user is clean and sober. Rather, "enabling" is positive reinforcement for using, or more commonly, interfering with its natural negative consequences. Some therapists encourage initial changes in the CSO's behavior through a sampling procedure introduced in the Community Reinforcement Approach model. This technique teaches a CSO to "sample" a new behavior for a limited period or a number of times in order to give the process a chance to work (Azrin et al., 1982; Meyers & Smith, 1995; Miller & Page, 1991; Smith & Meyers, 1995). Thus a reluctant CSO might be asked to experiment with introducing positive reinforcement at nonusing times, and to observe whether it creates any movement toward the ultimate goal of reducing the user's alcohol or drug use.

A checklist of the skills required before implementing the use of positive reinforcement with the substance user follows:

1. The CSO can describe the concept and has identified appropriate positive reinforcers.
2. The CSO has the capability of delivering suitable reinforcers, as demonstrated in role-plays and by practicing first with another family member or friend.
3. The CSO has discussed possible resentment for being expected to give rewards to someone who has caused so much pain.

4. The CSO understands that the reward should be introduced only when the user is clean, sober and not hungover (Meyers & Smith, 1997; Meyers *et al.,* 1996).

5. The CSO is aware of a variety of possible consequences of this new behavior, and is prepared to address any problematic negative reactions.

One of the best ways for the therapist to teach the CSO about positive reinforcement is to utilize it throughout CRAFT sessions. In this manner the CSO is able to experience it firsthand, and to see many demonstrations of how and when it is delivered.

TIME OUT FROM POSITIVE REINFORCEMENT

In addition to teaching a CSO how to reward nonusing behavior, it is important to also explain the need for withdrawing positive reinforcement when the loved one *is* using. Time should be devoted to identifying some of the positive things that the CSO does for the substance user, and determining which ones would be appropriate and effective to withdraw. The goal would be to demonstrate to the user that a time out from positive reinforcement will occur if he or she chooses to use.

In most cases the CSO's presence is a positive reinforcer for the substance user. The CSO can capitalize on this by simply physically withdrawing from the loved one when alcohol or drugs have been used. The CSO would be trained to state in a clear and supportive way the reason for the change in behavior. One example is, "I love you and want to spend quality time with you, but when you drink, the time with you is not as much fun. So I'm not going to sit with you now because you're drinking. I think I'll go to the bedroom and read." Other CSOs make a point of sleeping in the guest room on the evenings that the loved one comes to bed under the influence. Some CSOs elect to withhold something other than just their presence. An example is the CSO who does not cook a special breakfast if the loved one gets up with a hangover. Regardless of the type of behavior that is changed, the CSO needs to be certain that it is one that will be missed by the user if it is withheld.

NATURAL CONSEQUENCES FOR USING

Another critical component of CRAFT is teaching the CSO how not to unintentionally reward drinking or drug using by interfering with the natural consequences of such behaviors. The therapist should gently point out ways in which the CSO may be unknowingly "supporting" the partner's using, such as by reheating dinner for a partner who has stopped at a bar on the way home from work, calling in sick for a loved one with a hangover, and making excuses to family members for negative drug-using behavior. In the event that a CSO has difficulty identifying actions that unintentionally are supporting drinking or drug using, a review of the consequences section of the functional analysis is sometimes helpful.

In preparing the CSO to allow the substance user to experience the natural, negative consequences for using behavior, four steps should be followed:

158   ROBERT J. MEYERS et al.

1. Have the CSO select one situation in which he or she inadvertently has been supporting the partner's using behavior.
2. Have the CSO consider what the natural consequences for the using behavior would be. For example, if the CSO did not step in and clean up the bathroom each time the loved one got sick during a binge, would the drinker have to clean it? If so, this might be an ideal situation for having the drinker face the natural consequences.
3. Explore any possible problematic repercussions for allowing the natural consequences, and devise a plan for following through.
4. Role-play how the CSO will explain to the user the decision to refrain from interfering with the occurrence of natural consequences for the substance use. The guidelines for verbal interchanges should be followed (refer to section, "Communication Training").

REINFORCERS FOR THE CSO

A major goal of CRAFT is to improve the quality of life for the CSO, regardless of whether the substance user ever enters treatment. The process begins with an examination of the CSO's current level of satisfaction in various life areas. The Happiness Scale that is utilized in the Community Reinforcement Approach (see Meyers & Smith, 1995) is one tool for obtaining such information efficiently. The next step is to introduce new reinforcers, such as social and recreational activities, to areas of low satisfaction. The CSO is encouraged to select a number of pleasurable activities independent of the substance user, and often a good place to start is through involvement with extended family members or close friends. In many cases CSOs have tried to hide their loved one's use and its negative consequences from others, and consequently have created a self-imposed exile from social functions. Because family and friends can be rewarding and supportive to a CSO, it is often worthwhile to encourage the CSO to rekindle old ties with these individuals. In the event that a CSO's work-related reinforcers are lacking, the therapist would discuss the opportunity for increasing the rewarding nature of a current job, or the value in trying a new position altogether.

SUGGESTION OF TREATMENT TO THE DRINKER OR DRUG USER

The CSO should be encouraged to invite the user to attend treatment only when the CSO feels comfortable and safe with the prospect, and has demonstrated the necessary skill to attempt it. The skill level can be determined upon observing role-play scenarios in which treatment is suggested. In some cases CSOs have limited verbal ability and are frightened at the prospect of openly discussing treatment with the loved one. However, they may embrace the idea of writing a letter or card that describes the program and invites the user to accompany them to treatment. Therapy time also should be devoted to identifying occasions when the user is apt to be more receptive to the invitation. For example, sometimes a substance user asks curiously about the CRAFT program once it becomes apparent that the CSO is in treatment. It also is common for a loved one to begin to question why a CSO's behavior has changed. These tend to be ideal times for the CSO to broach the topic of attending treatment. In the course of doing role-plays in which treatment is suggested, several should be rehearsed in which the user flatly refuses therapy. Since this is a natural part of the process, the CSO will need to learn to accept it as such, instead of as a personal failure.

RAPID INTAKE PROCEDURES

It is critical to lay the groundwork for a rapid intake of the substance user once the decision to enter treatment is made. The chances of treatment beginning at all will drop markedly if an ambivalent user is placed on a waiting list. Once the individual enters treatment, a behaviorally oriented program is recommended, since the philosophy and techniques will complement the CRAFT work that has already been done. The Community Reinforcement Approach (Azrin *et al.*, 1982; Hunt & Azrin, 1973; Meyers & Smith, 1995), which served as the foundation for the development of CRAFT, is one reasonable option.

Getting the loved one to enter treatment is really only the start, so the therapist will need to discuss the importance of the CSO staying active in the user's therapy. The structure of therapy may change, however, because some of the sessions may deal with the CSO and the substance user as a couple. The therapist should also prepare the CSO for the possibility that the user will enter treatment, only to drop out prematurely. Again the CSO should be reminded that CRAFT is an ongoing process. When a user leaves treatment early, it is just one step in the program, and more work needs to be done to encourage the individual to return.

CONCLUSION

Research over the years repeatedly has demonstrated the considerable difficulty in engaging and retaining in treatment an individual with substance abuse problems (Baekeland & Lundwall, 1975; Ellis, McCan, Price, & Sewell, 1992; Stark & Campbell, 1988). There is a growing body of evidence that concerned significant others can provide considerable leverage in convincing problem substance users to enter treatment. The support of the CSO also has been shown to aid in treatment retention and to increase the likelihood of treatment success. CRAFT was developed for training CSOs of alcohol- or drug-abusing loved ones to use behavioral techniques to decrease substance use and increase sober behavior. Preliminary analyses from a clinical trial of CRAFT suggest that this program is substantially more effective in engaging unmotivated problem drinkers in treatment than are the two approaches most commonly used for this purpose in the United States. Preliminary findings from another clinical trial suggest that the use of CRAFT techniques is highly effective for engaging resistant drug-abusing individuals as well. The data indicate that the CRAFT program merits additional scientific and clinical attention.

REFERENCES

Al-Anon Family Groups. (1965). *Al-Anon faces alcoholism*. New York: Author.
Atkinson, R. M., Tolson, R. L., & Turner, J. A. (1993). Factors affecting outpatient treatment compliance of older male problem drinkers. *Journal of Studies on Alcohol, 54*, 102–106.

Azrin, N. H. (1976). Improvements in the community reinforcement approach to alcoholism. *Behaviour Research and Therapy, 14,* 339–348.

Azrin, N. H., Sisson, R. W., Meyers, R. J., & Godley, M. D. (1982). Alcoholism treatment by disulfiram and community reinforcement therapy. *Journal of Behavior Therapy and Experimental Psychiatry, 3,* 105–112.

Baekeland, F., & Lundwall, L. (1975). Dropping out of treatment: A critical review. *Psychological Bulletin, 82,* 738–783.

Brennan, P. L., Moos, R. H., & Kelly, K. M. (1994). Spouses of late-life problem drinkers: Functioning, coping responses, and family contexts. *Journal of Family Psychology, 8,* 447–457.

Brown, T. G., Kokin, M., Seraganian, P., & Shields, N. (1995). The role of spouses of substance abusers in treatment: Gender differences. *Journal of Psychoactive Drugs, 27,* 223–229.

Carolyn W. (1984). *Detaching with love.* Minnesota: Hazelden.

Coleman, D., & Straus, M. (1983). Alcohol abuse and family violence. In E. Gottheil, K. Druley, T. Skoloda, & H. Waxman (Eds.), *Alcohol, drug abuse and aggression* (pp. 104–124). Springfield, IL: Thomas.

Collins, R. L., Leonard, K. E., & Searles, J. S. (1990). *Alcohol and the family: Research and clinical perspectives.* New York: Guilford.

Cunningham, J. A., Sobell, L. C., Sobell, M. B., & Kapur, G. (1995). Resolution from alcohol treatment problems with and without treatment: Reasons for change. *Journal of Substance Abuse, 7,* 365–372.

Dittrich, J. E., & Trapold, M. A. (1984). A treatment program for the wives of alcoholics: An evaluation. *Bulletin of the Society of Psychologists in Addictive Behaviours, 3,* 91–102.

Edwards, M. E., & Steinglass, P. (1995). Family therapy treatment outcomes for alcoholism. The effectiveness of marital and family therapy [Special issue]. *Journal of Marital and Family Therapy, 21,* 475–509.

Ellis, B. H., McCan, I., Price, G., & Sewell, C. M. (1992). The New Mexico treatment outcome study: Evaluating the utility of existing information systems. *Journal of Health Care for the Poor and Underserved, 3,* 138–150.

Galanter, M. (1993). Network therapy for substance abuse: A clinical trial. Psychotherapy for the addictions [Special issue]. *Psychotherapy, 30,* 251–258.

Gondolf, E. W., & Foster, R. A. (1991). Wife assault among VA alcohol rehabilitation patients. *Hospital and Community Psychiatry, 42,* 74–79.

Hingson, R., Mangione, T., Meyers, A., & Scotch, N. (1982). Seeking help for drinking problems: A study in the Boston metropolitan area. *Journal of Studies on Alcohol, 43,* 271–288.

Humphreys, K., Moos, R. H., & Finney, J. W. (1996). Life domains, Alcoholics Anonymous, and the role of incumbency in the 3-year course of problem drinking. *Journal of Nervous and Mental Disease, 184,* 475–481.

Hunt G. M., & Azrin, N. H. (1973). A community-reinforcement approach to alcoholism. *Behaviour Research and Therapy, 11,* 91–104.

Johnson, V. E. (1986). *Intervention: How to help those who don't want help.* Minneapolis, MN: Johnson Institute.

Leonard, K. E., & Jacob, T. (1988). Alcohol, alcoholism, and family violence. In V. B. Van Hasselt, R. L. Morrison, A. S. Bellack, & M. Hersen (Eds.), *Handbook of family violence* (pp. 383–406). New York: Plenum.

Liddle, H. A., & Dakof, G. A. (1995). Efficacy of family therapy for drug abuse: Promising but not definitive. The effectiveness of marital and family therapy [Special issue]. *Journal of Marital and Family Therapy, 21,* 511–543.

Liepman, M. R., Nirenberg, T. D., & Begin, A. M. (1989). Evaluation of a program designed to help family and significant others to motivate resistant alcoholics into recovery. *American Journal of Drug and Alcohol Abuse, 15,* 209–221.

Loneck, B., Garrett, J. A., & Banks, S. M. (1996). A comparison of the Johnson intervention with four other methods of referral to outpatient treatment. *American Journal of Drug and Alcohol Abuse, 22,* 233–246.

Meyers, R. J., & Smith, J. E. (1995). *Clinical guide to alcohol treatment: The Community Reinforcement Approach.* New York: Guilford.

Meyers, R. J., & Smith, J. E. (1997). Getting off the fence: Procedures to engage treatment-resistant drinkers. *Journal of Substance Abuse Treatment.*

Meyers, R. J., Dominguez, T. P., & Smith, J. E. (1996). Community reinforcement training with concerned others. In V. B. Van Hasselt & M. Hersen (Eds.), *Sourcebook of psychological treatment manuals for adult disorders* (pp. 257–294). New York: Plenum.

Miller, W. R., & Page, A. C. (1991). Warm turkey: Other routes to abstinence. *Journal of Substance Abuse Treatment, 8*, 227–232.

Miller, W. R., & Rollnick, S. (1991). *Motivational interviewing: Preparing people to change addictive behavior.* New York: Guilford.

Orford, J., & Harwin, J. (1982). *Alcohol and the family.* London: Croom Helm.

Paolino, T. J., & McCrady, B. S. (1977). *The alcoholic marriage: Alternative perspectives.* New York: Grune & Stratton.

Project MATCH Research Group. (1997). Matching alcoholism treatments to client heterogeneity: Project MATCH posttreatment drinking outcomes. *Journal of Studies on Alcohol, 58*, 7–29.

Room, R. (1987, August). *The U.S. general population's experience with responses to alcohol problems.* Paper presented at the Alcohol Epidemiology Section of the International Congress on Alcohol and Addictions, Aix-en-Provence, France.

Sisson, R. W., & Azrin, N. H. (1986). Family-member involvement to initiate and promote treatment of problem drinkers. *Journal of Behavior Therapy and Experimental Psychiatry, 17*, 15–21.

Smith, J. E., & Meyers, R. J. (1995). The community reinforcement approach. In R. Hester & W. Miller (Eds.), *Handbook of alcoholism treatment approaches: Effective alternatives* (2nd ed., pp. 251–266). New York: Pergamon.

Stark, M. J., & Campbell, B. K. (1988). Personality, drug use, and early attrition from substance abuse treatment. *American Journal of Drug and Alcohol Abuse, 14*, 475–487.

Stith, S. M., Crossman, R. K., & Bischof, G. P. (1991). Alcoholism and marital violence: A comparative study of men in alcohol treatment programs and battered treatment programs. *Alcoholism Treatment Quarterly, 8*, 3–20.

Straus, M. A. (1979). Measuring intrafamily conflict and violence: The Conflict Tactics (CT) Scales. *Journal of Marriage and the Family, 41*, 75–88.

Thomas, E. J., & Santa, C. A. (1982). Unilateral family therapy for alcohol abuse: A working conception. *American Journal of Family Therapy, 10*, 49–58.

Thomas, E. J., Santa, C., Bronson, D., & Oyserman, D. (1987). Unilateral family therapy with the spouses of alcoholics. *Journal of Social Service Research, 10*, 145–162.

Thomas, E. J., Yoshioka, M. R., Ager, R. D., & Adams, K. B. (1993). *Experimental outcomes of spouse intervention to reach the uncooperative alcohol abuser: Preliminary report.* Manuscript submitted for publication.

Thomas, E. J., Yoshioka, M. R., & Ager, R. D. (1994). Spouse Enabling Inventory. In J. Fischer & K. Corcoran (Eds.), *Measures for clinical practice: A source book: Vol. 1. Couples, families and children* (2nd ed., pp. 177–178). New York: Free Press.

Velleman, R., Bennett, G., Miller, T., Orford, J., Rigby, K., & Tod, A. (1993). The families of problem drug users: A study of 50 close relatives. *Addiction, 88*, 1281–1289.

12

Finding the Right Approach

MARGARET E. MATTSON

INTRODUCTION

While it is known that many individuals suffering from addictive disorders bene-fit from treatment, no single approach has been shown to be superior for all those needing care. It has been suggested that triaging, or matching, clients to treatments based on their particular needs and characteristics might significantly improve outcome. The potential of the "matching hypothesis" has been of particular inter-est in the treatment of alcohol use disorders, prompting researchers and clinicians to search for assignment rules to individualize treatment selection. The consider-able literature on patient–treatment matching in alcohol disorders treatment pro-vides a useful example to illustrate the rationale and status of the matching hypothesis and is the focus of this chapter.

A problem that clinicians involved with treating those afflicted with alcohol use disorders confront daily is how to choose from among a variety of treatment options for patients who typically present with a wide range of complex personal characteristics, histories, and clinical features. How does one find the right ap-proach when faced with a problem for which there is no "magic bullet" or "one size fits all" prescriptive approach? Recent findings on matching patients with al-cohol use disorders to treatments in light of the results from Project MATCH (a large clinical trial whose first results were published in 1997) and other recent re-search literature are reviewed. The objective is to provide clinicians with a re-search basis for decision making regarding patient–treatment matching. A brief history of how the present keen interest in treatment matching of patients with al-cohol use disorders evolved is discussed first. Second, a summary of the main findings of Project MATCH is reviewed; third, highlights of recent reports in the

MARGARET E. MATTSON • Treatment Research Branch, National Institute on Alcohol Abuse and Alcoholism, Bethesda, Maryland 20892.

Treating Addictive Behaviors, 2nd ed., edited by Miller and Heather. Plenum Press, New York, 1998.

matching literature; and last, a synthesis of messages for clinicians derived from the current research base.

HISTORICAL PERSPECTIVE ON MATCHING

THE FOUNDATIONS

The idea of matching is not new; it was first proposed in the alcohol treatment area in the 1940s (Bowman & Jellinek, 1941) and is common to other fields such as psychiatry, medicine, and education. As thinking concerning the treatment of alcoholism evolved, matching came to be regarded as the missing ingredient in the treatment selection process (Finney & Moos, 1986; Glaser, 1980; Skinner, 1981). The premise was that its addition could enhance outcomes above and beyond what could be accomplished by simply choosing generally effective treatments and paying attention to generic curative elements such as support, rapport, and communication from the therapist. This notion was fostered by more than a dozen studies published in the 1970s and early 1980s suggesting that a variety of patient features—demographic, drinking relating factors, intrapersonal characteristics, and interpersonal factors—appeared to "match" with particular treatments. This literature is summarized in several reviews (Lindstrom, 1992; Mattson & Allen, 1991; Mattson et al., 1994; Miller, 1989).

Despite some methodological shortcomings of the early database, the concept excited the field and held promise not only for improving patient outcomes but also for making more effective use of scarce resources as reimbursement polices and other economic forces invaded the field of addictions treatment. During the 1980s and early 1990s, methodologic advances occurred in addictions clinical research and a host of more sophisticated matching studies were reported, further strengthening the hope for matching as a clinical tool (Mattson et al., 1994). An important force was two major reports from the Institute of Medicine calling for definitive and systematic research on this pressing question. (Institute of Medicine, 1989, 1990).

PROJECT MATCH ENTERS THE ARENA

In 1989, the National Institute of Alcohol Abuse launched a multisite clinical trial, Project MATCH, with the expectation that it would be the largest, most statistically powerful, and most methodologically rigorous psychotherapy trial ever undertaken. The objective was to subject the matching hypothesis to its most stringent evaluation to date. Project MATCH based its research questions on the previous foundation of published studies and the latest knowledge of treatments believed to be generally effective and suitable for delivery both in a multisite clinical trial and in actual clinical practice.

The details of the rationale and design of Project MATCH have been published (Donovan & Mattson, 1994; Project MATCH Research Group, 1993). Briefly, the study tested promising patient–treatment combinations involving 21 patient characteristics and three treatments: Twelve Step Facilitation (TSF), Motivational Enhancement Therapy (MET), and Cognitive Behavioral Therapy (CBT). The treatments were described in three published therapists' manuals and their delivery was carefully specified and supervised (Kadden *et al.,* 1992; Miller, Zweben, DiClemente, & Rychtarik, 1992; Nowinski, Baker, & Carroll, 1992). Drinking outcomes and other indicators of function were assessed every 3 months for 1 year after the conclusion of the 3-month treatment period. A subset (outpatients only) were recontacted 39 months after treatment. The two primary drinking outcome measures were percent days abstinent and drinks per drinking day. A total of 1,726 patients were treated in two settings referred to as the "outpatient" and "aftercare" situations, with the latter group entering Project MATCH after the completion of a more intensive residential or day treatment.

RESULTS FROM PROJECT MATCH

MATCHING RESULTS

The initial results of Project MATCH (Longabaugh for the Project MATCH Research Group, 1997; Project MATCH Research Group, 1997a; Project MATCH Research Group, 1997b; Project MATCH Research Group, in press) were quite surprising to many and challenged the role of patient–treatment matching in the treatment of alcoholism. Contrary to the expectations raised from the supporting literature base, large and uniform effects for matches with single patient characteristics did not emerge. Many hypothesized matches were not supported and those found were, for the most part, of rather modest magnitude and often varied over time, between arms of the trial, and for the two primary outcome measures.

Of the 21 patient variables studied, the four with matching effects deemed more plausible were those involving, in the outpatient arm, *psychiatric severity, client anger, social network support for drinking,* and, in the aftercare arm, *alcohol dependence.* Other patient variables (e.g., motivational readiness to change, meaning seeking, self-efficacy, antisocial personality disorder, and social support) showed indications of matching either within treatment or during the posttreatment period but were less straightforward in interpretation because of their variability over time or the fact that some of the interactions were opposite to the direction predicted; these variables are not discussed here.

Patients in the outpatient arm with low *psychiatric severity* treated with TSF had more abstinent days as compared to those treated with CBT, a differential as high as 10% for several months during the follow-up period. The largest difference occurred 6 months after the end of treatment, when clients without concomitant psychopathology had 87% days abstinent in TSF versus 73% in CBT (Project MATCH Research Group, 1997a).

MET was postulated to be more effective for clients with higher *anger* scores presumably because of its nonconfrontive nature. MET clients in the outpatient study who were high in anger were abstinent more often than clients receiving the other treatments (a differential of 9%; i.e., 85% vs. 76%) and drank less intensely when they did drink. Low-anger clients fared better in CBT and in TSF as compared to MET. The effect persisted throughout the 1 year after treatment and was also present at the 39-month follow-up. This finding was the most consistent matching result across time. (Longabaugh for the Project MATCH Group, 1997; Project MATCH Research Group, 1997b; Project MATCH Research Group, in press).

As predicted, clients with a *social network supportive of drinking* did better in TSF than in MET. This difference was not apparent in the first year after treatment, emerging among the outpatients at 3 years. TSF patients reported abstinence on 83% of days versus 66% for the MET patients. This difference of 17 percentage points was the largest size effect observed in Project MATCH. The effects appear due to a steady decline among clients with high drinking support in the MET group after the end of treatment, whereas those in the TSF group maintained their gains. An influential factor may be differences in levels of AA attendance, with attendance levels higher in the TSF group than in the MET group. (Longabaugh for the Project MATCH Research Group, 1997; Project MATCH Research Group, 1997b).

It had been hypothesized that clients high in *alcohol dependence* would do better in TSF while those lower in that trait would benefit more from CBT. Since TSF is a treatment that puts greater emphasis on total abstinence, it was postulated to be more effective with highly dependent clients than either CBT (which taught skills to deal with "slips") or MET (which focused on clients' own decision making to motivate them to become abstinent). Aftercare clients low in alcohol dependence had better outcomes when treated with CBT than TSF (i.e., abstinence on 96% of posttreatment days vs. 89%). However, at higher levels of dependence, the better treatment choice was TSF (i.e., 94% vs. 84% days abstinent). The effect was consistent for the posttreatment period of 15 months. (Longabaugh for Project MATCH Research Group, 1997; Project MATCH Research Group, 1997b).

In summary, the results of the testing a priori matching hypotheses showed several matches of modest to moderate magnitude, often with variability over time, outcome measures, and arm of the study. These results suggest that matching clients on several of the attributes tested in Project MATCH to one of the three treatments appears to enhance outcomes to a degree, with the most robust of the confirmed effects constituting a moderate difference of 17 percentage points in abstinent days. Viewpoints differ on how clinically important these single characteristic effects are, although, overall, the findings do not suggest that major changes in triaging procedures are warranted.

Main Effects

Apart from these matching effects, Project MATCH also sheds light on the important question of how clients fare after treatment, both overall and for the three treatments individually. Patients in all three treatment conditions demonstrated major improvements in drinking, as well as other areas of functioning such as depression, use of illicit drugs, and liver enzyme status. Overall, MATCH clients were abstaining over 85% of the days throughout the year following treatment and alcohol consumption decreased fivefold. Even those not successful in maintaining abstinence who continued to drink experienced a substantial reduction in alcohol consumption. In general, effects for the three treatments were similar, with the exception that 10% more of the outpatients receiving TSF attained complete abstinence over the 1-year follow-up period compared with the other two treatments. Also, more aftercare patients were able to sustain complete abstinence throughout the year after treatment than the outpatients, despite the fact that the aftercare patients entered the study with more alcohol dependence symptoms.

OTHER RECENT MATCHING STUDIES

Although no other studies the size of Project MATCH have been mounted, articles dealing with matching and ways to tailor treatment selection continue to appear in the literature. A few potentially fruitful areas have been identified, although larger-scale replication is clearly necessary before any clinical implications can be drawn. Recent studies involving matching to AA, pharmacologic agents, alcoholic typology, and level of care are briefly summarized in the following sections.

ALCOHOLICS ANONYMOUS

It has been observed that although a large number of AA attenders drop out of the program within one year, those who remain tend to do very well (McCrady & Delaney, 1995). Several reports, reviewed by Galaif and Sussman (1995), indicate that only about 5% to 13% of treated alcoholics maintain an "enduring" relationship with AA. According to the 1990 AA membership survey, 65% of those responding reported sobriety for at least 1 year (Alcoholics Anonymous, 1990). Thus, it may be that AA affiliation and success involves a process of self-selection, or self-matching.

A question currently being researched is "Who joins AA and what factors predict success?" (Tonigan & Hiller-Sturmhofel, 1994). Some progress has been made in identifying affiliators of AA which may provide clues to more effective matching of clients to self-help programs. For example, a metanalysis led Emrick, Tonigan, Montgomery, and Little (1993) to conclude that the characteristics associated with joining AA were history of using external supports to stop drinking, loss of control over drinking, more heavy drinking, and obsessive-compulsive involvement with drinking.

Galaif and Sussman (1995) conclude that AA is unlikely to appeal to those uncomfortable disclosing in group situations and with the religious tone of AA, those who desire controlled drinking as a goal, and the dually diagnosed in need of psychologically based treatment. Greater AA involvement modestly predicted improvements in drinking outcome (Emrick *et al.*, 1993), although this may be more true of males than females (Tonigan & Hiller-Sturmhofel, 1994). It has been emphasized that study of affiliator characteristics should be approached carefully because AA cannot be seen as a single entity despite its many unifying principles, due to the great heterogeneity in philosophy and membership composition across AA groups. (Tonigan, Ashcroft, & Miller, 1995).

Glaser (1995) simplifies current advice to clinicians in two principles: (1) Because we do not know what constitutes a mismatch, no one should be required to attend AA, and (2) because we do not know what constitutes a match, everyone should be encouraged to try AA. Galaif and Sussman (1995) hypothesize that those desiring immediate support, affiliation with others, a structured program of recovery emphasizing spirituality, and abstinence as the goal may be good candidates for

AA. Variation in the last two of these areas may point to referral to secular organizations for sobriety as reasonable alternatives.

DRUGS AS ADJUNCTIVE AGENTS AND POTENTIAL MATCHING TARGETS

A variety of studies, reviewed by Kranzler, Mason, Pettinati, and Anton (in press), Kranzler, McLellan, and Bohn (1995), Litten and Allen (1991, 1992), and Litten, Allen, and Fertig (1996) support the role of pharmacologic agents as aids in treatment of alcoholism. Recent interest has focused on naltrexone (O'Malley, 1995a; Volpicelli, Volpicelli, & O'Brien, 1995). Data from studies of the efficacy of naltrexone as an adjunct in the treatment of alcohol use disorders were subjected to subsequent post hoc analyses (Jaffe et al., 1996; O'Malley, 1995b). These results opened the issue of matching subgroups of patients to drug and psychosocial combinations and posed the question, Do patients with certain baseline characteristics react more favorably to the combinations than those without these characteristics? One analysis (Jaffe et al., 1996) found that placebo treated subjects with high craving scores or low cognitive abilities had poorer outcomes than subjects low in craving or high in cognitive abilities. In contrast, both groups of subjects had similar improved response when treated with naltrexone. If these results can be replicated, naltrexone may prove especially useful as an adjunct in patients with significant alcohol craving and poor learning ability. Other potential interactions between patient characteristics and pharmacologic agents await further research in this area.

MATCHING USING CLIENT PROFILES VERSUS SINGLE CHARACTERISTICS

Most work on matching has involved single patient characteristics which interact with a particular treatment to produce differential effects. Work by Litt, Babor, DelBoca, Kadden, and Cooney (1992) suggested that there might be "type" matches involving combinations of characteristics: that is, Type A alcoholics had better outcomes with an interactional form of therapy and Type B, with coping skills. However, when Project MATCH extended this test, no evidence for matching was found. Post hoc testing involving patient profiles or combinations of characteristics is planned for the Project MATCH data set. Until further data emerge, there is little guidance for the clinician on this topic, although interest in matching clients based on their overall profile of needs for ancillary services is emerging. (See Chapter 13, this volume.)

MATCHING TO LEVEL OF CARE VERSUS A SINGLE MODALITY

It has been suggested that matching to level of care may be beneficial, involving use of placement criteria, or algorithms, to match patients to a particular level of care. This is similar to the notion of stepped care, a common approach in biomedical practice, for example, in the treatment of hypertension. In this approach if the initial level of care is insufficient, the intensity of care is increased or alternative care or services offered (Sobell & Sobell, 1995). Sobell and Sobell point out the applicability of this method to the substance abuse field in that it reserves the more intensive (and hence more costly) services for the more difficult cases.

Levels of care have been defined as "those settings that offer discrete treatment intensities, structure, and restrictiveness" (Gastfriend & McLellan, in press). The matching question is, "Which patients experience the best outcomes from different levels of care?" Gastfriend and McLellan trace the historical evolution of a body of such prescriptive guidelines, driven to a large extent during the 1980s by cost pressures and managed care (Gastfriend & McLellan, 1997; Sobell & Sobell, 1995). Two examples of such algorithms for matching to levels of care are the Cleveland Criteria (developed by Hoffman, Halikas, & Mee-Lee, 1987) and the American Society of Addiction Medicine Criteria (Hoffman, Halikas, Mee-Lee, & Weedman, 1991). The appeal of such criteria is intuitive and the implications for potential cost savings obvious. However, solid experimental validation of the effectiveness of the assignment criteria is lacking, despite a growing incorporation into practice settings (Gastfriend & McLellan, 1997). Adequate testing of such matching criteria would require large and heterogeneous populations, an effort not underway systematically, although smaller-scale studies have been attempted. For example, McKay, McLellan, and Alterman (1992) in a retrospective study contrasted alcohol- and cocaine-abusing patients in a V.A. hospital who received an intensive outpatient program with patients who were properly matched to intensive outpatient according to the Cleveland Criteria. There was little difference in retention and outcome between those matched versus those mismatched.

CLINICAL MESSAGES: TO MATCH OR NOT TO MATCH?

Taking into account the body of matching literature, including the results of Project MATCH, which attempted to replicate virtually every matching effect reported in the literature, what suggestions may be given to the clinician?

Matching does not appear to be vital to effective treatment. Developing a priori algorithms for assigning patients to different treatments seems thus far not to dramatically increase the overall efficacy of treatment. Rather than being a compelling requirement for effective treatment as previously thought, matching is an additional consideration the clinician should weigh in the treatment selection process.

This suggests, on the one hand, that if a provider has limited resources and training and can offer only one well-proven approach, there is no reason to feel apologetic. But by the same token, there is no justification to insist that the same approach be required for all clients. The view of AA that it is "not for everyone" is applicable to treatment philosophy generally. Extending the thoughts of Glaser (1995), we might take the view that since we do not know what constitutes a match, we should not be compelled to take a particular approach, and, likewise, because we do not know what constitutes a mismatch, we should be encouraged to explore the range of treatment options currently available.

Furthermore, the clinician should be prepared to assist the client, as needed, in a process of informed decision making to evaluate the range of options the field has to offer. The clinician and client need to know about the overall efficacy of approaches available within the system or community through which the client seeks care (see Chapter 15, this volume). In Project MATCH, for example, the three treatments achieved comparable long- and short-term outcomes, which suggests that if any of the three treatments is given with skill as conducted in Project MATCH, the treatment would yield similar improvement in drinking. In addition, matching effects found in Project MATCH, although not strongly prescriptive, are reasonable considerations in evaluating the appropriateness of a therapy. Clinicians should evaluate each case individually and consider the "matched" treatment if it is available. For example, TSF may be considered for outpatient clients without concomitant psychopathology, or who have a social support network that supports their continued drinking, and for those aftercare clients who have more severe alcohol dependency, Likewise, for those outpatients high in anger, MET may be considered, or CBT for those lower in dependency. Although there is less supportive data, other findings from Project MATCH may be helpful starting points.

Finally, the practitioner should project a positive and supportive attitude to the patient embarking on therapy by (1) commending the decision to enter treatment, (2) stressing the likely beneficial effects, and (3) conveying the notion that although a particular treatment may work for many people, if it is not effective in a particular case, there are other possibilities to pursue. Encouragement can be along the lines of "We don't know whether this approach will be the best one for you. But if you give it a good try and find it's not working for you, don't be discouraged or blame yourself. There are other approaches we can try until we find what works for you." Further, the clinician need not "steer the ship alone" and feel compelled to decide for the patient, nor adopt the parental model of "I know what is best for you." An informal partnership approach may be more productive.

Finding the right approach is a *process* and, often, a *partnership,* in which persistence, support, and sound knowledge all play a role in finding the approach that works best for each client. We offer clients the best chance of recovery, perhaps, by providing then with a range of viable options and helping them to make informed, self-directed choices. Helping clients to find the right approach for them is one of the best services we can provide.

Acknowledgments

The author appreciates the helpful guidance of Dr. William Miller, the reviews and comments of Dr. Richard Longabaugh and Dr. Richard Fuller, and thanks Ms. Veronica Wilson for her fine manuscript preparation assistance.

REFERENCES

Alcoholics Anonymous. (1990). *Alcoholics Anonymous 1989 membership survey.* New York: Alcoholics Anonymous World Services.

Bowman, K. M., & Jellinek, E. M. (1941). Alcohol addiction and its treatment. *Quarterly Journal of Studies on Alcohol, 2,* 98–176.

Donovan, D. M., & Mattson, M. E. (Eds.). (1994). Alcoholism treatment matching research: Methodological and clinical approaches. *Journal of Studies on Alcohol* (Suppl. No. 12), 171.

Emrick, C. D., Tonigan, J. S., Montgomery, H., & Little, L. (1993). Alcoholics Anonymous: What is currently known? In B. S. McCrady & W. R. Miller (Eds.), *Research on Alcoholics Anonymous: Opportunities and alternatives* (pp. 41–76). New Brunswick, NJ: Rutgers Center of Alcohol Studies.

Finney, J., & Moos, R. (1986). Matching patients with treatments: Conceptual and methodological issues. *Journal of Studies on Alcohol, 47,* 122–134.

Galaif, E. R., & Sussman, S. (1995). For whom does Alcoholics Anonymous work? *International Journal of the Addictions, 30*(2), 161–184.

Gastfriend, D. R., & McLellan, A. T. (1997). Treatment matching: Theoretical basis and practical implications. *Medical Clinics of North America, 81*(4), 946–966.

Glaser, F. G. (1980). Anybody got a match? Treatment research and the matching hypothesis. In G. Edwards & M. Grants (Eds.), *Alcoholism treatment in transition* (pp. 178–196). Baltimore: University Park Press.

Glaser, F. G. (1995). Matchless? Alcoholics Anonymous and the matching hypothesis. In B. S. McCrady & W. R. Miller (Eds.), *Research on Alcoholics Anonymous: Opportunities and alternatives* (pp. 379–395). New Brunswick, NJ: Alcohol Research Documentation, Inc., Rutgers Center of Alcohol Studies.

Hoffman, N., Halikas, J., & Mee-Lee, D. (1987). *The Cleveland Admission, Discharge and Transfer Criteria: Model for chemical dependency treatment programs.* Cleveland, OH: Northern Ohio Chemical Dependency Treatment Consortium.

Hoffman, N., Halikas, J., Mee-Lee, D., & Weedman, R. (1991). *ASAM—Patient placement criteria for the treatment of psychoactive substance use disorders* (1st ed.). Washington, DC: American Society of Addiction Medicine.

Institute of Medicine. (1989). *Prevention and treatment of alcohol problems: Research opportunities.* Report of a study by a Committee of the Institute of Medicine, Division of Mental Health and Behavioral Medicine. Washington, DC: National Academy Press.

Institute of Medicine. (1990). *Broadening the base of treatment for alcohol problems.* Washington, DC: National Academy Press.

Jaffe, A. J., Rounsaville, B., Chang, G., Schottenfeld, R. S., Meyer, R. E., & O'Malley, S. S. (1996). Naltrexone, relapse prevention, and supportive therapy with alcoholics: An analysis of patient treatment matching. *Journal of Consulting and Clinical Psychology, 64*(5), 1044–1053.

Kadden, R. P., Carrol, K., Donovan, D., Cooney, N., Monti, P., Abrams, D., Litt, M., & Hester, R. (1992). Cognitive-behavioral coping skills therapy manual: A clinical research guide for therapists treating individuals with alcohol abuse and dependence. Washington, DC: Project MATCH Monograph Series, Vol. 3, DHHS Pub. No. (ADM) 92-1895.

Kranzler, H. R., McLellan, A. T., & Bohn, M. J. (1995). Pharmacotherapies for alcoholism: Theoretical and methodological perspectives. In H. R. Kranzler (Ed.), *Pharmacology of alcohol abuse: Handbook of experimental pharmacology* (Vol. 114, pp. 513–537). New York: Springer-Verlag.

Kranzler, H. R., Mason, B. J., Pettinati, H. M., & Anton, R. F. (1997). Methodological issues in pharmacotherapy trials with alcoholics. In M. Hertman & D. Feltner (Eds.), *Clinical trials of CNS drugs* (pp. 213–245). New York: New York University Press.

Lindstrom, L. (1992). *Managing alcoholism: Matching clients to treatment.* New York: Oxford University Press.

Litt, M. D., Babor, T. F., DelBoca, F. K., Kadden, R. M., & Cooney, N. L. (1992). Types of alcoholics: II. Application of an empirically derived typology to treatment matching. *Archives of General Psychiatry, 49*, 609–614.

Litten, R. Z., & Allen, J. P. (1991). Pharmacotherapies for alcoholism: Promising agents and clinical issues. *Alcoholism: Clinical and experimental research, 15*(4), 620–633.

Litten, R. Z., & Allen, J. P. (1992). Research advances in pharmacotherapy for alcoholism. In R. R. Watson (Ed.), *Alcohol abuse treatment* (pp. 65–86). Totowa, NJ: Humana.

Litten, R. Z., Allen, J., & Fertig, J. (1996). Pharmacotherapies for alcohol problems: A review of research with focus on developments since 1991. *Alcoholism: Clinical and Experimental Research 20*(5), 859–876.

Longabaugh, R., for the Project MATCH Research Group. (1997, June). Secondary hypotheses: Results from Project MATCH. Paper presented at the annual meeting of the Research Society for Alcoholism, San Francisco.

Mattson, M. E., & Allen, J. P. (1991). Research on matching alcoholic patients to treatments: Findings, issues, and implications. *Journal of Addictive Diseases, 11*(2), 33.

Mattson, M. E., Allen, J. P., Longabaugh, R., Nickless, C. J., Connors, G. J., & Kadden, R. M. (1994). A chronological review of empirical studies matching alcoholic clients to treatment. *Journal of Studies on Alcohol, 12*, 16–29.

McCrady, B. S., & Delaney, S. I. (1995). Self-help groups. In R. K. Hester & W. R. Miller (Eds.), *Handbook of alcoholism treatment approaches: Effective alternatives* (pp. 160–175). Needham Heights, MA: Allyn & Bacon.

McKay, J. R., McLellan, A. T., & Alterman, A. I. (1992). An evaluation of the Cleveland criteria for inpatient treatment of substance abuse. *American Journal of Psychiatry, 149*(9), 1212–1218.

Miller, W. R. (1989). Matching individuals with interventions. In R. K. Hester & W. R. Miller (Eds.), *Handbook of alcoholism treatment approaches* (pp. 261–271). New York: Pergamon.

Miller, W. R., & Hester, R. K. (1986). Matching problem drinkers with optimal treamtments. In W. R. Miller & N. Hester (Eds.), *Treating addictive behaviors: Processes of change* (pp. 175–203). New York: Pergamon.

Miller, W. R., Zweben, A., DiClemente, C., & Rychtarik, R. (1992). *Motivational Enhancement Therapy manual: A clinical research guide for therapists treating individuals with alcohol abuse and dependence.* Washington, DC: Project MATCH Monograph Series, Vol. 2, DHHS Pub. No. (ADM) 92-1894.

Nowinski, J., Baker, S., & Carroll, K. (1992). *Twelve Step Facilitation Therapy manual: A clinical research guide for therapists treating individuals with alcohol abuse and dependence.* Washington, DC: Project MATCH Monograph Series, Vol. 1, DHHS Pub. No (ADM) 92–1893.

O'Malley, S. S. (1995a). Integration of opioid antagonists and psychosocial therapy in the treatment of narcotic and alcohol dependence. *Journal of Clinical Psychiatry, 56*(7), 30–38.

O'Malley, S. S. (1995b). Strategies to maximize the efficacy of naltrexone for alcohol dependence. In L. S. Onken, J. D. Blaine, & J. J. Boren (Eds.), *Integrating behavioral therapies with medications in the treatment of drug dependence* (NIDA Research Monograph 150, pp. 53–64). Rockville, MD: National Institute on Drug Abuse.

Project MATCH Research Group. (1993). Project MATCH: Rationale and methods for a multisite clinical trial matching patients to alcoholism treatment. *Alcohol: Clinical and Experimental Research 17*(6), 1130–1145.

Project MATCH Research Group. (1997). Matching Alcoholism Treatments to Client Heterogenity: Project MATCH posttreatment drinking outcomes. *Journal of Studies on Alcohol, 58*(1), 7–29.

Project MATCH Research Group. (1997a). Project MATCH secondary a priori hypotheses. *Addiction, 92*(12), 1671–1698.

Project MATCH Research Group. Matching Alcoholism Treatments to Client Heterogenity: Project MATCH three-year drinking outcomes (in press).

Skinner, H. A. (1981). Different strokes for different folks. In R. F. Meyer, T. F. Babor, B. C. Gleuck, J. H. Jaffe, J. E. O'Brien, & J. R. Stabenau (Eds.), *Differential treatment for alcohol abuse* (pp. 349–376). Evaluation of the alcoholic: Implications for research, theory, and treatment. (NIAAA Research Monograph No. 5, USDHHS Publ. No. [ADM] 81-1033, 1984). Washington, DC: American Psychiatric Press.

Sobell, M. B., & Sobell, L. C. (1995). Controlled drinking after twenty-five years: How important was the great debate? *Addiction, 90*(9), 1149–1153.

Tonigan, J. S., & Hiller-Sturmhofel, S. (1994). Alcoholics Anonymous: Who benefits? *Alcohol Health and Research World, 18*(4), 308–310.

Tonigan, J. S., Ashcroft, F., & Miller, W. R. (1995). AA group dynamics and 12-step activity. *Journal of Studies on Alcohol, 56*(6), 616–621.

Volpicelli, J. R., Volpicelli, L. A., & O'Brien, C. P. (1995). Medical management of alcohol dependence: Clinical use and limitations of naltrexone treatment. *Alcohol and Alcoholism, 30*(6), 789–798.

13

Deciding where to Start
Working with Polyproblem Individuals

JAMES R. MCKAY AND A. THOMAS MCLELLAN

INTRODUCTION

Some individuals who enter treatment for alcohol or drug abuse have relatively few serious problems other than those that are the direct result of excessive alcohol or drug use. An example of such a patient might be an alcoholic without significant comorbid medical or psychiatric problems who is somewhat depressed and quite embarrassed, but has family members and an employer who are committed to providing support during the recovery process. Other substance abusers may have accompanying problems, but of the sort that are likely to resolve rather easily if abstinence is achieved and maintained. For example, a physician with a prescription drug habit may have legal and marital difficulties, but there is a reasonably good chance that these problems will clear up relatively quickly if the physician is able to stop using drugs.

However, significant numbers of individuals seeking treatment for substance abuse have a host of serious problems that will not necessarily remit or moderate even if abstinence is achieved. This is particularly true for public sector patients, who may have few or no financial resources, poor employment skills, a history of legal problems, and medical or psychiatric problems that have not been adequately treated in the past (McLellan & Weisner, 1996). Even individuals with considerable financial resources may have serious medical, psychiatric, or family problems that, if left untreated, could interfere with each phase of the recovery

JAMES R. McKAY • Department of Psychiatry, University of Pennsylvania, Philadelphia, Pennsylvania 19104.   A. THOMAS McLELLAN • Department of Psychiatry, University of Pennsylvania, and Philadelphia Department of Veterans Affairs Medical Center, Philadelphia, Pennsylvania 19104.

Treating Addictive Behaviors, 2nd ed., edited by Miller and Heather. Plenum Press, New York, 1998.

process. The purpose of this chapter is to outline important issues to consider when initiating treatment with individuals with serious comorbid problems. We refer to these as "polyproblem" patients.

The approach that we advocate involves the *concurrent* treatment of these problems with the alcohol and drug focused care and striving to match particular treatment services to the specific additional problems manifested by individual patients. With this approach, professional treatment services in areas such as medical or psychiatric care are *added* to standard addictions treatment for those individuals who have comorbid problems in these areas. It should be noted that this represents an approach different from "matching" patients to treatment as attempted in Project MATCH, the recent large-scale multisite study sponsored by the National Institute on Alcohol Abuse and Alcoholism (Project MATCH Research Group, 1997). The goal in that study was to identify characteristics of patients that would predict the best response to three outpatient substance abuse interventions: motivational enhancement, cognitive-behavioral treatment, and 12-step facilitation. While these three treatments were conceptually quite different, all were focused exclusively on alcohol drinking. None of the three conditions attempted to match adjunctive, specialized services to additional problems. The Project MATCH approach therefore focused on matching client characteristics to different types of substance abuse–focused treatment, rather than to different services added to a core substance abuse treatment protocol.

In this chapter, we briefly review the sorts of comorbid problems clinicians are likely to see at the point of treatment intake. Instruments that can be used to assess problem severity in multiple areas are described. Rationales for initial clinician decisions related to the need for detoxification and the choice of initial treatment setting are presented and discussed. Research that has examined the impact of providing comprehensive treatment services or of matching additional services to particular comorbid problem areas is presented, and the strengths and limitations of this approach to treating polyproblem individuals is discussed. Finally, the issue of the point at which it is best to provide additional services is addressed, although there is a relative paucity of research findings on this topic.

TYPICAL PROBLEMS IN THE POLYPROBLEM
SUBSTANCE ABUSER

Medical, economic, psychiatric, family, and legal problems often appear in conjunction with substance abuse (McLellan & Gastfriend, 1996; McLellan *et al.*, 1994), and the majority of patients who seek help for one substance use disorder also have diagnosable problems with other substances of abuse. For example, many cocaine dependent individuals have a comorbid alcohol use disorder and heroin users may also abuse cocaine, alcohol, and benzodiazepines. Other combinations of problems have been observed in substance abusers. Substance abusers with severe employment problems have also been shown to have high rates of chronic medical and psychiatric problems and high current problem severities in these areas (McKay, McLellan, Durell, Ruetsch, & Alterman, 1998). Some, if not all, of these co-occurring difficulties can interfere with alcohol and drug rehabilitation and increase the likelihood of posttreatment relapse.

Co-occurring psychiatric and family or social problems have been particularly well studied and have been consistent predictors of poorer response to treatment and worse posttreatment outcomes (Moos, Finney, & Cronkite, 1990). However, with regard to psychiatric comorbidity, it appears to be important to distinguish between current severity level and lifetime incidence of a disorder. Whereas higher levels of current symptom severity (i.e., past 30 days) typically predict worse outcomes (Carroll, Rounsaville, & Gawin, 1991; Carroll, Power, Bryant, & Rounsaville, 1993; McLellan, Luborsky, Woody, Druley, & O'Brien, 1983), the presence of a lifetime diagnosis of major depression or anxiety disorders has actually been associated with better outcomes in several studies of cocaine abusers (Carroll et al., 1993; Carroll et al., 1994; McKay, Alterman, et al., 1997).

ASSESSMENT INSTRUMENTS

Several assessment instruments are useful for determining the number and severity of co-occurring problems in treatment-seeking substance abusers. The Addiction Severity Index (ASI) (McLellan, Luborsky, Woody, & O'Brien, 1980; McLellan et al., 1992) is probably the most widely used instrument of this type. The ASI is a 45- to 60-minute structured interview that yields information on problem severites in seven areas: alcohol, drug, medical, employment, legal, family and social, and psychiatric. Some items address symptom severity, whereas others assess level of functioning. After completing each section of the intake-baseline version of the ASI, the interviewer assigns a severity score that provides a subjective indication of whether additional treatment in that area is needed. The intake-baseline and follow-up versions of the ASI also generate composite scores for each area that assess problem severity in the preceding 30 days and can be used to monitor changes over time. The ASI has good test–retest, interrater, and internal consistency reliabilities, and each section has demonstrated evidence of concurrent and predictive validity (McLellan et al., 1980, McLellan et al., 1985). New ASI subscales that appear to have even stronger psychometric properties have also been derived in a population of methadone maintenance patients (McDermott et al., 1996).

A second multidimensional assessment instrument, the Opiate Treatment Index (OPI; Darke, Hall, Wodak, Heather, & Ward, 1992), which was developed in Australia, can be used to measure problems in areas of particular relevance to opiate addicts. This instrument measures six domains: drug use, HIV risk-taking behavior, social functioning, criminality, physical health, and psychological adjustment. The OPI was modeled to some degree after the ASI, and most sections of the instrument correlate moderately with relevant ASI scales and other sources of data such as collateral reports and urinalysis. Initial work on the psychometric properties of the OTI has indicated that the subscales of the instrument possess moderate to excellent reliability (Darke et al., 1992).

The Recovery Attitude and Treatment Evaluator (RAATE) (Mee-Lee, 1988) is another multidimensional interview-based instrument that was developed to facilitate placement in different levels of care. The RAATE assesses the following areas: degree of resistance to treatment, degree of resistance to continuing care, acuity of biomedical problems, acuity of psychiatric problems, and extent of social and family problems unsupportive to recovery. Initial studies have indicated that the subscales of both the clinical and research versions of the RAATE possess moderate to good interrater and internal consistency reliabilties and are relatively independent (Najavits *et al.*, 1997). However, no information is yet available on the predictive validity of the RAATE. Information on problems often experienced by substance abusers, which can be helpful in matching additional services to specific problems, can be obtained with the Brief Drinker Profile (Miller & Marlatt, 1987).

Several instruments designed to assess psychiatric problems can also be useful in determining which patients require specialized psychiatric services. For example, the Symptom Checklist 90 (SCL-90; DeRogatis, Lipman, & Covi, 1973) provides information on symptom severity in nine areas, including interpersonal sensitivity, depression, anxiety, hostility, paranoid ideation, and psychoticism. The Beck Depression Inventory (Beck, Ward, Mendelson, Mock, & Erbaugh, 1961) is a brief self-report questionnaire that provides somewhat more comprehensive information about depression symptoms. The California Psychological Inventory (CPI) Socialization subscale (Gough, 1987) can be useful for assessing antisocial tendencies. These questionnaires are widely used and have good psychometric properties.

It may be useful to obtain *DSM-IV* (American Psychiatric Association, 1994) Axis I diagnostic information on substance abusing patients who appear to have comorbid psychiatric problems, particularly if psychotropic medication is being considered. Several structured interviews are available that yield comprehensive information on Axis I disorders, including the Structured Clinical Interview for DSM (SCID; First, Spitzer, Gibbon, & Williams, 1996) and Diagnostic Interview Schedule (DIS; Robins, Helzer, Croughan, & Ratcliff, 1981). For most disorders, these interviews provide data on current (past 30 days) as well as lifetime occurrences. This can be useful in trying to determine whether a current psychiatric problem, such as depression, is independent of substance use. The limitations of structured diagnostic interviews are that they require a fair amount of training to administer properly, are relatively lengthy, and have diminished psychometric properties when used with substance abusing populations.

MATCHING SERVICES TO PROBLEMS

The approach to patient–treatment "matching" that has received the greatest attention from substance abuse treatment researchers involves attempting to identify the characteristics of individual patients that predict the best response to different forms of substance abuse treatment (e.g., cognitive-behavioral vs. 12-step, or inpatient vs. outpatient) (Mattson *et al.*, 1994; Project MATCH Research Group, 1997). Another approach to matching is to assess patients' problem severity at treatment admission in a range of areas and then add other adjunctive treatment services as indicated to the standard substance abuse treatment protocol (McLellan & Gastfriend, 1996; McLellan, Grissom, Zanis, & Brill, 1997). This approach has the potential to be particularly helpful for the polyproblem substance abuser, as most substance abuse–focused interventions are not intended also to address serious co-occurring problems in other areas. In this section, we review research on the impact of services designed to facilitate initial stabilization, address psychiatric and interpersonal problems, and improve outpatient treatment for more severe cocaine addiction. Several studies that have evaluated comprehensive interventions that provide services in a number of areas will also be reviewed.

One important issue that must be addressed when attempting to match services to problems is the timing of these additional interventions; in other words, the point at which they should be provided. Unfortunately, there is surprisingly little research on this issue from which conclusions can be drawn. In the absence of a strong research literature, we believe that the most defensible guideline is that comorbid problems should be addressed relatively quickly when they are likely to either lead to early treatment dropout or interfere in some other way with patients' ability to immediately benefit from substance abuse treatment. Problems that do not meet either of these conditions can safely be addressed at a later point in the treatment process.

INITIAL STABILIZATION OF THE POLYPROBLEM PATIENT

Detoxification

One of the first decisions faced by clinicians is whether detoxification is necessary and if so, whether it can be accomplished safely on an outpatient basis. Although a complete discussion of detoxification is beyond the scope of this chapter, a few remarks are in order concerning detoxification and the polyproblem patient. Generally speaking, the co-occurrence of medical and psychiatric problems raises the likelihood that a detoxification will be necessary (or at least a period of physiological stabilization), as does the use of multiple substances of abuse. This is because these problems complicate withdrawal and can increase the risk of serious problems such as seizure or cardiac distress. In the case of polysubstance abuse, it is possible that the drug of choice might not require detoxification but a secondary abused substance might. For example, a "primary" crack cocaine user may not be concerned with his alcohol use, but an assessment of recent quantity and frequency of alcohol consumption may lead to the conclusion that an alcohol detoxification is necessary. Furthermore, most co-occurring problems have the potential to interfere with an outpatient detoxification, which might mean that the relative merits of an inpatient detoxification should be considered. For example, patients with severe current psychiatric or family problems may not be able to reliably take their detoxification medications outside of an inpatient or residential facility. Therefore, although research has generally shown that outpatient detoxification can be as effective as inpatient care for many alcohol patients (Hayashida *et al.*, 1989), the outpatient setting for practical reasons may be inadequate for some polyproblem substance abusers.

Levels of Care

After it has been determined whether the polyproblem substance abuser requires detoxification, the next decisions faced by the clinician are choice of treatment setting and intensity or frequency of treatment during the first phase of rehabilitation. If a highly structured, controlled living environment appears warranted, treatment can be provided in a hospital if the patient requires close medical monitoring (i.e., inpatient care) or in a residential facility in other cases. If inpatient or residential care is not necessary, various intensities of outpatient treatment can be considered, including day hospital (5 days per week), intensive outpatient (3 days per week), and standard outpatient (1 to 2 days per week). Many research studies, including Project MATCH, have shown that substance abusers can achieve substantial reductions in alcohol or drug use with relatively low-intensity, brief outpatient treatments, such as one therapy session per week for 12 weeks or four sessions over 12 weeks (Project MATCH Research Group, 1997). However, this type of treatment may not be adequate for some polyproblem substance abusers, particularly outside the context of a research study, where patients receive additional support and monitoring through contacts with research staff.

Most reviews of the relative effectiveness of inpatient versus outpatient treatment have concluded that for the majority of alcoholics, outpatient treatment produces outcomes that are as good as those achieved with inpatient or residential care (Annis, 1986; Miller & Hester, 1986). One randomized study with cocaine abusers also reported equivalent outcomes for inpatient and intensive outpatient treatment (Alterman *et al.*, 1994). On the other hand, alcoholic patients in the aftercare condition of Project MATCH, most of whom received inpatient or residential treatment prior to outpatient treatment, had better drinking outcomes than those who received outpatient treatment alone (Project MATCH Research Group, 1997). Furthermore, a recent review that included nonrandomized studies found a modest advantage for inpatient over outpatient treatment at up to 3 months postintake (Finney, Hahn, & Moos, 1996).

Two methodological issues are important to consider when evaluating research on inpatient versus outpatient treatment and the applicability of this research to treatment placement decisions for the polyproblem patient. First, because patients with acute medical or psychiatric problems or a history of severe psychiatric problems such as schizophrenia are frequently screened out of research studies, it has been difficult to make use of research results to determine the point at which comorbid problems become serious enough to justify inpatient or residential treatment. This is an important question for future research. Second, most comparisons of inpatient and outpatient rehabilitation have looked at outcomes that are at least 3 months postdischarge. Although longer-term outcomes are certainly important, study designs that focus exclusively on distal outcomes may ignore one of the main benefits of inpatient care: the early stabilization of patients so that they may be better engaged and integrated into outpatient treatment. For example, in the general psychiatry area, inpatient care is now used primarily to stabilize patients so that they can be treated effectively on an outpatient basis. When inpatient care serves this function, the most appropriate outcome measures for determining efficacy are reduction in acute symptoms and successful engagement and retention in outpatient care—not symptom severity 3 months later.

The American Society of Addiction Medicine (ASAM) has developed placement criteria for various levels of substance abuse treatment that have at least the potential to aid clinicians in determining which polyproblem patients require inpatient care at the beginning of treatment (ASAM, 1996). Under the ASAM system, placement recommendations are determined by ratings in two medical problem areas and four psychosocial problem areas. Although the degree of detail provided by the ASAM criteria clearly exceeds that included in any other placement system, some dimensions suffer from a lack of specificity concerning how individual components should be operationalized and assessed and how recent a problem has to be to be considered "current." Furthermore, very little empirical research has been done on the actual predictive validity of the criteria. The only published outcome study to date (McKay, Cacciola, McLellan, Alterman, & Wirtz, 1997) found little evidence to support the predictive validity of the psychosocial dimensions of the criteria for placing individuals with alcohol or cocaine use disorders in inpatient or intensive outpatient treatment. Results indicated that patients who were correctly matched to treatment setting according to ASAM did not have better outcomes than those who were incorrectly placed. However, there was some evidence that polyproblem cocaine patients had marginally better short-term outcomes if they received inpatient care rather than the intensive outpatient program (IOP).

Although concern for the safety of the patient is always an issue with substance abusers, it takes on a higher priority with polyproblem individuals. Therefore, initial clinical decisions regarding need for detoxification and treatment setting and intensity assume greater importance. In the absence of compelling research findings regarding which polyproblem patients require hospital or residential care at the beginning of treatment, perhaps the best approach is to consider whether the patient is in immediate danger from self or others, or in need of medical or psychiatric care that cannot reasonably be provided on an outpatient basis. Patients with acute and severe co-occurring problems, such as suicidality, active psychosis or mania, or extreme domestic violence, should initially be treated in a controlled environment where their co-occurring problems can be stabilized to some degree prior to outpatient treatment. A more structured initial phase of treatment may also be required for what is perhaps the most difficult group of patients to work with: those with both low motivation for change (Chapter 9, this volume) and acute polyproblems.

PSYCHIATRIC PROBLEMS

Substance abusers with comorbid psychiatric problems may be particularly good candidates for specialized services, in the form of professionally delivered psychotherapy, psychotropic medication, greater treatment intensity or structure, or a combination of all three. For example, recent studies suggest that tricyclic antidepressants and the selective serotonergic medication fluoxetine may reduce both drinking and depression levels in alcoholics with major depression (Cornelius et al., 1997; Mason, Kocsis, Ritvo, & Cutler, 1996; McGrath et al., 1996). Similarly, the anxiolytic buspirone may reduce drinking in alcoholics with a comorbid anxiety disorder (Kranzler et al., 1994). Highly structured relapse prevention interventions may also be more effective in decreasing cocaine use, as compared to less structured interventions, in cocaine abusers with comorbid depression (Carroll, Nich, & Rounsaville, 1995).

Woody and colleagues (1983) have evaluated the value of individual psychotherapy when added to paraprofessional counseling services in the course of methadone maintenance treatment. In that study patients were randomly assigned to receive standard drug counseling alone (DC group) or drug counseling *plus* one of two forms of professional therapy: supportive-expressive psychotherapy (SE) or cognitive-behavioral psychotherapy (CB) over a 6-month period. Results showed that patients receiving psychotherapy showed greater reductions in drug use, more improvements in health and personal function, and greater reductions in crime than those receiving counseling alone. Stratification of patients according to their levels of psychiatric symptoms at intake showed that the main psychotherapy effect was in those with greater than average levels of psychiatric symptoms. That is, patients with low symptom levels made considerable gains with counseling alone and there were no differences between groups. However, patients with more severe psychiatric problems showed few gains with counseling alone but substantial improvements with the addition of the professional psychotherapy.

There has been some debate over the optimal timing of pharmacological interventions to address co-occurring psychiatric problems. The fact that many of the patients who display symptoms of depression or anxiety at admission to treatment experience an improvement in these symptoms following a few weeks of abstinence suggests that decisions about medication should be put off until at least several weeks of abstinence have been achieved, unless there is clear evidence that the mood disorder is primary or at least independent of the substance use disorder (Cornelius et al., 1997; McGrath et al., 1996; Schuckit, 1985). However, a recent study yielded modest evidence to support the use of antidepressants after 1 week of abstinence with primary alcoholics who have secondary depression (Mason et al., 1996), which indicates that additional work is needed in this area before a consensus can be achieved on how quickly to medicate symptoms of depression. Patients who are actively psychotic or in a manic episode should be evaluated immediately by a psychiatrist for medication and possible hospitalization.

INTERPERSONAL PROBLEMS

Controlled studies that have evaluated couples therapy for alcoholism have generally found that this intervention produces improvements in both drinking and marital satisfaction, particularly when behavioral couples therapy (BCT) is used (Miller et al., 1995; O'Farrell, 1995). A recent study also found that substance abusers who received BCT in addition to individual outpatient treatment had better drug use and relationship outcomes than those who received individual treatment only (Fals-Stewart, Birchler, & O'Farrell, 1996). These results suggest that BCT may be a useful addition to other forms of treatment for substance abusers who are currently in relationships.

Unfortunately, there is little research evidence to indicate which substance abusers will benefit to the greatest degree from couples treatment. Obviously, the patient must have a significant other who is willing to participate in the treatment. Most of the other factors found to predict completion of couples therapy for alcoholism are the same factors that predict retention in most forms of treatment (O'Farrell, 1995). With regard to substance use outcomes, one study found that couples relapse prevention delivered as aftercare was more effective than a no-treatment control condition, particularly for patients with more severe alcohol and marital problems at entrance to treatment (O'Farrell, Choquette, & Cutter, in press). Another study found that the effectiveness of couples therapy varied as a function of complex interactions involving the patient's degree of investment in relationships, degree of support for abstinence from significant others, and planned number of conjoint sessions (Longabaugh, Wirtz, Beattie, Noel, & Stout, 1995).

Although little if any research has specifically addressed the issue of when to provide couples treatment, there is evidence to indicate that either couples therapy or the involvement of significant others can be effective as a means of engaging substance abusers in treatment (Chapter 11, this volume), during the primary treatment experience (Fals-Stewart *et al.*, 1996; Miller *et al.*, 1995), or as part of aftercare (O'Farrell *et al.*, in press). Therefore, when patients have significant interpersonal problems and a spouse or other family members who are willing to participate in conjoint treatment, couples or family therapy should be provided relatively early in treatment.

SEVERE COCAINE ADDICTION

Another kind of substance abuser that can pose particular problems for outpatient treatment is the cocaine dependent patient who either presents for treatment with a severe cocaine problem or who is unable to achieve remission from cocaine dependence early in outpatient treatment. Several randomized studies suggest that highly structured cognitive-behavioral treatment is particularly efficacious with such individuals. For example, two outpatient studies with cocaine abusers showed that those with more severe cocaine problems at intake had significantly better cocaine use outcomes if they received structured relapse prevention rather than interpersonal or clinical management treatments (Carroll *et al.*, 1991; Carroll *et al.*, 1994). In a third study, cocaine dependent patients who continued to use cocaine during a 4-week IOP had much better cocaine use outcomes if they subsequently received aftercare that included a combination of group therapy and a structured relapse prevention protocol delivered through individual sessions rather than aftercare that consisted of group therapy alone (McKay, Alterman, *et al.*, 1997).

ADDING COMPREHENSIVE SERVICES

The impact of adding additional, professionally delivered treatment services to a basic methadone program was investigated by McLellan and colleagues (McLellan, Arndt, Metzger, Woody, & O'Brien, 1993). In this study, patients were randomly assigned to receive (a) methadone only; (b) methadone plus standard counseling; or (c) methadone and counseling plus on-site medical, psychiatric, employment, and family therapy services (the "enhanced" condition). Although these additional services were not "matched" to patients on an individual basis, most of the patients in the study were polydrug abusers with relatively high problem severity levels in other areas. On most outcome measures, the best results were obtained in the enhanced condition, followed by methadone plus counseling, and methadone alone. Improvements in the enhanced condition were significantly better than those in the methadone plus counseling condition in the areas of employment, alcohol use, criminal activity, and psychiatric status.

Another comprehensive treatment intervention designed to address problems in several areas of functioning is the community reinforcement approach, or CRA (Meyers & Smith, 1995). In addition to substance abuse–focused interventions such as functional analysis of drinking antecedents and disulfiram, CRA includes basic skills training, a job club, social and recreational counseling, access to a substance-free "social club," and marital therapy. The overall goal of this intervention is to make sobriety more rewarding than substance use. Studies have consistently found CRA to be an effective treatment (Miller *et al.*, 1995). With regard to polyproblem individuals, a recent study found that CRA was more effective than standard treatment for homeless alcoholics (Smith, Meyers, & Delaney, in press). The results from the McLellan, Arndt, and colleagues (1993) and CRA studies described previously demonstrate the potential value of providing additional professional treatment services to polyproblem substance abusers, even when these services are not "matched" to specific problems at the level of the individual patient (see Chapter 11, this volume).

The most direct and comprehensive test of the effectiveness of the matching services to problems approach was conducted by McLellan and colleagues (1997) in two inpatient and two outpatient private treatment facilities utilized by an employee assistance program (EAP). At intake, patients ($N = 130$) were placed in one of the four programs, assessed with the ASI, and randomized to either the standard or matched services conditions. In the standard condition, the treatment program received information from the intake ASI, and personnel were instructed to treat the patient in the "standard manner, as though there were no evaluation study ongoing." The programs were instructed not to withhold any standard services from the patients in the standard condition. Patients who were randomly assigned to the matched services condition were also placed in one of the four treatment programs and ASI information was forwarded to the program. Programs agreed to also provide at least three individual sessions to patients in this condition in the areas of employment, family and social relations, or psychiatric health delivered by a professionally trained staff person to improve functioning when a patient evidenced a significant degree of impairment in one or more of these areas at intake. For example, a patient whose intake ASI revealed significant impairments in the areas of social and psychiatric functioning would receive at least six individual sessions, three by a psychiatrist and three by a social worker.

The standard and matched patients were compared on a number of measures, including number of services received while in treatment, treatment completion rates, 6-month improvements in the seven problem areas assessed by the ASI, and other key outcomes at 6 months. The following results were obtained. First, matched patients received significantly more psychiatric and employment services than standard patients, but not more family and social services or alcohol and drug services. Second, matched patients were more likely to complete treatment (93% vs. 81%), and showed more improvement in the areas of employment and psychiatric functioning than the standard patients. Third, while matched and standard patients had sizable and equivalent improvements on most measures of alcohol and drug use, matched patients were less likely to be retreated for substance abuse problems during the 6-month follow-up. These findings suggest that matching treatment services to co-occurring problems can improve outcomes in key areas and may also be cost-effective by reducing the need for subsequent treatment due to relapse.

OTHER PROBLEMS

Two other problems that are found frequently in substance abusers are employment difficulties and comorbid dependence on nicotine. There is reason to believe that substance abusers who have employment problems can benefit from counseling to improve their job finding and retention skills, and such counseling was built into the McLellan and colleagues (1997) EAP study and is part of CRA. However, because unemployment is not likely to prevent substance abusers from initially engaging in treatment or to interfere in some way with that treatment, problems in this area can be addressed at a later point in treatment. With regard to nicotine dependence, it is obviously better for overall health reasons that substance abusers stop using tobacco products. However, there is some evidence to suggest that mandatory smoking cessation for substance abusers in treatment may be counterproductive and that substance abusers are more receptive to such interventions after they have achieved a period of abstinence (Monti, Rohsenow, Colby, & Abrams, 1995). The issue of smoking cessation for substance abusers is comprehensively addressed in Chapter 18 (this volume).

STRENGTHS AND LIMITATIONS OF THE MATCHING SERVICES TO PROBLEMS APPROACH

It is difficult to argue against the face validity of a treatment approach for polyproblem substance abusers that stresses the importance of providing additional services to address co-occurring medical, economic, psychiatric, family, and legal problems. After all, effective substance abuse–focused interventions such as cognitive behavioral therapy or 12-step facilitation (Project MATCH Research Group, 1997), no matter how well delivered, are not designed to address serious problems in other areas. If left untreated, co-occurring problems can increase risk for poor treatment response and poor posttreatment outcome. And in some cases, it may be impossible even to initiate treatment for a substance abuse problem until treatment for a severe co-occurring problem has been provided. In addition to benefits for the patients, the matching services to problems approach can also reduce stress levels in clinicians who treat polyproblem individuals, provided that a team approach to treatment is taken and regular lines of communication are established between clinicians involved with a case.

The primary limitation of this approach concerns the potential lack of resources in a time of health care cost containment. Funding may not be available to substance abuse treatment providers for adjunctive services in areas such as medical and psychiatric care, unless the level of problem severity is high enough that these co-occurring disorders can be considered "primary." Recent research has shown that even well-funded, private substance abuse programs vary widely in the number and frequency of adjunctive services they provide (McLellan, Grissom, *et al.,* 1993), which may reflect differences between programs in the funding available for such services. Obviously, it is impossible to match services to problems if the appropriate services are not available. The scarcity of resources underlies the need for accurate assessment and diagnosis of co-occurring problems, so as to ensure that patients who are more in need of such services will stand a better chance of receiving them. Outcomes for the polyproblem individual are likely to be enhanced if the clinician can serve not only as a therapist, but also as a case manager and patient advocate in negotiations with individuals or organizations that control access to care for co-occurring problems.

Another potential problem with the matching services to problems approach is that even when adjunctive services are available in the community, they may not be offered at the clinic or agency in which the patient is receiving substance abuse-focused treatment. In cases where patients have to go to other agencies to obtain additional services, there is a greater chance of attrition due to logistical problems or flagging motivation. This is a strong argument for combining substance abuse treatment with a broader array of services, which is sometimes referred to as "one-stop shopping," in settings where a more interdisciplinary approach can be taken for the treatment of the polyproblem individual.

REFERENCES

Alterman, A. I., O'Brien, C. P., McLellan, A. T., August, D. S., Snider, E. C., Droba, M., Cornish, J. W., Hall, C. P., Raphaelson, A. H., & Schrade, F. X. (1994). Effectiveness and costs of inpatient and day hospital cocaine rehabilitation. *Journal of Nervous and Mental Disease, 182,* 157–163.

American Psychiatric Association. (1994). *Diagnostic and statistical manual of mental disorders* (4th ed.). Washington, DC: Author.

American Society of Addiction Medicine. (1996). *Patient placement criteria for the treatment of substance-related disorders* (2nd ed.) (ASAM PPC-II). Chevy Chase, MD: Author.

Annis, H. M. (1986). Is inpatient rehabilitation cost effective? Con position. *Advances in Alcohol and Substance Abuse, 5,* 175–190.

Beck, A. T., Ward, C. H., Mendelson, M., Mock, J. E., & Erbaugh, J. K. (1961). An inventory to measure depression. *Archives of General Psychiatry, 4,* 561–571.

Carroll, K. M., Rounsaville, B. J., & Gawin, F. H. (1991). A comparative trial of psychotherapies for ambulatory cocaine abusers: Relapse prevention and interpersonal psychotherapy. *American Journal of Drug and Alcohol Abuse, 17,* 229–247.

Carroll, K. M., Power, M. D., Bryant, K., & Rounsaville, B. J. (1993). One-year follow-up status of treatment-seeking cocaine abusers: Psychopathology and dependence severity as predictors of outcome. *Journal of Nervous and Mental Disease, 181,* 71–79.

Carroll, K. M., Rounsaville, B. J., Gordon, L. T., Nich, C., Jatlow, P., Bisighini, R. M., & Gawin, F. H. (1994). Psychotherapy and pharmacotherapy for ambulatory cocaine abusers. *Archives of General Psychiatry, 51,* 177–187.

Carroll, K. M., Nich, C., & Rounsaville, B. J. (1995). Differential symptom reduction in depressed cocaine abusers treated with psychotherapy and pharmacotherapy. *Journal of Nervous and Mental Disease, 183,* 251–259.

Cornelius, J. R., Salloum, I. M., Ehler, J. G., Jarrett, P. J., Cornelius, M. D., Perel, J. M., Thase, J. E., & Black, A. (1997). Fluoxetine in depressed alcoholics: A double-blind, placebo controlled trial. *Archives of General Psychiatry, 54,* 700–705.

Darke, S., Hall, W., Wodak, A., Heather, N., & Ward, J. (1992). Development and validation of a multidimensional instrument for assessing outcome of treatment among opiate users: The Opiate Treatment Index. *British Journal of Addiction, 87,* 733–742.

DeRogatis, L. R., Lipman, R. S., & Covi, L. (1973). The SCL-90: An outpatient psychiatric rating scale. *Psychopharmacological Bulletin, 9,* 13–28.

Fals-Stewart, W., Birchler, G. R., & O'Farrell, T. J. (1996). Behavioral couples therapy for male substance abusing patients: Effects on relationship adjustment and drug-using behavior. *Journal of Consulting and Clinical Psychology, 64,* 959–972.

Finney, J. W., Hahn, A. C., & Moos, R. H. (1996). The effectiveness of inpatient and outpatient treatment of substance abuse: The need to focus on mediators and moderators of setting effects. *Addiction, 91,* 1773–1796.

First, M. B., Spitzer, R. L., Gibbon, M., & Williams, J. B. W. (1996). *Structured Clinical Interview for DSM-IV Axis I Disorders.* New York: Biometrics Research Department, New York State Psychiatric Institute.

Gough, H. (1987). *California Psychological Inventory Administrator's Guide.* Palo Alto, CA: Consulting Psychologists' Press.

Hayashida, M., Alterman, A. I., McLellan, A. T., O'Brien, C. P., Purtill, J. J., Volpicelli, J. R., Raphaelson, A. H., & Hall, C. P. (1989). Comparative effectiveness and costs of inpatient and outpatient detoxification of patients with mild-to-moderate alcohol withdrawal syndrome. *New England Journal of Medicine, 320,* 358–365.

Kranzler, H. R., Burleson, J. A., Del Boca, F. K., Babor, T. F., Korner, P., Brown, J., & Bohn, M. J. (1994). Buspirone treatment of anxious alcoholics: A placebo-controlled trial. *Archives of General Psychiatry, 51,* 720–731.

Longabaugh, R., Wirtz, P. W., Beattie, M. C., Noel, N., & Stout, R. (1995). Matching treatment focus to patient social investment and support: 18 month follow-up results. *Journal of Consulting and Clinical Psychology, 63,* 296–307.

Mason, B. J., Kocsis, J. H., Ritvo, E. C., & Cutler, R. B. (1996). A double-blind, placebo-controlled trial of desipramine for primary alcohol dependence stratified on the presence or absence of major depression. *Journal of the American Medical Association, 275,* 761–767.

Mattson, M. E., Allen, J. P., Longabaugh, R., Nickless, C. J., Connors, G. J., & Kadden, R. M. (1994). A chronological review of empirical studies matching alcoholics to treatment. *Journal of Studies on Alcohol* (Suppl. 12), 16–29.

McDermott, P. A., Alterman, A. I., Brown, L., Zaballero, A., Snider, E. C., & McKay, J. R. (1996). Construct refinement and confirmation for the intake Addiction Severity Index scales. *Psychological Assessment: A Journal of Consulting and Clinical Psychology, 8,* 182–189.

McGrath, P. J., Nunes, E. V., Stewart, J. W., Goldman, D., Agosti, V., Ocepek-Welikson, K., & Quitkin, F. M. (1996). Imipramine treatment of alcoholics with primary depression: A placebo-controlled clinical trial. *Archives of General Psychiatry, 53,* 232–240.

McKay, J. R., Cacciola, J., McLellan, A. T., Alterman, A. I., & Wirtz, P. W. (1997). An initial evaluation of the psychosocial dimensions of the ASAM criteria for inpatient and day hospital substance abuse rehabilitation. *Journal of Studies on Alcohol, 58,* 239–252.

McKay, J. R., Alterman, A. I., Cacciola, J. S., Rutherford, M. R., O'Brien, C. P., & Koppenhaver, J. (1997). Group counseling vs. individualized relapse prevention aftercare following intensive outpatient treatment for cocaine dependence: Initial results. *Journal of Consulting and Clinical Psychology 65,* 778–788.

McKay, J. R., McLellan, A. T., Durell, J., Ruetsch, C., & Alterman, A. I. (1998). Characteristics of recipients of Supplemental Security Income (SSI) benefits for drug addicts and alcoholics. *Journal of Nervous and Mental Disease, 186,* 172–180.

McLellan, A. T., & Gastfriend, D. (1996). Treatment matching: Theoretical basis and practical implications. In J. Samet & M. Stein (Eds.), *Medical Clinics of North America* (pp. 241–256). New York: Saunders.

McLellan, A. T., & Weisner, C. (1996). Achieving the public health potential of substance abuse treatment: Implications for patient referral, treatment "matching" and outcome evaluation. In W. Bickel & R. DeGrandpre (Eds.), *Drug policy and human nature* (pp. 310–338). Philadelphia: Wilkins and Wilkins.

McLellan, A. T., Luborsky, L., Woody, G. E., & O'Brien, C. P. (1980). An improved evaluation instrument for substance abuse patients: The Addiction Severity Index. *Journal of Nervous and Mental Disease, 168,* 26–33.

McLellan, A. T., Luborsky, L., Woody, G. E., Druley, K. A., & O'Brien, C. P. (1983). Predicting response to alcohol and drug abuse treatments: Role of psychiatric severity. *Archives of General Psychiatry, 40,* 620–625.

McLellan, A. T., Luborsky, L., Cacciola, J., Griffith, J., Evans, F., Barr, H., & O'Brien, C. P. (1985). New data from the Addiction Severity Index: Reliability and validity in three centers. *Journal of Nervous and Mental Disease, 173,* 412–423.

McLellan, A. T., Cacciola, J., Kushner, H., Peters, F., Smith, I., & Pettinati, H. (1992). The fifth edition of the Addiction Severity Index: Cautions, additions, and normative data. *Journal of Substance Abuse Treatment, 9,* 199–213.

McLellan, A. T., Arndt, I. O., Metzger, D. S., Woody, G. E, & O'Brien, C. P. (1993). The effects of psychosocial services in substance abuse treatment. *Journal of the American Medical Association, 269,* 1953–1959.

McLellan, A. T., Grissom, G. R., Brill, P., Durell, J., Metzger, D. S., & O'Brien, C. P. (1993). Private substance abuse treatments: Are some programs more effective than others? *Journal of Substance Abuse Treatment, 10,* 243–254.

McLellan, A. T., Alterman, A. I., Metzger, D. S., Grissom, G., Woody, G. E., Luborsky, L., & O'Brien, C. P. (1994). Similarity of outcome predictors across opiate, cocaine and alcohol treatments: Role of treatment services. *Journal of Consulting and Clinical Psychology, 62,* 1141–1158.

McLellan A. T., Grissom, G., Zanis, D., & Brill, P. (1997). Problem–service "matching" in addiction treatment: A prospective study in four programs. *Archives of General Psychiatry, 54,* 730–735.

Mee-Lee, D. (1988). An instrument for treatment progress and matching: The Recovery Attitude and Treatment Evaluator (RAATE). *Journal of Substance Abuse Treatment, 5,* 183–186.

Meyers, R. J., & Smith, J. E. (1995). *Clinical guide to alcohol treatment: The Community Reinforcement Approach.* New York: Guilford.

Miller, W. R., & Hester, R. K. (1986). Inpatient alcoholism treatment: Who benefits? *American Psychologist, 41,* 794–805.

Miller, W. R., & Marlatt, G. A. (1987). *Manual supplement for the Brief Drinker Profile, Follow-up Drinker Profile, and Collateral Interview Form.* Odessa, FL: Psychological Assessment Resources.

Miller, W. R., Brown, J. M., Simpson, T. L., Handmaker, N. S., Bien, T. H., Luckie, L. F., Montgomery, H. A., Hester, R. K., & Tonigan, J. S. (1995). What works? A methodological analysis of the alcohol treatment outcome literature. In R. K. Hester & W. R. Miller (Eds.), *Handbook of alcoholism treatment approaches* (2nd ed., pp. 12–44). Needham Heights, MA: Allyn & Bacon.

Monti, P. M., Rohsenow, D. J., Colby, S. M., & Abrams, D. B. (1995). Smoking among alcoholics during and after treatment: Implications for models, treatment strategies, and policy. In J. B. Fertig & J. P. Allen (Eds.), *Alcohol and tobacco: From basic science to clinical practice* (pp. 187–206). Bethesda, MD: National Institute on Alcohol Abuse and Alcoholism.

Moos, R. H., Finney, J. W., & Cronkite, R. C. (1990). *Alcoholism treatment: Context, process, and outcome.* New York: Oxford University Press.

Najavits, L. M., Gastfriend, D. R., Nakayama, E. Y., Barber, J. P., Blaine, J., Frank, A., Muenz, L. R., & Thase, M. (1997). A measure of readiness for substance abuse treatment: Psychometric properties of the RAATE-R interview. *American Journal on Addictions, 6,* 74–82.

O'Farrell, T. J. (1995). Marital and family therapy. In R. K. Hester & W. R. Miller (Eds.), *Handbook of alcoholism treatment approaches* (2nd ed., pp. 195–220). Needham Heights, MA: Allyn & Bacon.

O'Farrell, T. J., Choquette, K. A., & Cutter, H. S. G. (in press). Couples relapse prevention sessions after behavioral marital therapy for male alcoholics: Outcomes during the three years after starting treatment. *Journal of Studies on Alcohol.*

Project MATCH Research Group. (1997). Matching alcoholism treatments to client heterogeneity: Project MATCH posttreatment drinking outcomes. *Journal of Studies on Alcohol, 58,* 7–29.

Robins, L. N., Helzer, J. E., Croughan, J., & Ratcliff, K. S. (1981). The NIMH Diagnostic Interview Schedule: Its history, characteristics, and validity. *Archives of General Psychiatry, 38,* 381–389.

Schuckit, M. A. (1985). The clinical implications of primary diagnostic groups among alcoholics. *Archives of General Psychiatry, 42,* 1043–1049.

Smith, J. E., Meyers, R. J., & Delaney, H. D. (in press). The Community Reinforcement Approach with homeless alcohol-dependent individuals. *Journal of Consulting and Clinical Psychology.*

Woody, G., Luborsky, L., McLellan, A. T., O'Brien, C. P., Beck, A. T., Blaine, J., Herman, I., & Hole, A. (1983). Psychotherapy for opiate addicts: Does it help? *Archives of General Psychiatry, 40,* 1639–1645.

IV

Facilitating Change

Historically, addiction professionals have most often focused their attention on behavior change. Once an individual is ready for change, what are the options? Chapters 15 through 19 are condensed literature reviews for five specific addictive behaviors: alcohol problems, other drug problems, eating disorders, tobacco smoking, and problem gambling. The focus in these chapters is on clear guidance for clinicians, giving best advice based on current research evidence. Chapter 20 offers research-based clinical guidance on involving the family in treatment.

It is important to remember, however, that formal treatment is but a small part of the picture of change. Many individuals recover from addictive behaviors without formal therapeutic intervention. One of the fundamental insights of the transtheoretical model is, in fact, that the stages and processes of change are similar whether it occurs inside or outside a treatment context. Chapter 14, which opens this section, reviews natural change processes and outlines a program for facilitating a self-guided approach. The other bookend for this section, Chapter 21, is a practitioners' guide to the ubiquitous 12-step groups that represent the most common source of help for addictive behaviors in some nations. These mutual-help groups can be thought of not only as an alternative to treatment, but also as an adjunct to it, particularly when the practitioner knows how to combine approaches.

Together, these chapters outline an impressive menu of options for those seeking to change addictive behaviors. Although we do not yet have sufficient wisdom about how to assign clients to treatments, there is certainly reason for optimism in the range of approaches with documented efficacy. The idea of "one size fits all" treatment is being replaced by the knowledge that if one approach doesn't work, others are available. The rapidly growing menu of effective options is yet another significant change in the addiction field since our first edition.

14

Guiding Self-Change

MARK B. SOBELL AND LINDA C. SOBELL

NATURAL RECOVERY: RECOVERY WITHOUT
FORMAL HELP OR TREATMENT

Recovery from substance abuse problems without treatment has been well documented for cigarettes (Fiore *et al.,* 1990; Orleans *et al.,* 1991; Schacter, 1982), different drugs (e.g., cocaine and heroin; Biernacki, 1986; Shaffer & Jones, 1989; Waldorf, Reinarman, & Murphy, 1991), and alcohol (L. C. Sobell, Sobell, Toneatto, & Leo, 1993; L. C. Sobell, Cunningham, & Sobell, 1996; Tuchfeld, 1981). For example, one of the most noteworthy longitudinal studies of natural recovery was by Robins and her colleagues (Robins, Davis, & Goodwin, 1974), who followed veterans of the Vietnam War. Of the many veterans who had been addicted to heroin in Vietnam, only 5% continued to be addicted in the first year after returning home. Further, over the first 3 years after their return, only 12% became readdicted, and usually only for a short time. Because only a third of the veterans addicted to heroin had received even simple detoxification and very few entered treatment upon returning, it appears that the large majority stopped narcotic use on their own. Despite documentation of the phenomenon of natural recovery, the general public and many addictions counselors are either skeptical about or do not believe that someone with a substance abuse problem can change on their own (Cunningham, Sobell, & Chow, 1993; Rush & Allen, 1997).

One possible reason that there is little recognition of natural recoveries is that individuals who exhibit severe forms of the disorder have occupied public attention. The phenomenon of addiction, at least alcohol problems (Cahalan, 1987), looks very different when viewed at a population level rather than focusing on those who enter treatment. Epidemiological studies have shown that severely

MARK B. SOBELL AND LINDA C. SOBELL • Center for Psychological Studies, Nova Southeastern University, Fort Lauderdale, Florida 33314.

Treating Addictive Behaviors, 2nd ed., edited by Miller and Heather. Plenum Press, New York, 1998.

dependent individuals constitute a very small portion of those with alcohol problems (Institute of Medicine, 1990). It would be expected that recoveries without treatment would be more prevalent among individuals with less severe problems, because such individuals often respond well to nonintensive interventions (M. B. Sobell & Sobell, 1993b). The fact that individuals who enter treatment tend to have more serious problems than those who do not enter treatment often blinds us to the fact that there are multiple pathways to recovery—including treatment, self-help groups like AA, and natural recovery or self-change. This chapter describes research that has been conducted on self-change, or natural recovery, and how those findings can influence community and treatment interventions for alcohol and drug problems.

There are important reasons for studying natural recoveries. For example, a sizable percentage of people with substance abuse problems never seek treatment; in the alcohol field the ratio of untreated to treated alcohol abusers has been estimated to range from 3:1 to 13:1 (Nathan, 1989; Roizen, Cahalan, & Shanks, 1978). The major reasons that substance abusers give for not entering traditional treatment programs are the *stigma* associated with being labeled, their belief that their problem is not serious enough to warrant attention (i.e., traditional programs are often too intense and too demanding for individuals who are not severely dependent), and their wish to handle their problem on their own (reviewed in Chiauzzi & Liljegren, 1993; Cunningham, Sobell, Sobell, Agrawal, & Toneatto, 1993). If we are to develop interventions that are perceived as attractive and to be sought out rather than avoided, it is important to understand why substance abusers do not seek treatment.

Another reason for studying natural recoveries is that available treatments are only relatively small determinants of long-term outcomes (Moos, Finney, & Cronkite, 1990). Also, little is known about how to successfully match individuals to treatments. Studies that have gathered data on the reasons for natural recoveries, although few in number and often suffering from methodological problems, still are instructive in trying to understand the processes by which recoveries come about. Knowledge derived from such studies can be useful in developing treatments, as this chapter illustrates.

With regard to how natural recoveries occur, considerable attention has been devoted to the role of life events (e.g., see L. C. Sobell, Sobell, & Toneatto, 1992), mostly described in global terms, such as changes in family milieu, vocation, or health. Some investigators have noted, however, the association of recovery with less prominent factors, termed "strangely trivial" factors by Knupfer (1972). Despite the intuitive appeal of event-related explanations of recoveries, a controlled design is needed to draw conclusions about causal relationships. For example, because changes in factors such as vocational and marital status may frequently occur in the lives of substance abusers, the fact that certain life events may have occurred around the time of recovery may be merely coincidence, not causation.

To investigate causal relationships, we undertook a controlled study for which the methodology is only briefly described (L. C. Sobell *et al.*, 1992). Individuals who had recovered from an alcohol problem without treatment were solicited by media advertisements. They had to have been recovered for at least 3 years and had to be able to provide collateral informants to verify that they had a problem and that they had recovered. A control group of alcohol abusers was also solicited who had had an alcohol problem for at least 5 years, had not received treatment, and were willing to be interviewed. Persons who had recovered were interviewed about events that had occurred during the year leading up to their recovery. Control subjects were interviewed about events that had occurred during a control year (for details see L. C. Sobell et al., 1992).

One major finding of the study was that when a control group was used for evaluating life events, significant relationships were not found between life events and recovery. Two other major findings are noteworthy. First, about a third of recoveries were reported to be immediate and often event related (e.g., traumatic event, health problem, religious conversion). Changes initiated in this manner are readily understood. But the most common way that recovery occurred (57% of cases) was by a process that we have described as a cognitive appraisal, meaning that subjects reported that their initiation of change was preceded by a process of their evaluating the pros and cons of changing their drinking and eventually becoming committed to change. Often some small and not uncommon event was perceived by the subjects to be related to the recovery, similar to events noted by Knupfer (1972) as "strangely trivial." A cognitive appraisal process has also been reported by other investigators studying the natural recoveries process with alcohol and drug abusers (Biernacki, 1986; Klingemann, 1992; Ludwig, 1985; L. C. Sobell et al., 1996; Toneatto et al., 1994; Waldorf et al., 1991).

Recoveries associated with cognitive evaluations as opposed to recoveries precipitated by discrete events are of particular interest as such recoveries have implications for clients in treatment and for individuals who want to change on their own but do not want to enter treatment. If a cognitive appraisal process (e.g., a balance sheet evaluating the pros and cons of continuing to use and not use) facilitates the resolution of substance abuse problems, then outcomes for such individuals might be improved by having them engage in an appraisal of their substance use. The intent would be (1) to accentuate or make more salient the costs of the person's use, (2) when possible, to lessen the perceived rewards of their use, (3) to make apparent the benefits of change or recovery, and (4) to identify potential obstacles to change, that is, the costs of changing. Applying this approach, individuals formulate their concerns about their alcohol and drug use as a payoff matrix or balance sheet of "pros" and "cons" for different courses of action. A decisional balance process has been used successfully with smokers and for weight loss (reviewed in L. C. Sobell, Cunningham, Sobell, Agrawal et al., 1996).

Although a cognitive appraisal process could have relevance for treatment, understanding how it develops is important in terms of implementing such a process in an intervention. A possible explanation has been suggested by Baumeister (1996) as a process he calls the crystallization of discontent. Baumeister speculates that (1) people engage in cognitive activities with a purpose of making sense of their lives and experiences, and (2) there is a natural tendency to maintain homogeneity in order to minimize distress that accompanies threats to our well-being. Thus, Baumeister hypothesizes, with some empirical support, that people ordinarily tend to minimize costs and exaggerate benefits of their ongoing roles and relationships, while tending to defuse potential threats. The crystallization of discontent involves people coming to view some aspects of their world differently. Similar to what we think of as insight, some focal event starts a process of linking together perceptions of costs, problems, and other undesirable features of a situation such that people perceive the situation differently—"so that a broad pattern of dissatisfaction and shortcoming is discerned" (p. 294). Thus, the same complex of events and other features that previously served to maintain a positive relationship are now reorganized as providing reason for discontent, thereby leading to a commitment to change. This hypothesized process of crystallization of discontent has the advantage of explaining how individuals come to reappraise the costs and benefits of their drinking, and why "seemingly trivial" events are sometimes reported as triggering the reappraisal process.

In terms of coping strategies for maintaining recovery, the literature is scant but consistent. The greatest single factor associated with maintaining recoveries for alcohol abusers is that of social support or a positive milieu, particularly from friends and family (L. C. Sobell et al., 1993). For drug abusers, the most common strategy for avoiding relapse has been to remove themselves from the environment where drugs are used and to break off social relationships with friends who use drugs (Waldorf et al., 1991).

Besides showing that the majority of natural recoveries occur for individuals who are mild to moderately dependent on alcohol and drugs, almost all of the natural recovery studies for alcohol problems indicate that there are two distinct pathways to recovery—abstinence and moderate drinking (L. C. Sobell et al., 1992; L. C. Sobell, Cunningham, & Sobell, 1996). There is also some evidence that some individuals who once had a drug problem return to nonproblem drug use (Biernacki, 1986; Waldorf et al., 1991). Last, most alcohol abusers who return to moderate drinking on their own also appear to be less dependent on alcohol at the start, a finding similar to that for individuals in alcohol treatment studies who moderate their drinking (M. B. Sobell & Sobell, 1995). The remainder of this chapter describes how natural recovery research can influence treatment and community interventions. We use as examples two lines of research we have been conducting for the past several years.

FOUNDATIONS OF GUIDED SELF-CHANGE TREATMENT

Guided self-change (GSC) treatment is a brief motivational intervention designed for use with individuals who have alcohol and drug problems. Developed in the early 1980s, it was influenced by several convergent lines of research.

Research on natural recoveries was one of several influences in the development of guided self-change (GSC) treatment, and it has led to refinements in GSC treatment as we have learned more about self-change. Although GSC treatment is now used with individuals who abuse drugs other than alcohol, its development started with the search for effective and efficient interventions for problem drinkers, individuals who have alcohol problems but who are not severely dependent on alcohol. Considerable research has found that individuals with less serious problems considerably outnumber those with severe problems (Institute of Medicine, 1990; M. B. Sobell & Sobell, 1993a, 1993b).

Concurrent with the identification of problem drinkers as a major population in need of services, considerable evidence also had accumulated demonstrating that alcohol problems are not inexorably progressive (Pattison, Sobell, & Sobell, 1977; M. B. Sobell & Sobell, 1987, 1993a). Conventional wisdom has long viewed individuals with low levels of alcohol problems as in the "early stages" of an irreversible progression from mild to severe "alcoholism." That view formed the basis for using the same treatment for all individuals with alcohol problems, even if their problems were not severe. Epidemiological research, however, has found that it is common for individuals to move into and out of periods of alcohol problems of varying severity separated by periods of either not drinking or of drinking without problems (Cahalan, 1987; Cahalan & Room, 1974). Besides demonstrating that alcohol problems were not progressive, this research suggested that, as in other areas of health care, persons with less serious problems typically need less intensive treatment than those with more serious problems.

Another important influence on the development of the GSC treatment was the well-known clinical trial of treatment versus advice by Edwards and his colleagues in England (Edwards *et al.,* 1977). That study found that the treatment outcomes of male alcohol abusers who were randomly assigned to a standard treatment program (individualized care that could have included inpatient and outpatient treatment and Antabuse®) were no different than for those who had been randomly assigned to a single session of advice or counseling. A corollary finding was that subjects whose problems were less severe did better during their second year of follow-up if they had been treated by the single session of advice or counseling, whereas those with more serious problems did better if they had received the standard treatment (Orford, Oppenheimer, & Edwards, 1976). This finding was readily accepted by many in the field, probably because it made sense that individuals who had fewer problems had more resources available to aid their recovery. Because the single advice or counseling session appeared to have enhanced subjects' commitment to change and their confidence that they could change with minimal help, it could be characterized as a motivational intervention. In summary, it appeared that problem drinkers would do well in a brief motivational intervention. Two other lines of research also supported this conclusion.

Adding further strength to the utility of motivational interventions was work by Prochaska and his colleagues on stages of change (DiClemente & Prochaska, 1982; Prochaska, 1983), and Miller's formulation of motivational enhancement as a focus of treatment (Miller, 1983, 1985). This research suggested that examining and increasing an individual's motivation to change could be an important intervention itself. Among the components postulated by Miller to increase motivation were motivational interviewing and the provision of personalized feedback.

Finally, the development of GSC treatment was also greatly influenced by research on alcohol treatment goals, and the formulation by Bandura (1996), of a social learning theory that hypothesized that allowing goal choice could be an important procedure for increasing an individual's commitment to a goal. As discussed elsewhere (M. B. Sobell & Sobell, 1995), the findings of research on alcohol treatment goals and outcomes can be summarized as follows: (1) Severely dependent alcohol abusers recover predominantly through abstinence; (2) alcohol abusers not severely dependent on alcohol recover predominantly through moderation; and (3) outcome type and dependence severity appear to be independent of treatment advice. Thus, not only is severity of dependence (rather than treatment goal advice) the best predictor of whether one will achieve an abstinence or moderation recovery, but goal advice seems to have little relevance. If goal assignment makes no difference and allowing choice increases commitment to change, an important component of a brief motivational treatment would be to allow clients to select their own goals.

INITIAL GUIDED SELF-CHANGE PROCEDURES

The first GSC intervention consisted of an assessment followed by two 90-minute sessions. The initial study evaluated the treatment with and without a cognitive relapse prevention component (M. B. Sobell & Sobell, 1993a; M. B. Sobell, Sobell, & Leo, 1990). Because not all clients will have a positive outcome from any given treatment, an important component of a brief treatment is to include provisions for dealing with problems encountered after treatment. Relapse prevention, with its focus on the maintenance of treatment effects (Marlatt & George, 1984), was an obvious choice for maintaining the strength of behavior change over time.

Relapse prevention has traditionally been thought of as embracing two major components: (1) identification of high risk situations and skills training for dealing with those situations without drinking, and (2) cognitive components focusing on thoughts about relapse. For the first study, it was hypothesized that the cognitive components of relapse prevention would lead to more robust outcomes. These procedures encouraged clients to adopt the perspective that relapses may occur following treatment, and that although relapses are unfortunate, how one deals with them is important. Clients were told that relapses should (1) be interrupted as soon as possible in order to minimize consequences, (2) be considered as learning experiences that identify previously unrecognized high-risk situations or inadequate methods of coping, and (3) not be attributed to personal failings (which promote a low sense of self-efficacy) but rather to situational factors that can be dealt with successfully in the future.

The study ($N = 100$) compared two groups: Problem drinkers were randomly assigned to either behavioral counseling (BC) or to behavioral counseling plus cognitive relapse prevention (RP). Both conditions had the following components: (1) an assessment; (2) within-treatment drinking data gathered by the time-line followback method (L. C. Sobell & Sobell, 1992); (3) subjects provided with advice but allowed to select their own treatment goals; (4) treatments involving brief readings and homework assignments that asked subjects to identify high-risk situations related to their drinking and to develop options and action plans for dealing with those situations; and (5) treatments using motivational strategies to increase clients' commitment to change. The treatment was designed to encourage clients to take responsibility for formulating and enacting their own plans for change.

The difference between the BC and RP treatments was that the session content and portions of the readings included the cognitive relapse prevention components for group RP but were absent for group BC. All clients could also receive additional sessions at their request. A detailed description of the treatment rationale and procedures has been published elsewhere (M. B. Sobell & Sobell, 1993a).

The major finding from this initial study was that while subjects in both groups improved very significantly from pre- to posttreatment, there were no significant differences between the groups. The total reduction in reported alcohol consumption was 53.8% compared with the year preceding treatment. This degree of reduction is consistent with that reported for other brief interventions with problem drinkers (e.g., Graber & Miller, 1988; Sanchez-Craig, Spivak, & Davila, 1991; Sanchez-Craig & Wilkinson, 1989). The fact that the group treated with the cognitive relapse prevention components did not fare any better than the behavioral counseling group is consistent with recent evidence that relapse prevention concepts may have greater applicability for more severely impaired substance abusers than for those less severely impaired (Carroll, 1996).

Because the reductions in drinking found in this study were in the same general range as those in other studies of brief interventions, the question arises as to how the GSC intervention differs from other approaches. The answers, we believe, relate to (1) its appeal to clients—it intrudes very little on their lifestyles—and (2) its empowerment of clients to take responsibility and credit for their change. Research has shown that problem drinkers tend to resist confrontational treatments (Miller, Benefield, & Tonigan, 1993). The GSC treatment was well liked by the vast majority of subjects in this study, with 97% saying that the treatment should continue to be made available. Consistent with the philosophy of GSC, 73% said that their outcome was "very much" attributable to themselves (M. B. Sobell & Sobell, 1993a).

Finally, although this study did not find that adding a relapse prevention component to the treatment resulted in better outcomes, the relapse prevention procedures were included in future trials of GSC because the therapists found it awkward to conduct treatment without reference to relapse prevention concepts, and those procedures fit well with the other treatment procedures and required no additional time in treatment (M. B. Sobell & Sobell, 1993a).

REFINEMENTS AND EXTENSIONS OF GUIDED SELF-CHANGE TREATMENT

The second study that used the GSC treatment evaluated the influence of social support on enhancing treatment outcome. One way that social support could be integrated into the GSC treatment as a maintenance factor was in relation to the relapse prevention components. It was hypothesized that spouses could play a critical role in helping their partners cope with high-risk drinking situations and in helping them cope with relapses that may occur. The clients in this study were restricted to married alcohol abusers who were willing to have their spouses involved in their treatment. Because 52% of the clients in the first study felt that the treatment was too brief (M. B. Sobell & Sobell, 1993a), the treatment was extended to four 60-minute sessions (an increase of 1 hour in contact time). With the exception of adding self-monitoring of drinking during treatment, the treatment components for all clients were identical to the relapse prevention condition in the first study but spread out over four sessions. Clients could also receive additional sessions at their request.

The study ($N = 56$) used a randomized two-group design. The two groups, natural social support (NSS) and directed social support (DSS), differed only in the procedures used with spouses. In both conditions the clients' spouses attended two 60-minute sessions with a therapist who was not the therapist for their spouse. Clients' spouses received readings similar to those provided to the clients, but modified to reflect a theme of helping one's spouse rather than helping one-self. The focus of the spouse counseling sessions was to provide the spouses with an understanding of the clients' treatment program and to provide the spouses with a realistic perspective for viewing recovery from alcohol problems. The NSS condition controlled for the amount of clinical contact with spouses in the two groups. For spouses in the NSS condition, the readings were similar to those read by the clients except that they were phrased from a third-person perspective. Spouses in the NSS condition were not given any explicit instructions to be sup-portive of their partners' changes. Therefore, any social support received by the clients in this condition was "natural," as it did not occur as the result of recom-mendations made to the spouse as part of the treatment program.

The intent of the DSS condition was to have the spouse become an agent of change with an emphasis on the role that the spouse could play in the partner's af-tercare. In other words, we sought to facilitate their provision of social support. Thus, the readings for spouses in the DSS condition suggested that they could be supportive by helping the partner (i.e., client) identify high-risk drinking situa-tions, devise and carry out plans for dealing with such situations, and construc-tively deal with relapses (i.e., stop the slip as soon as possible, construe it as a learning rather than a failure experience).

As in the first study, clients in both spouse groups showed very significant decreases in drinking from 1 year pretreatment to 1 year posttreatment. Although there were no significant differences in drinking outcomes between treatment groups, there was a significant interaction between treatment condition and self-efficacy. Clients who had low self-efficacy scores as measured by the Situational Confidence Questionnaire (Annis & Graham, 1988) had a greater reduction in days when they drank only 5 to 9 drinks if their spouse was in the DSS than the NSS group. This suggests that spousal support may be particularly important for clients who lack confidence in their own ability to recover.

Interestingly, in this study 69% of the subjects and 65% of the spouses rated the amount of treatment as sufficient at 2-year follow-up (the remainder said the amount was too little). Thus, although the proportion of clients satisfied with the amount of treatment was greater than in the first study, about one third still felt they needed a longer intervention.

Although our previous work has shown that problem drinkers preferred to se-lect their own goals (M. B. Sobell, Sobell, Bogardis, Leo, & Skinner, 1992), it was not known whether clients' significant others would agree that goal choice was a preferred procedure. In this study, when the clients were asked if they had just en-tered treatment would they prefer to select their own goal or have it selected by their therapist, 91% said they would prefer to select their own goal, 3% said they would prefer to have the therapist select their goal, and the remaining 6% had no opinion. At follow-up, almost all (97%) of the clients and 85% of their significant others felt that having clients select their own goal was a good thing. Only 4% of clients and 4% of their significant others felt that asking clients to select their own goal was not good. All clients from whom 2-year follow-up data were col-lected ($N = 32$) reported that they felt their drinking was either no longer a prob-lem (31%) or less of a problem (69%) than before treatment. Their spouses ($N = 26$) largely agreed: 23% said it was no longer a problem, 73% said it was less of a problem, and 4% said it was unchanged. The majority of clients (69%) as well as their spouses (56%) rated the clients as being most responsible for their outcome. As in the first study, this was consistent with the GSC orientation that encouraged clients to accept responsibility for their change.

The next study evaluated two extensions of the GSC treatment: (1) to a group therapy format, and (2) to drug abusers (clients who had injected drugs or used heroin were excluded). The study was a randomized controlled trial using a large sample: 232 alcohol abusers and 55 drug abusers who had voluntarily sought treatment. Individual therapy consisted of four 60-minute sessions. In both conditions clients were told that they would be contacted by telephone by their therapist for aftercare at 1 and 3 months following their last scheduled treatment session. As in previous GSC trials, clients were able to request additional sessions.

The treatment was basically the same as for clients in the spouse support study, with two additions: (1) a decisional balance reading and exercise were added (L. C. Sobell, Cunningham, Sobell, Agrawal, *et al.*, 1996), and (2) clients were provided with feedback and advice regarding their drinking, drug use, and high-risk situations during the past year using information obtained from the timeline followback interview (L. C. Sobell & Sobell, 1992) and from a variation of the Situational Confidence Questionnaire (SCQ; Annis & Graham, 1988; L. C. Sobell, Cunningham, Sobell, Agrawal, *et al.*, 1996). The decisional balance exercise was given to the clients at the end of their assessment and they were asked to bring the completed exercise to their first treatment session. From Baumeister's (1996) perspective the decisional balance exercise can be hypothesized as facilitating the crystallization of discontent. The timeline followback and SCQ feedback were given to clients at the first and second sessions, respectively. For clients in the group therapy condition the procedures were the same as in individual therapy, but topics were discussed in a round-robin fashion with the therapists responsible for promoting the use of group process and participation by all members (L. C. Sobell, Sobell, Brown, & Cleland, 1995).

In terms of drinking or drug use outcomes there were no significant differences between the individual and group treatment conditions. For alcohol clients, the results paralleled those of earlier studies. There were significant increases in abstinent days, significant decreases in very heavy and heavy drinking days, and little change in the number of limited drinking days (L. C. Sobell *et al.*, 1995). Although the vast majority of clients chose a reduced drinking rather than abstinence goal, the major way their drinking changed from pretreatment to posttreatment was that heavier drinking days diminished and abstinent days increased (M. B. Sobell, Buchan, & Sobell, 1996). For drug abusers, the main outcome measure was abstinent days. Similar to the pattern of alcohol abusers, drug abusers' days of abstinence increased significantly from pretreatment to posttreatment with no significant difference between the individual and group conditions.

In terms of client satisfaction, only 19% of the individual therapy clients felt the amount of treatment was not sufficient. This may reflect the effect of the aftercare telephone call procedures for addressing clients' concerns about the brevity of the treatment. Although 43% of the group therapy clients felt the amount of treatment was too little, this subjective perception must be evaluated in the context that there were no significant differences in outcomes between the formats. Finally, cost comparisons showed that providing treatment in a group format achieved a cost savings of 42% over the cost of providing individual treatment, and there was an eightfold difference in appointments missed by clients in the individual ($N = 210$ sessions) as compared to the group ($N = 25$ sessions) condition.

CROSS-CULTURAL EXTENSIONS AND EVALUATIONS OF GUIDED SELF-CHANGE TREATMENT

The GSC intervention and related materials have been translated into Spanish and evaluated in a controlled trial in Mexico (Ayala-Velazquez, Cardenas, Echeverria, & Gutierrez, 1995). The study was originally intended as a replication of the individual versus group format GSC study. The group format condition, however, could not be replicated in the Mexican study. The investigators attributed this difficulty to the reluctance of Mexican males (who constituted the vast majority of clients) to discuss their personal problems in a group format. The results for clients in the individual treatment condition paralleled those found in previous studies of GSC. Besides replicating the research findings, the Mexican study is important because the GSC materials were translated into Spanish and field tested. Currently, there are plans to disseminate the GSC treatment more widely in Mexico. Finally, although not yet the topic of a controlled trial, GSC materials have been translated into Swedish and the treatment is currently being disseminated among primary care medical settings in Sweden (personal communication, S. Andreasson, 1996).

FOSTERING SELF-CHANGE: AN INTERVENTION TO FACILITATE NATURAL RECOVERIES IN THE COMMUNITY

The most recent extension of GSC is not as traditional treatment, but rather as a community-level intervention. It constitutes an effort to increase the prevalence of recoveries in the community without using formal help or treatment. The Fostering Self-Change project being conducted in Toronto (L. C. Sobell, Cunningham, Sobell, Agrawal, et al., 1996) takes elements from the GSC treatment procedures (e.g., decisional balance exercise; Brief Situational Confidence Questionnaire; timeline drinking advice and feedback) and makes them available by mail to individuals in the community who wish to change their drinking on their own. Individuals volunteer for the study by responding to media solicitations and are sent assessment materials. After the materials are completed and returned by mail, the respondents in the experimental condition are sent a set of personalized feedback materials relating to their drinking levels, high-risk situations, and motivation for change (see L. C. Sobell, Cunningham, Sobell, Agrawal, et al., 1996, Appendix A). Respondents assigned to the control group are sent two educational pamphlets rather than personalized feedback. The sample consists of 825 respondents recruited primarily through newspaper advertisements that state: "Thinking about changing your drinking? Do you know that 75% of people change their drinking on their own? Call for free mail-out materials." If this minimal-intensity mailed out intervention is successful, such a procedure would allow large numbers of people to be served at a relatively low cost.

FUTURE DIRECTIONS

There are several ways that the GSC intervention may be extended in the future: (1) identifying client factors (individual difference variables) that predict who will do well in the treatment and who will do poorly, (2) extending the treatment to more severely dependent alcohol abusers, (3) continuing to explore extensions of the approach to individuals who abuse drugs other than alcohol, and (4) determining the relative efficacy of the various components of the treatment.

Although the extension of the approach to more severely dependent individuals might seem inconsistent with research on brief interventions, recent research suggests that such an extension is fully warranted (reviewed in M. B. Sobell, Breslin, & Sobell, 1998). Brief interventions and motivational interventions were developed when severity of dependence was considered to be an important predictor of treatment needs. This context was supported by the findings of Orford and colleagues (1976), who found that males who had low severity problems did better with a single session of advice or counseling than with a more intensive package of care, and that those whose problems were more severe did better in intensive treatment. For this and other reasons, including that it "made sense," brief interventions have been used almost exclusively with problem drinkers. Two recent reports, however, suggest that this needs to be reevaluated. Edwards and Taylor (1994) published a further analysis of the findings reported by Orford and his colleagues in 1976. This further analysis found no evidence of an interaction between severity of dependence and treatment intensity. The second report, using a much larger sample, was from Project MATCH, a large multicenter clinical trial that compared three interventions: Twelve-Step Facilitation, Cognitive-Behavioral Coping Skills, and Motivational Enhancement Treatment. The first two treatments involved 12 sessions; the Motivational Enhancement Treatment had only 4 sessions. Again no differences were found relating severity of dependence to differential treatment effectiveness (Project MATCH Research Group, 1997).

These recent developments suggest that brief interventions may be as helpful as other treatments even for more severely dependent alcohol abusers. Using approaches such as GSC as part of a stepped-care approach would provide a safety net for clients who do not respond well to brief treatment, and would maximize the benefits of brief treatment. Stepped care refers to a set of principles for health care provision that govern the services provided for most health problems. According to a stepped-care approach, choice of the initial treatment provided for an individual should be based on three principles:

1. Assessment and treatment should be individualized. Different types and intensities of assessments and treatments should be used depending on the presenting problem and other client characteristics.
2. The recommended treatment should be the one that is least intensive but likely to resolve the problem. More intensive treatments are reserved for more extreme problems.
3. Recommended treatments should be consistent with the contemporary research literature. (M. B. Sobell & Sobell, in press)

Implementing these principles would suggest that in many cases the first attempt at change should involve self-change, followed by increasingly intensive interventions if less intensive interventions fail. From this perspective, barring extenuating circumstances, attempting recovery without treatment should be a stepped option in an effective and efficient approach to health care system.

Finally, GSC treatment could be tested with adolescents. This is because it is well known that adolescents place high value on self-determination and independence. The GSC approach offers such empowerment, and more directive approaches could be reserved for adolescents who do not show positive change when given the opportunity to guide their own change.

ACKNOWLEDGMENTS

Preparation of this chapter was supported in part by a grant (AA08593) from the National Institute on Alcohol Abuse and Alcoholism.

REFERENCES

Annis, H. M., & Graham, J. M. (1988). *Situational Confidence Questionnaire (SCQ 39): User's guide.* Toronto, Ontario, Canada: Addiction Research Foundation.

Ayala-Velazquez, H., Cardenas, C., Echeverria, L., & Gutierrez, M. (1995). Initial results of an autocontrol program for problem alcoholics in Mexico. *Salud Mental, 18,* 18–24.

Bandura, A. (1986). *Social foundations of thought and action: A social cognitive theory.* Englewood Cliffs, NJ: Prentice Hall.

Baumeister, R. F. (1996). The crystallization of discontent in the process of major life change. In T. F. Heatherton & J. L. Weinberger (Eds.), *Can personality change?* (pp. 281–297). Washington, DC: American Psychological Association.

Biernacki, P. (1986). *Pathways from heroin addiction recovery without treatment.* Philadelphia: Temple University Press.

Cahalan, D. (1987). Studying drinking problems rather than alcoholism. In M. Galanter (Ed.), *Recent developments in alcoholism* (Vol. 5, pp. 363–372). New York: Plenum.

Cahalan, D., & Room, R. (1974). *Problem drinking among American men.* New Brunswick, NJ: Rutgers Center of Alcohol Studies.

Carroll, K. M. (1996). Relapse prevention as a psychosocial treatment: A review of controlled clinical trials. *Experimental and Clinical Psychopharmacology, 4,* 46–56.

Chiauzzi, E. J., & Liljegren, S. (1993). Taboo topics in addiction treatment: An empirical review of clinical folklore. *Journal of Substance Abuse Treatment, 10,* 303–316.

Cunningham, J. A., Sobell, L. C., & Chow, V. M. C. (1993). What's in a label? The effects of substance types and labels on treatment considerations and stigma. *Journal of Studies on Alcohol, 54,* 693–699.

Cunningham, J. A., Sobell, L. C., Sobell, M. B., Agrawal, S., & Toneatto, T. (1993). Barriers to treatment: Why alcohol and drug abusers delay or never seek treatment. *Addictive Behaviors, 18,* 347–353.

DiClemente, C. C., & Prochaska, J. O. (1982). Self-change and therapy change of smoking behavior: A comparison of processes of change in cessation and maintenance. *Addictive Behaviors, 7,* 133–142.

Edwards, G., & Taylor, C. (1994). A test of the matching hypothesis: Alcohol dependence, intensity of treatment, and 12-month outcome. *Addiction, 89,* 553–561.

Edwards, G., Orford, J., Egert, S., Guthrie, S., Hawker, A., Hensman, C., Mitcheson, M., Oppenheimer, E., & Taylor, C. (1977). Alcoholism: A controlled trial of "treatment" and "advice." *Journal of Studies on Alcohol, 38,* 1004–1031.

Fiore, M. C., Novotny, T. E., Pierce, J. P., Giovani, G. A., Hatziandreu, E. J., Newcomb, P. A., Surawicz, T. S., & Davis, R. M. (1990). Methods used to quit smoking in the United States. *Journal of the American Medical Association, 263,* 2760–2765.

Graber, R. A., & Miller, W. R. (1988). Abstinence or controlled drinking goals for problem drinkers: A randomized clinical trial. *Psychology of Addictive Behaviors, 2*, 20–33.

Institute of Medicine. (1990). *Broadening the base of treatment for alcohol problems.* Washington, DC: National Academy Press.

Klingemann, H. K. H. (1992). Coping and maintenance strategies of spontaneous remitters from problem use of alcohol and heroin in Switzerland. *International Journal of the Addictions, 27*, 1359–1388.

Knupfer, G. (1972). Ex-problem drinkers. In M. Roff, L. Robins, & H. Pollack (Eds.), *Life history research in psychopathology* (Vol. 2, pp. 256–280). Minneapolis: University of Minnesota Press.

Ludwig, A. M. (1985). Cognitive processes associated with "spontaneous" recovery from alcoholism. *Journal of Studies on Alcohol, 46*, 53–58.

Marlatt, G. A., & George, W. H. (1984). Relapse prevention: Introduction and overview of the model. *British Journal of Addiction, 79*, 261–273.

Miller, W. R. (1983). Motivational interviewing with problem drinkers. *Behavioural Psychotherapy, 11*, 147–172.

Miller, W. R. (1985). Motivation for treatment: A review with special emphasis on alcoholism. *Psychological Bulletin, 98*, 84–107.

Miller, W. R., Benefield, R. G., & Tonigan, J. S. (1993). Enhancing motivation for change in problem drinking: A controlled comparison of two therapist styles. *Journal of Consulting and Clinical Psychology, 61*, 455–461.

Moos, R. H., Finney, J. W., & Cronkite, R. C. (1990). *Alcoholism treatment: Context, process, and outcome.* New York: Oxford University Press.

Nathan, P. E. (1989). Treatment outcomes for alcoholism in the U. S.: Current research. In T. Lørberg, W. R. Miller, P. E. Nathan, & G. A. Marlatt (Eds.), *Addictive behaviors: Prevention and early intervention* (pp. 87–101). Amsterdam/Lisse: Swets & Zeitlinger.

Orford, J., Oppenheimer, E., & Edwards, G. (1976). Abstinence or control: The outcome for excessive drinkers two years after consultation. *Behaviour Research and Therapy, 14*, 409–418.

Orleans, C. T., Schoenbach, V. J., Wagner, E. H., Quade, D., Salmon, M. H., Pearson, D. C., Fielder, J., Porter, L. Q., & Kaplan, B. H. (1991). Self-help quit smoking interventions: Effects of self-help materials, social support instructions, and telephone counseling. *Journal of Consulting and Clinical Psychology, 59*, 439–448.

Pattison, E. M., Sobell, M. B., & Sobell, L. C. (1977). *Emerging concepts of alcohol dependence.* New York: Springer.

Prochaska, J. O. (1983). Self-changers versus therapy versus Schachter [Letter to the editor]. *American Psychologist, 38*, 853–854.

Project MATCH Research Group. (1997). Matching alcoholism treatments to client heterogeneity: Project MATCH posttreatment drinking outcomes. *Journal of Studies on Alcohol, 58*, 7–29.

Robins, L. N., Davis, D. H., & Goodwin, D. W. (1974). Drug use by U.S. army enlisted men in Vietnam: A follow-up on their return home. *American Journal of Epidemiology, 99*, 235–249.

Roizen, R., Cahalan, D., & Shanks, P. (1978). Spontaneous remission among untreated problem drinkers. In D. B. Kandel (Ed.), *Longitudinal research on drug use: Empirical findings and methodological issues* (pp. 197–221). Washington, DC: Hemisphere.

Rush, B., & Allen, B. A. (1997). Attitudes and beliefs of the general public about treatment for alcohol problems. *Canadian Journal of Public Health, 88*, 41–43.

Sanchez-Craig, M., & Wilkinson, D. A. (1989). Brief treatments for alcohol and drug problems: Practical and methodological issues. In T. Løberg, W. R. Miller, P. E. Nathan, & G. A. Marlatt (Eds.), *Addictive behaviors: Prevention and early intervention* (pp. 233–252). Amsterdam/Lisse: Swets & Zeitlinger.

Sanchez-Craig, M., Spivak, K., & Davila, R. (1991). Superior outcome of females over males after brief treatment for the reduction of heavy drinking: Replication and report of therapist effects. *British Journal of Addiction, 86*, 867–876.

Schacter, S. (1982). Recidivism and self-cure of smoking and obesity. *American Psychologist, 37*, 436–444.

Shaffer, H. J., & Jones, S. B. (1989). *Quitting cocaine: The struggle against impulse.* Lexington, MA: Lexington Books.

Sobell, L. C., & Sobell, M. B. (1992). Timeline follow-back: A technique for assessing self-reported alcohol consumption. In R. Z. Litten & J. Allen (Eds.), *Measuring alcohol consumption: Psychosocial and biological methods* (pp. 41–72). Towota, NJ: Humana.

Sobell, L. C., Sobell, M. B., & Toneatto, T. (1992). Recovery from alcohol problems without treatment. In N. Heather, W. R. Miller, & J. Greeley (Eds.), *Self-control and the addictive behaviors* (pp. 198–242). New York: Maxwell/MacMillan.

Sobell, L. C., Sobell, M. B., Toneatto, T., & Leo, G. I. (1993). What triggers the resolution of alcohol problems without treatment? *Alcoholism: Clinical and Experimental Research, 17,* 217–224.

Sobell, L. C., Sobell, M. B., Brown, J., & Cleland, P. A. (1995, November). *A randomized trial comparing group versus individual Guided Self-Change treatment for alcohol and drug abusers.* Poster presented at the 29th annual meeting of the Association for Advancement of Behavior Therapy, Washington, DC.

Sobell, L. C., Cunningham, J. A., & Sobell, M. B. (1996). Recovery from alcohol problems with and without treatment: Prevalence in two population surveys. *American Journal of Public Health, 86,* 966–972.

Sobell, L. C., Cunningham, J. C., Sobell, M. B., Agrawal, S., Barin, D. R., Leo, G. I., & Singh, K. N. (1996). Fostering self-change among problem drinkers: A proactive community intervention. *Addictive Behaviors, 21,* 817–833.

Sobell, M. B., & Sobell, L. C. (1987). Conceptual issues regarding goals in the treatment of alcohol problems. In M. B. Sobell & L. C. Sobell (Eds.), *Moderation as a goal or outcome of treatment for alcohol problems: A dialogue* (pp. 1–37). New York: Haworth.

Sobell, M. B., & Sobell, L. C. (1993a). *Problem drinkers: Guided self-change treatment.* New York: Guilford.

Sobell, M. B., & Sobell, L. C. (1993b). Treatment for problem drinkers: A public health priority. In J. S. Baer, G. A. Marlatt, & R. J. McMahon (Eds.), *Addictive behaviors across the lifespan: Prevention, treatment, and policy issues* (pp. 138–157). Beverly Hills, CA: Sage.

Sobell, M. B., & Sobell, L. C. (1995). Controlled drinking after 25 years: How important was the great debate? *Addiction, 90,* 1149–1153.

Sobell, M. B., & Sobell, L. C. (in press). Stepped care for alcohol problems: An efficient method for planning and delivering clinical services. In J. A. Tucker, D. A. Donovan, & G. A. Marlatt (Eds.), *Changing addictive behavior.* New York: Guilford.

Sobell, M. B., Sobell, L. C., & Leo, G. I. (1990, November). *Guided self-management for problem drinkers: An evaluation of the unique contribution of a relapse prevention perspective.* Poster session presented at the 24th annual meeting of the Association for Advancement of Behavior Therapy, San Francisco.

Sobell, M. B., Sobell, L. C., Bogardis, J., Leo, G. I., & Skinner, W. (1992). Problem drinkers' perceptions of whether treatment goals should be self-selected or therapist-selected. *Behavior Therapy, 23,* 43–52.

Sobell, M. B., Buchan, G., & Sobell, L. C. (1996, November). *Relationship of goal choices by substance abusers in Guided Self-Change treatment to subject characteristics and treatment outcome.* Poster presented at the 30th annual meeting of the Association for Advancement of Behavior Therapy, New York.

Sobell, M. B., Breslin, C. F., & Sobell, L. C. (1998). Project MATCH: The time has come . . . to talk of many things. *Journal of Studies on Alcohol, 59,* 124–125.

Toneatto, T., Sobell, L. C., Rubel, E., Leo, G. I., Sobell, M. B., & Agrawal, S. (1994, November). *Comparing untreated recovery in cocaine and alcohol abusers.* Poster presented at the 28th annual meeting of the Association for Advancement of Behavior Therapy, San Diego.

Tuchfeld, B. S. (1981). Spontaneous remission in alcoholics: Empirical observations and theoretical implications. *Journal of Studies on Alcohol, 42,* 626–641.

Waldorf, D., Reinarman, C., & Murphy, S. (1991). *Cocaine changes: The experience of using and quitting.* Philadelphia: Temple University Press.

15

A Wealth of Alternatives

Effective Treatments for Alcohol Problems

WILLIAM R. MILLER, NICHOLE R. ANDREWS,
PAULA WILBOURNE, AND MELANIE E. BENNETT

PROGRESS IN TREATMENT EFFECTIVENESS

The science of healing is progressing at a remarkable pace. Major advances have been made within the past decade in the treatment of many chronic health problems including cancer, depression, diabetes, and heart disease. One assumes, when seeking medical care, that health professionals keep abreast of current research and new developments, and will offer current treatments that are most likely to be beneficial.

The early history of medicine, of course, was one of prescribing remedies with no scientific basis, which in some cases helped (mostly through placebo effects) and in other cases harmed (Shapiro, 1971). Gradually, as health sciences emerged and established reliable methods for testing the efficacy of treatments, medical practice came to be informed by scientific evidence, although many other factors still influence the delivery of health care. Malpractice includes the delivery of a treatment known to be ineffective or harmful.

For a variety of reasons, treatment for alcohol and other drug problems has been slower to respond to emerging scientific evidence. Dr. Enoch Gordis, Director of the U.S. National Institute on Alcohol Abuse and Alcoholism (NIAAA), has observed that

> in the case of alcoholism, our whole treatment system, with its innumerable therapies, armies of therapists, large and expensive programs, endless conferences,

WILLIAM R. MILLER, NICHOLE R. ANDREWS, PAULA WILBOURNE, AND MELANIE E. BENNETT
• Department of Psychology, University of New Mexico, Albuquerque, New Mexico 87131.

Treating Addictive Behaviors, 2nd ed., edited by Miller and Heather. Plenum Press, New York, 1998.

innovation and public relations activities is founded on hunch, not evidence, and not on science. . . . To determine whether a treatment accomplishes anything we have to know how similar patients who have not received the treatment fare. Perhaps untreated patients do just as well. This would mean that the treatment does not influence outcome at all. Perhaps treated patients do worse; that is, perhaps the treatment is really harmful in unexpected ways so that patients who are not treated get better more often. Perhaps even if the treatment is helpful, a little bit of it is just as useful as a lot of it. (Gordis, 1987, p. 582)

This gap between research and practice may be due, in part, to a history of specialist treatment provided by those whose training did not emphasize scientific method. Indeed, prior to the 1970s, most U.S. health professionals showed little inclination to treat alcoholism, and humanitarian care was provided almost exclusively by recovering paraprofessionals and peers. The founding of NIAAA in 1970 began a period of growing professional interest, training, and scientific research to address alcohol problems. In the ensuing three decades there has been a dramatic increase in the volume and quality of research providing new knowledge immediately relevant to effective treatment. Unfortunately, this knowledge is often published only in scientific journals and has been relatively inconvenient for the busy clinician to access.

This chapter is meant to provide a concise summary of the current state of knowledge from research on the treatment of alcohol problems. More detailed reviews can be found in other sources (e.g., Finney & Monahan, 1996; Hester & Miller, 1995; Institute of Medicine, 1990; O'Farrell, 1993). The emphasis here is on practical implications of current research.

MESA GRANDE: SUMMARIZING THE OUTCOME LITERATURE

For two decades our research group has been compiling and preparing narrative reviews of treatment outcome studies (Miller & Hester, 1980, 1986a) including specialized reviews of client–treatment matching (Miller & Hester, 1986c), motivational interventions (Miller, 1985; Miller & Rollnick, 1991), and effects of treatment length, cost, and setting (Holder, Longabaugh, Miller, & Rubonis, 1991; Miller & Hester, 1986b). More recently we have conducted metanalyses of studies of brief interventions (Bien, Miller, & Tonigan, 1993), and Alcoholics Anonymous (Emrick, Tonigan, Montgomery, & Little, 1993; Tonigan, Toscova, & Miller, 1996).

The most ambitious review project by far, however, has been a methodological review of controlled clinical trials of treatments for alcohol problems. Three groups have been pursuing this task (Finney & Monahan, 1996; Mattick & Jarvis, 1992; Miller et al., 1995). Our efforts in New Mexico have focused on the construction of a large table (hence the Mesa Grande Project) detailing the methodological quality and findings of controlled outcome studies. We have chosen to focus on controlled trials—those in which compared groups of clients are equated before treatment, usually by randomization, so that they start treatment on equal footing. Although it has limitations, the randomized clinical trial is generally recognized as the gold standard in demonstrating the efficacy of a medication or treatment, providing credible evidence that observed benefits are attributable to specific effects of the treatment(s) being studied. Because it is usually unacceptable to leave clients untreated, most of these studies have compared different kinds of treatment with each other, or have evaluated the addition of a special component or therapy to treatment as usual. In our most recently published review (Miller *et al.*, 1995), a total of 219 studies were identified and rated. To these we have added 85 more trials, raising the total of reviewed studies to 302 (two new studies displaced earlier reports), comprising the outcomes of treatment for 59,833 clients with alcohol problems. (The full list of rated studies is available from the first author.)

The methods used to compile this review have been detailed elsewhere (Miller *et al.*, 1995), and are described only briefly here as a context for our findings. Through manual and computer searches we identified controlled trials comparing at least two equated treatment (or control) conditions and reporting posttreatment outcomes on at least one measure of drinking or related problems. We are confident that we have identified most trials available through 1996 in the English language, and we have included studies in other languages as our abilities allowed. Unpublished studies were incorporated when a full report was available. Two independent raters judged the quality of study methodology on each of 12 specific dimensions, resulting in a maximum possible Methodological Quality Score (MQS) of 17. Reviewers then compared their ratings, reconciling discrepancies against the original manuscript(s) and, when available, with information obtained from study authors.

Outcome Logic Scores (OLS) were also determined for each study by a similar process, following procedures specified in a coding manual (available from the first author). We identified treatment modalities for which specific outcomes could be inferred logically from each study design. For example, if a two-group study compared Treatment A with Treatment A + B, the additive efficacy of Treatment B could be inferred by comparing the groups, but no judgment could be made regarding the efficacy of Treatment A, which was given to all clients in the study. Study designs were classified as providing positive evidence (+1) or strong positive evidence (+2), negative evidence (−1) or strong negative evidence (−2) for each imputable modality. Null findings (e.g., failure to find a significant superiority of one treatment over other treatment(s) with which it was compared) resulted in the weaker (−1) negative evidence score, whereas stronger negative studies (e.g., inferiority to another treatment, or no difference from an untreated control) resulted in a −2 OLS. Some studies permitted imputation of an OLS for more than one modality. A few controlled studies (13, or 4%) were designed in such a way that no modality OLS could be inferred.

MQS and OLS were then multiplied for each study. This allowed us to weight each study's contribution according to its methodological quality. A well-designed study (MQS = 15) providing strong evidence of a positive effect for a specific treatment modality (OLS = +2) would contribute +30 points to the evidence score for that modality. A weaker study (MQS = 6) yielding no evidence of efficacy for a modality (OLS = −1) would subtract evidence points (−6) from that modality's total. We then summed the cross-product points from all of the studies providing evidence on a specific treatment modality to derive its Cumulative Evidence Score (CES), shown in Table 1. The CES can thus be thought of as the balance of evidence regarding the efficacy of each treatment approach. A highly positive score reflects a large volume of studies with predominantly positive evidence. A highly negative score reflects a large volume of studies that offer primarily negative evidence. An

TABLE 1
Summary of Evidence for the Efficacy of Specific Treatment Methods

Modality	% Clinical	MQS	N+	N−	CES
Treatment methods with three or more outcome studies					
Brief intervention	46	12.68	19	9	+221
Motivational enhancement	54	13.31	10	3	+145
Social skills training	88	10.94	11	6	+120
Community reinforcement approach	75	13.25	4	0	+80
GABA agonist medication	100	12.00	3	0	+72
Opioid antagonist medication	100	11.00	3	0	+66
Behavior contracting	100	10.40	4	1	+64
Client-centered therapy	80	10.40	4	1	+47
Aversion therapy (nausea)	100	10.05	3	3	+36
Marital therapy (cognitive-behavioral)	100	12.86	4	3	+34
Behavioral self-control training	68	12.94	17	17	+25
Cognitive therapy	86	10.26	3	4	+22
Aversion therapy (apnea)	100	9.66	2	1	+18
Covert sensitization	100	10.88	3	5	+18
Acupuncture	100	9.67	2	1	+14
Antidipsotropic—disulfiram	100	10.76	10	11	+09
Self-help manual	60	12.00	2	3	+01
Aversion therapy (electrical)	100	11.13	7	9	−03
Marital therapy (other)	100	12.25	4	4	−11
Placebo medication	100	13.00	1	2	−27
Stress management	80	11.00	1	4	−29
Lithium medication	100	11.43	3	4	−32
Functional analysis	67	12.00	0	3	−36
Relapse prevention	75	11.75	5	11	−37
Self-monitoring	100	13.00	1	2	−37
Antidepressant (SSRI)	36	8.45	5	6	−38
Hypnosis	100	10.25	0	4	−41
Psychedelic medication	100	9.88	2	6	−45
Antidipsotropic—calcium carbamide	100	10.00	0	3	−52
Antidepressant medication (non-SSRI)	100	8.75	0	4	−59
"Standard" treatment	80	10.20	1	4	−67
Milieu therapy	93	11.00	3	11	−78
Anxiolytic medication	100	8.25	3	9	−79
Videotape self-confrontation	100	10.29	0	7	−84
Alcoholics Anonymous (mandated)	80	11.40	1	4	−90
Antidipsotropic—metronidazole	100	9.64	1	10	−102
Relaxation training	69	10.81	3	13	−135
Confrontational counseling	67	11.67	0	9	−155
Psychotherapy	86	11.21	2	12	−163
General alcoholism counseling	84	11.20	2	17	−226
Educational lectures/films	35	9.68	4	27	−364
Treatment methods with only one or two outcome studies					
Sensory deprivation	0	10.00	2	0	+40
Biofeedback	100	13.00	2	0	+38
Cue exposure	100	10.00	2	0	+32
Developmental counseling	0	14.00	1	0	+28
Meditation	100	12.00	1	0	+24
Assessment only	0	11.00	1	0	+22
Dopamine antagonist	100	11.00	1	0	+22
Sedative—hypnotic medication	100	11.00	1	0	+22

TABLE 1 (*Continued*)

Modality	% Clinical	MQS	N+	N–	CES
Feedback	0	10.00	1	0	+20
Unilateral family therapy	0	10.00	1	0	+20
Case management	100	11.00	1	0	+11
Exercise	50	10.50	1	1	+09
Twelve-step facilitation	100	17.00	1	1	00
Tobacco cessation	100	6.00	0	1	–06
Minnesota Model	100	11.50	1	1	–10
Surveillance	100	11.00	0	1	–11
Neurotherapy	100	12.00	0	1	–12
Problem solving	100	12.00	0	1	–12
Legal interventions	0	11.00	0	1	–22
BAC discrimination training	100	12.00	0	2	–24
Choice of treatments	50	8.00	1	1	–24
Beta blocker medication	100	13.00	0	1	–26
Serotonin agonist medication	50	11.50	0	2	–34
Antipsychotic medication	100	9.00	0	2	–36
Dopamine agonist medication	100	9.00	0	2	–36
Placebo medication	100	11.00	0	2	–44

intermediate score may reflect a smaller volume of studies, or a larger number of studies with conflicting evidence. To avoid drawing conclusions from too few studies, we have separated in Table 1 those modalities with only one or two studies conducted to date. Obviously, there are many other treatment methods not mentioned at all in Table 1, for which not even a single controlled trial has been published. In addition to the CES for each modality, Table 1 shows the total number of positive (N+) and negative (N–) studies reviewed, and the average (mean) MQS (range = 0–17) for all studies of the modality, reflecting overall quality of evidence. Finally, we rated the severity of the client population being treated in each study. Ratings of 1 or 2 were given to nonclinical populations, such as those identified in medical care settings but not seeking treatment for alcohol problems. Ratings of 3 or 4 were given to clinical populations with clear evidence of significant alcohol problems (3) or dependence (4). The "% Clinical" column of Table 1 reflects the percentage of rated studies in which the treatment method was tested with a clinical population (3 or 4).

Some caveats are in order here. First, it is no simple matter to construct a summary such as that contained in Table 1. Many difficult qualitative decisions must be made, such as how to categorize treatment modalities to which one assigns particular studied therapies. The interpretation of Table 1 out of its qualitative context is thus hazardous. Beyond the more detailed methodology (Miller *et al.*, 1995), we provide in later sections our own qualitative reflections on the clinical implications of our review to date.

Furthermore, the weight that one gives to these data depends on one's rules of evidence (Miller & Hester, 1989). Some simply dismiss clinical research that conflicts with their own judgment and opinions. Some are concerned that controlled trials present only part of the picture, and seek to integrate evidence from uncontrolled outcome studies as well (Finney & Monahan, 1996; Miller & Hester, 1980). It is not uncommon for conclusions from uncontrolled studies to conflict with those of controlled trials. For example, it is a frequent observation that the longer people remain in treatment, the better their outcomes. Yet in controlled trials where clients are randomly assigned to longer versus shorter, or to more versus less intensive treatment for alcohol problems, differences in outcomes are seldom observed (Bien *et al.*, 1993; Institute of Medicine, 1990; Miller & Hester, 1986b). One's prior belief that "more is better" may be altered by this evidence, or may incline one to dismiss controlled trials as flawed and to embrace the testimony of uncontrolled studies. We have explicitly relied upon the findings of controlled (primarily randomized) clinical trials as a standard in estimating the efficacy of different treatments.

CLINICAL IMPLICATIONS OF OUTCOME EVIDENCE

ARE DIFFERENT TREATMENTS TRULY DIFFERENT?

One seemingly obvious conclusion from examination of Table 1 is that treatment approaches differ substantially in their demonstrated efficacy. In general, clients treated by consistently supported methods such as social skills training (+120) and the community reinforcement approach (+80) would be expected to benefit far more than those given educational lectures and films (−364), from which benefit has rarely been observed in controlled trials. This is not to say that all clients benefit from social skills training, or that no client ever benefits from educational lectures and films. It is a matter of relative probabilities.

This stands in contrast to a common impression that it makes little difference which method one provides or receives in treatment for alcohol problems. Project MATCH Research Group (1997), for example, found relatively few differences in outcomes from three carefully controlled treatments that were intentionally designed to differ dramatically in philosophy and execution. Roughly half of the clinical trials included in this review similarly found no significant differences between compared treatments. Such null findings, particularly from a large trial such as Project MATCH, can lead to a general cynicism that treatment method matters not at all, and that outcomes are determined by other factors such as client attributes and social environment.

On the other hand, about half of all controlled clinical trials *have* observed a significant outcome difference between compared treatments, and such positive findings have not been linked to either higher or lower methodological quality of studies (Miller *et al.*, 1995). The field thus seems to have a glass half full and half empty. It *does* often make a difference which treatment method a client receives, even in the controlled conditions of a clinical trial. Yet in other controlled trials, treatments that were expected to be very different have had similar outcomes.

To be sure, treatment method is not the *only*, and often not even the *primary* determinant of client outcomes. The relative contributions of treatment and extra-treatment factors are further complicated by their interaction. In the presence of potent treatments, individual differences would be expected to exert less relative influence on outcomes than in placebo treatments. Again, it is a matter of relative probabilities. No treatment works for everyone, and no single study is conclusive. If one gives credence to the *cumulative* evidence of clinical trials, however, it would seem sensible to emphasize in treatment those approaches found toward the top of Table 1, and to invest fewer resources in treatment methods with negative scores. Furthermore, where possible, it would seem sensible to have available a variety of empirically supported options. This should give clients the best chance of benefiting from treatment. Meanwhile, the search should continue for extratreatment determinants of outcome and the way these interact with factors in the content and delivery of treatment.

ENGAGING THE CLIENT'S OWN RESOURCES

The two modalities at the top of Table 1 could have been combined, and indeed have been collapsed in prior reviews (e.g., Holder *et al.*, 1991). They reflect the fact that even relatively brief counseling (1 to 4 sessions) is rather consistently found to be superior to no treatment or to placement on a waiting list, with benefits that endure over one or more years of follow-up (Bien *et al.*, 1993). This should not in itself be surprising, but it does require thought as to what may be happening in the context of brief intervention. Typically this approach involves no skill training, no medication, no aversive conditioning, and nothing ordinarily thought of as psychotherapy. Yet reliable behavior change occurs and endures, often with magnitude similar to that associated with more extensive treatments.

Six elements are frequently, though not invariably, present in effective brief interventions (Bien *et al.*, 1993; Miller & Sanchez, 1994; cf. Chapter 9, this volume), and are summarized by the acronym FRAMES. *Feedback* regarding the client's personal situation is often provided, based on systematic assessment of drinking and related problems at an initial visit and often at follow-up visits as well. This is not to be confused with providing general education about alcohol and its consequences (found at the very bottom of Table 1). The client's own *Responsibility* for change is emphasized, acknowledging that no one else can decide, force, or achieve behavior change for the client, who is free to change or to continue as before. Nevertheless, clear *Advice* to change is always given, sometimes with a *Menu* of alternative courses of action. As discussed later in this chapter, an *Empathic* counseling style is characteristic, as well as building client *Self-Efficacy* or optimism for the ability to achieve beneficial change. A blending of these six components is typical in reports of brief interventions that trigger change in problem drinking.

It is plausible that brief intervention impacts the client's perception or motivation, which sets in motion a self-directed process of change (Miller, 1997; Sobell & Sobell, 1993). Therapeutic methods identified in Table 1 as Motivational Enhancement explicitly focus on eliciting the client's intrinsic motivation for change (Miller & Rollnick, 1991; Miller, Zweben, DiClemente, & Rychtarik, 1992). The underlying view is that change is ultimately in the hands of the client, who has unique skills and resources to draw upon once a commitment to change is made. This philosophy is shared more generally by client-centered approaches, which also appear with a positive CES, and by other treatments not yet evaluated in controlled trials, such as solution-focused therapy (Berg & Miller, 1992). This is quite a different tone from the implicit view that treatment is something imparted from therapist to client (such as insight, knowledge, wisdom, or skills). Evoking the client's own motivation, wisdom, and resources is not, of course, incompatible with other strategies described here. It is noteworthy that the stages and processes of change appear to be quite similar whether occurring within or outside the context of treatment (Prochaska, DiClemente, & Norcross, 1992), and that therapy may therefore be a process of evoking and facilitating natural change processes (Sobell & Sobell, 1993; Tough, 1982). A more thorough discussion of motivational counseling strategies can be found in Chapter 9 (this volume).

TEACHING COPING SKILLS

A second strongly supported treatment strategy involves teaching clients behavioral coping skills for sober living. Effective treatment here has often focused on more *general* skills for successful living and relationships (such as communication and assertion skills), rather than on more specific skills for avoiding substance use. Prospective studies of relapse point to coping skills as a key element in maintaining sobriety. Active coping styles are prognostic of more favorable outcomes, whereas avoidant coping strategies are associated with higher risk of relapse (e.g., Miller, Westerberg, Harris, & Tonigan, 1996). Within this perspective, substance abuse may itself be viewed as a coping strategy, albeit not a very effective one in most cases, and prone to detrimental side effects. "Alcohol is not a problem for me," the saying goes, "it is a solution."

Social skills training is strongly supported in nearly all reviews of alcohol treatment outcome research. Social support has been found to be a robust predictor of sobriety (e.g., Project MATCH Research Group, 1997), and the ability to establish rewarding interpersonal relationships seems to be an important factor in preventing and reversing problematic drinking. Well-tested therapist guidelines are available for social skills training with problem drinkers (Kadden *et al.,* 1992; Monti, Abrams, Kadden, & Cooney, 1989).

Also prominent in reviews of effective treatment methods is the community reinforcement approach (CRA), originally introduced by Nathan Azrin and his colleagues (Azrin, Sisson, Meyers, & Godley, 1982; Hunt & Azrin, 1973). Based on operant learning theory, CRA seeks to change the client's social environment so that positive reinforcement is freely available without alcohol, whereas drinking leads to a "time out" or reduction in reinforcement. Emphasis is placed on developing rewarding employment, leisure activities, and relationships that do not involve alcohol or other drugs. A key is helping each client to find and become involved in what is more reinforcing, more valued, more dear to them than drinking. Whenever possible, significant others are engaged in CRA treatment as well, because they hold important sources of positive reinforcement for the client. CRA procedures for therapists have been well described by Meyers and Smith (1995).

The teaching of skills for managing one's own drinking behavior has also been evaluated. Simple strategies of behavior contracting have been found helpful—setting clear goals and establishing self-rewards for their achievement. Behavioral self-control training has been the subject of more controlled trials (34 as of this review) than any other treatment strategy for alcohol problems. Many of the "negative" trials here arise from the frequent finding that therapist-directed self-control training yields outcomes similar to those for a client self-directed approach working with written guidelines for self-control (Hester, 1995). It appears that *both* therapist-directed and self-directed self-control training reduce problematic drinking (cf. Harris & Miller, 1990).

Although coping skill training methods have often been called "cognitive-behavioral," there is substantially stronger support for teaching behavioral coping strategies than for cognitive restructuring. Evaluated separately, cognitive therapies attain a modest positive score (+22, with three positive and four negative studies), as compared with +120 for social skills training. "Relapse prevention" approaches focused on cognitive retraining show, on balance, a negative CES (−37). It is important to note here that the term "relapse prevention" has taken on such broad meanings that it represents a general change goal more than a specific treatment strategy. Marlatt's approach has long encompassed social skills training and active behavioral coping strategies (Marlatt & Gordon, 1985). Other methods have focused heavily on cognitive constructs such as self-efficacy (Annis, 1986). After two decades, Gorski's popular CENAPS approach (Gorski & Miller, 1982) still has not, to our knowledge, been subjected to a single controlled trial.

USING MEDICATIONS AS ADJUNCTS

The use of medications in treating alcoholism has had a rocky history. Treatment programs endorsing a "drug-free" philosophy have often shunned the use of psychiatric medications as a crutch or substitute for alcohol. At another extreme, the 1960s witnessed a series of studies of hallucinogens as therapeutic agents for alcoholism (CES = −45). Even the antibiotic metronidazole was used for two decades to treat alcoholism following unsubstantiated reports of its effectiveness (CES = −102). More recently, antidepressants, neuroleptics, lithium, and anxiolytic agents have all been tested without much in the way of encouraging results (all CES values negative).

An interesting puzzle is posed by the antidipsotropic agents—those that induce illness if the client drinks. The only such agent used in the United States, and the only one to be extensively evaluated, is disulfiram (Antabuse®), with 10 positive and 11 negative trials (CES = +9). There appears to be a clear deterrent placebo effect for clients who are told they are taking disulfiram, but the additional specific effect of the medication is usually modest, with best effects shown by those clients who faithfully take their prescribed doses (Fuller *et al.*, 1986). Relatedly, disulfiram has been found to suppress drinking more reliably when additional methods are used to ensure that it is taken.

Other medications have yielded more promising results. Naltrexone (Revia®), an opioid antagonist, has been found to reduce drinking and craving, and appears to be a useful adjunct in treating alcohol problems, although the high current cost of this medication has deterred its use. Acamprosate, a GABA agonist, has also shown encouraging results as a treatment adjunct in European outcome trials.

WORKING WITH RELATIONSHIPS

Family therapy has been a popular component of addiction treatment programs since the 1970s. As with relapse prevention, there is a definitional problem here, because family therapy is defined (as for billing purposes) simply by the presence of other family members in the treatment session. What is actually *done* with the family has varied widely.

Outcome research currently supports most strongly a behavioral approach, and here most studies have been devoted to marital or couples therapy rather than family therapy. That is, in most studies the client and spouse or partner have been treated together, without other family members present. Behavioral marital or family therapy emphasizes the teaching of skills to improve communication and behavior change negotiation, and works to increase the level of positive reinforcement exchanged by the couple—elements familiar from the community reinforcement approach described above. Including the spouse or partner in behavioral treatment has been found to enhance sobriety and improve relationship quality. Again, excellent therapist guidelines are available (e.g., O'Farrell, 1993). Relatively little is known about the efficacy of systemic, structural, and other family therapy approaches in treating alcohol problems, or about the benefits of including the larger family (rather than only the spouse or partner) in treatment.

A more recent strategy that shows promise is *unilateral* family therapy, which most often involves working through concerned significant others when the problem drinker is unmotivated for treatment (Meyers, Dominguez, & Smith, 1995). Patterns of reinforcement and communication can be altered within the family by working with even one cooperative member, and this provides an avenue for helping and engaging the unmotivated drinker. Unfortunately, the most popular unilateral intervention method, promoted by the Johnson Institute, has not yet been evaluated in a published controlled trial.

LESS SUPPORTED APPROACHES

What can be learned from the bottom of Table 1, if one accepts the evidence that these treatment approaches do not produce reliable change in drinking and related problems? It is striking that some of what have been central components in traditional American treatment programs are represented here. The lack of benefit from a treatment method is not a conclusive test of its underlying theory of etiology, nor does therapeutic efficacy prove the validity of a treatment's underlying conceptual framework. However, evidence regarding what works (and what does not) can provide at least indirect support for hypothesized mechanisms in the development and resolution of alcohol problems. (Such evidence is strengthened when treatment studies include direct tests of processes and causal chains predicted to underlie change.) The striking lack of support for the value of educational lectures and films about alcohol, for example, suggests that clinical alcohol problems are not the result of a knowledge deficit. (One must be careful here, in that "education" is a broad term that could encompass many of the behavioral skill training strategies described above.) Studies are also fairly consistent in finding little beneficial impact on drinking of psychodynamic psychotherapies, confrontational approaches, or undifferentiated individual alcoholism counseling or group psychotherapy. Though they have intuitive appeal, relaxation training and stress management are not well supported as beneficial components of treatment, adding to growing doubts that stress reduction is a key motivation for problematic drinking. No benefit has been shown for hypnosis. Although there may be pragmatic reasons for hospitalization or residential supervision (e.g., suicidal risk, homelessness, medical illness), there is little evidence that removal to an inpatient milieu yields greater benefit than can be accomplished on an outpatient basis with proper treatment methods.

Alcoholics Anonymous (AA) is widely lauded as an aid in recovery, and research does point to a positive association between AA involvement and abstinence (Emrick *et al.*, 1993; Montgomery, Miller, & Tonigan, 1995). Yet AA philosophy has also become intertwined with treatment approaches and etiologic models that are not part of (and in some cases are inconsistent with) the precepts and traditions of AA (Miller & Kurtz, 1994). The only randomized trial of a 12-step facilitation therapy, to date, found it to be associated with outcomes at least as favorable as those for cognitive-behavioral and motivational enhancement therapies (Project MATCH Research Group, 1997). A test of a treatment method based on the AA philosophy is not, of course, an evaluation of AA itself. Most controlled trials to date have focused on the efficacy of *mandating* individuals to attend AA meetings. Here the evidence is quite consistent in showing that coerced attendance at AA meetings does not improve outcomes, a finding that questions the common American practice of ordering AA involvement through the courts or employee assistance programs. It must be noted that this finding is by no means an indication of the efficacy of AA when sought voluntarily, and that coerced involvement directly conflicts with precepts set forth in AA's own core literature (Miller & Kurtz, 1994).

OTHER IMPORTANT FINDINGS

Though reflected only indirectly in the studies of Table 1, there are other research findings that can inform clinical practice in important ways. We limit this closing discussion to three such findings.

EMPATHY

There is strong evidence that within any given treatment approach or program, clients fare significantly better or worse depending on the particular therapist with whom they work (Najavits & Weiss, 1994). This is so even when clients are randomly assigned to therapists, eliminating possible biases in case assignment. What accounts for such therapist differences?

Several studies point to therapist empathy as a key factor in clients' long-term outcomes. This is not empathy in the sense of being able to *identify with* alcoholics by virtue of being in recovery oneself. Studies consistently show that personal recovery status neither increases nor decreases therapists' effectiveness in treating clients with alcohol problems. Rather, the type of therapist empathy associated with more favorable client outcomes is that described by Carl Rogers and his students: the ability to listen reflectively, clarify the client's meaning, and allow the client to continue experiencing his or her own processes without the imposition of the therapist's own material or judgments (Gordon & Edwards, 1995; Truax & Carkhuff, 1967; cf. Chapter 9, this volume). Clients show better short-term and long-term drinking outcomes when treated by therapists who display high levels of client-centered counseling skills.

ACTIVE INTEREST

Clients also benefit when therapists take an *active* interest in them. Even the intangible quality of believing in a client's ability to change can be a powerful self-fulfilling prophecy (Leake & King, 1977). For present purposes, we are referring to relatively specific and concrete expressions of caring. As shown in several studies, a simple handwritten note or telephone call after the first visit, or after a missed visit, can double or triple the likelihood that a client will return (Miller, 1985). When making a referral, the probability that a client will actually get there is dramatically increased by placing the call and making the appointment from the office, rather than just giving the client the phone number to call. In the U.S. alcohol field, such helpful actions have somehow become muddled with and inhibited by notions of "enabling" and "taking responsibility." The fact is that such simple acts of caring can substantially enhance motivation for and the likelihood of change (see Chapter 9, this volume).

ADHERENCE

Another very consistent finding, informative for clinicians, is that a client's *doing something* toward change is one of the best predictors of actual change in drinking. Just the taking of a step, the doing of something, may be more important than the specific content of the action. Clients who get more actively involved in AA tend to get better, although just going to meetings may not be enough (Montgomery *et al.*, 1995). Those who take their medication faithfully (even if it is a placebo) tend to get better. Those who do their therapy homework assignments tend to get better. This suggests two guidelines for therapists. First, keep clients actively involved in their own recovery. Avoid the implication that the therapy or therapist will somehow cure them if they endure passively. Just showing up is a start, but not enough. Second, help clients find what they are willing (even eager) to do toward their own recovery. Offer a menu of options, rather than prescribing one way that may not be attractive or acceptable. Do not focus on trying to make the client do what you think they need, but negotiate with the client what would be acceptable steps in the right direction. Inertia has two meanings: a body at rest tends to stay at rest, and a body in motion tends to stay in motion.

SUMMARY

This is a genuinely exciting time to be treating alcohol problems. Table 1 reflects a virtual armamentarium of options with good evidence of helpfulness. Although no one of these works for all or even most clients on first try, the fact is that in the long run most people with serious alcohol problems do resolve them and go on to live more stable and happy lives. The ways in which they do so are legion, and only a minority of them ever come for professional help. When they do, we have much to offer that is likely to be of benefit. A comprehensive treatment program can offer a variety of approaches chosen from those with sound scientific evidence of efficacy. Clients can be engaged actively in the selection and design of their own program of change. A helpful and honest message is, "We can work together to try what seems most likely to help you. If it works, great. If not, don't be discouraged or take it personally. It most likely would mean that we hadn't yet found the right approach for you. There are many different ways in which people change successfully, and I will stay with you until we find what works for you."

REFERENCES

Annis, H. M. (1986). A relapse prevention model for treatment of alcoholics. In W. R. Miller & N. Heather (Eds.), *Treating addictive behaviors: Processes of change* (pp. 407–433). New York: Plenum.

Azrin, N. H., Sisson, R. W., Meyers, R., & Godley, M. (1982). Alcoholism treatment by disulfiram and community reinforcement therapy. *Journal of Behavior Therapy and Experimental Psychiatry, 13,* 105–112.

Berg, I. K., & Miller, S. D. (1992). *Working with the problem drinker: A solution-focused approach.* New York: Norton.

Bien, T. H., Miller, W. R., & Tonigan, J. S. (1993). Brief interventions for alcohol problems: A review. *Addiction, 88,* 315–336.

Emrick, C. D., Tonigan, J. S., Montgomery, H., & Little, L. (1993). Alcoholics Anonymous: What is currently known? In B. S. McCrady & W. R. Miller (Eds.), *Alcoholics Anonymous: Opportunities and alternatives* (pp. 41–76). New Brunswick, NJ: Rutgers Center of Alcohol Studies.

Finney, J. W., & Monahan, S. C. (1996). The cost-effectiveness of treatment for alcoholism: A second approximation. *Journal of Studies on Alcohol, 57,* 229–243.

Fuller, R. K., Branchey, L., Brightwell, D. R., Derman, R. M., Emrick, C. D., Iber, F. L., James, K. E., Lacoursiere, R. B., Lee, K. K., Lowenstam, I., Maany, I., Neiderheider, D., Nocks, J. J., & Shaw, S. (1986). Disulfiram treatment of alcoholism: A Veterans Administration cooperative study. *Journal of Nervous and Mental Disease, 256,* 1449–1455.

Gordis, E. (1987). Accessible and affordable health care for alcoholism and related problems: Strategy for cost containment. *Journal of Studies on Alcohol, 48,* 579–585.

Gordon, T., & Edwards, S. (1995). *Making your patient your partner.* Westport, CT: Auburn House.

Gorski, T. T., & Miller, M. (1982). *Counseling for relapse prevention.* Independence, MO: Herald House–Independence Press.

Harris, K. B., & Miller, W. R. (1990). Behavioral self-control training for problem drinkers: Components of efficacy. *Psychology of Addictive Behaviors, 4,* 82–90.

Hester, R. K. (1995). Behavioral self-control training. In R. K. Hester & W. R. Miller (Eds.), *Handbook of alcoholism treatment approaches: Effective alternatives* (2nd ed., pp. 148–159). Boston: Allyn & Bacon.

Hester, R. K., & Miller, W. R. (1995). *Handbook of alcoholism treatment approaches: Effective alternatives* (2nd ed.). Boston: Allyn & Bacon.

Holder, H., Longabaugh, R., Miller, W. R., & Rubonis, A. V. (1991). The cost effectiveness of treatment for alcoholism: A first approximation. *Journal of Studies on Alcohol, 52,* 517–540.

Hunt, G. M., & Azrin, N. H. (1973). A community-reinforcement approach to alcoholism. *Behaviour Research and Therapy, 11,* 91–104.

Institute of Medicine. (1990). *Broadening the base of treatment for alcohol problems.* Washington, DC: National Academy Press.

Kadden, R., Carroll, K., Donovan, D., Cooney, N., Monti, P., Abrams, D., Litt, M., & Hester, R. (1992). *Cognitive-behavioral coping skills therapy manual.* Rockville, MD: National Institute on Alcohol Abuse and Alcoholism.

Leake, G. J., & King, A. S. (1977). Effect of counselor expectations on alcoholic recovery. *Alcohol Health and Research World, 11*(3), 16–22.

Marlatt, G. A., & Gordon, J. R. (1985). *Relapse prevention.* New York: Guilford.

Mattick, R. P., & Jarvis, T. J. (Eds.). (1992). *An outline for the management of alcohol problems: Quality assurance project.* Sydney, Australia: National Drug Abuse Research Centre.

Meyers, R. J., & Smith, J. E. (1995). *Clinical guide to alcohol treatment: The community reinforcement approach.* New York: Guilford.

Meyers, R. J., Dominguez, T., & Smith, J. E. (1995). Community reinforcement training with concerned others. In V. B. Hasselt & M. Hersen (Eds.), *Sourcebook of psychological treatment manuals for adults* (pp. 257–294). New York: Plenum.

Miller, W. R. (1985). Motivation for treatment: A review with special emphasis on alcoholism. *Psychological Bulletin, 98*, 84–107.

Miller, W. R. (in press). *Why do people change addictive behavior?* The 1996 H. David Archibald Lecture. *Addiction.*

Miller, W. R., & Hester, R. K. (1980). Treating the problem drinker: Modern approaches. In W. R. Miller (Ed.), *The addictive behaviors: Treatment of alcoholism, drug abuse, smoking, and obesity* (pp. 11–141). Oxford, England: Pergamon.

Miller, W. R., & Hester, R. K. (1986a). The effectiveness of alcoholism treatment methods: What research reveals. In W. R. Miller & N. Heather (Eds.), *Treating addictive behaviors: Processes of change* (pp. 121–174). New York: Plenum.

Miller, W. R., & Hester, R. K. (1986b). Inpatient alcoholism treatment: Who benefits? *American Psychologist, 41*, 794–805.

Miller, W. R., & Hester, R. K. (1986c). Matching problem drinkers with optimal treatments. In W. R. Miller & N. Heather (Eds.), *Treating addictive behaviors: Processes of change* (pp. 175–203). New York: Plenum.

Miller, W. R., & Hester, R. K. (1989). Inpatient alcoholism treatment: Rules of evidence and burden of proof. *American Psychologist, 44*, 1245–1246.

Miller, W. R., & Kurtz, E. (1994). Models of alcoholism used in treatment: Contrasting A.A. and other perspectives with which it is often confused. *Journal of Studies on Alcohol, 55*, 159–166.

Miller, W. R., & Rollnick, S. (1991). *Motivational interviewing: Preparing people for change.* New York: Guilford.

Miller, W. R., & Sanchez, V. C. (1994). Motivating young adults for treatment and lifestyle change. In G. Howard (Ed.), *Issues in alcohol use and misuse by young adults* (pp. 55–82). Notre Dame, IN: University of Notre Dame Press.

Miller, W. R., Zweben, A., DiClemente, C. C., & Rychtarik, R. G. (1992). *Motivational Enhancement Therapy manual: A clinical research guide for therapists treating individuals with alcohol abuse and dependence* (Vol. 2, Project MATCH Monograph Series). Rockville, MD: National Institute on Alcohol Abuse and Alcoholism.

Miller, W. R., Brown, J. M., Simpson, T. L., Handmaker, N. S., Bien, T. H., Luckie, L. F., Montgomery, H. A., Hester, R. K., & Tonigan, J. S. (1995). What works? A methodological analysis of the alcohol treatment outcome literature. In R. K. Hester & W. R. Miller (Eds.), *Handbook of alcoholism treatment approaches: Effective alternatives* (2nd ed., pp. 12–44). Boston: Allyn & Bacon.

Miller, W. R., Westerberg, V. S., Harris, R. J., & Tonigan, J. S. (1996). What predicts relapse? Prospective testing of antecedent models. *Addiction, 91* (Suppl.), S151–S172.

Montgomery, H. A., Miller, W. R., & Tonigan, J. S. (1995). Does Alcoholics Anonymous involvement predict treatment outcome? *Journal of Substance Abuse Treatment, 12*, 241–246.

Monti, P. M., Abrams, D. B., Kadden, R. M., & Cooney, N. L. (1989). *Treating alcohol dependence: A coping skills training guide.* New York: Guilford.

Najavits, L. M., & Weiss, R. D. (1994). Variations in therapist effectiveness in the treatment of patients with substance use disorders: An empirical review. *Addiction, 89*, 679–688.

O'Farrell, T. J. (Ed.). (1993). *Treating alcohol problems: Marital and family interventions.* New York: Guilford.

Prochaska, J. O., DiClemente, C. C., & Norcross, J. C. (1992). In search of how people change: Applications to addictive behaviors. *American Psychologist, 47*, 1102–1114.

Project MATCH Research Group. (1997). Matching alcoholism treatments to client heterogeneity: Project MATCH posttreatment drinking outcomes. *Journal of Studies on Alcohol, 58*, 7–29.

Shapiro, A. K. (1971). Placebo effects in medicine, psychotherapy, and psychoanalysis. In A. E. Bergin & S. L. Garfield (Eds.), *Handbook of psychotherapy and behavior change: An empirical analysis* (pp. 439–473). New York: Wiley.

Sobell, M. B., & Sobell, L. C. (1993). *Problem drinkers: Guided self-change treatment.* New York: Guilford.

Tonigan, J. S., Toscova, R., & Miller, W. R. (1996). Meta-analysis of the Alcoholics Anonymous literature: Sample and study characteristics moderate findings. *Journal of Studies on Alcohol, 57*, 65–72.

Tough, A. (1982). *Intentional changes.* Chicago: Follett.

Truax, C. B., & Carkhuff, R. R. (1967). *Toward effective counseling and psychotherapy.* Chicago: Aldine.

16

Treating Drug Dependence

Recent Advances and Old Truths

KATHLEEN M. CARROLL

INTRODUCTION: THE OLD TRUTHS

In the decade since the publication of the first edition of *Treating Addictive Behaviors,* much has changed in the treatment of drug abuse and dependence disorders. Most important, there is a much wider variety of effective psychotherapies and pharmacotherapies available to clinicians. For example, several new psychotherapeutic strategies have been developed and evaluated using the methods associated with the technology model of psychotherapy research (Waskow, 1984). The technology model requires specification of treatments in manuals as well as differentiation of the unique "active ingredients" of a treatment from its common, or shared, factors (Carroll & Rounsaville, 1990). Application of this model to psychosocial treatments for substance use has greatly enhanced investigators' ability to clearly define and then rigorously evaluate different therapies and thus to provide clearer information to the clinicians regarding what types of therapy may be most effective for treating substance use disorders. Several new pharmacotherapies are also available, the development of which has been closely linked to scientific advances in understanding the neurobiology of substance abuse, including neurotransmitter systems associated with the maintenance of drug dependence and brain changes associated with chronic use (O'Brien, 1996).

   Treatment of drug abuse and dependence has also advanced through greater recognition of commonalities across the substance use disorders. This included

KATHLEEN M. CARROLL   •   Division of Substance Abuse, Yale University, New Haven, Connecticut 06519.

Treating Addictive Behaviors, 2nd ed., edited by Miller and Heather. Plenum Press, New York, 1998.

codification of substance abuse and dependence disorders as essentially behavioral syndromes in *DSM-IV* (American Psychiatric Association, 1994), which deemphasized physical aspects of dependence such as tolerance and withdrawal. This opened the door for greater appreciation of the range of severity among individuals with drug use disorders, recognizing the importance of detecting and treating substance use disorders in their early stages, and expanding the breadth and role of treatment beyond management of withdrawal, stabilization, and treatment of comorbid disorders, and thus the need for an expanded repertoire of treatment options.

While many more treatment options are available, much has also remained the same and many of the general principles that applied to the treatment of drug abuse 10 years ago are relevant today.

Drug-Abusing Individuals Are Heterogeneous and Must Be Treated as Such

Given the diversity of drug-dependent individuals on important dimensions such as severity of drug dependence, type of substance use, nature and level of comorbid diagnoses and concurrent problems, readiness for change, and so on, the development of a single approach that is universally effective for any type of drug dependence is improbable. That is, even for our most effective treatment approaches, a great deal of variability in outcome is seen across different individuals.

Thus, an essential step in treatment planning remains a thorough pretreatment assessment to determine the appropriate treatment approach for the particular individual at the particular time. That is, while the empirical literature may guide clinicians to a range of treatments of proven efficacy, the selection of a particular treatment approach and the appropriate intensity of treatment remains largely a matter of clinical judgment and availability of resources.

Treatment Outcomes Should Be Multidimensional

The range of concurrent problems and disorders seen in most drug-dependent individuals dictates that while reduction in drug abuse is an important indicator of treatment success, improvement in drug use does not guarantee resolution of other psychosocial problems, and problems in these areas can impede the effectiveness of substance abuse treatment (McLellan, Luborsky, Woody, O'Brien, & Kron, 1981). Thus, it remains critical to address and monitor patients' functioning in a range of spheres, including employment, social, medical, legal, and psychiatric (McLellan *et al.*, 1994; Chapter 13, this volume).

Drug Dependence Is a Chronic Disorder Characterized by Relapse

While some individuals may become and remain fully abstinent after a single treatment episode, this is extremely rare. Drug-using careers are highly variable and characterized by heterogeneity in their course, with many individuals alternating periods of abstinence, relapse, low-intensity use, and high-intensity use. An approach that may have been suitable for a particular patient several years before may not be appropriate later (see Chapter 12, this volume).

No One Form of Treatment Is Universally Effective

The two major approaches to the treatment of drug dependence, psychotherapy and pharmacotherapy, differ in many ways. This includes, first, their time to effect change. Most pharmacotherapies achieve their effects quickly, whereas psychotherapies generally take longer to work but may have greater durability of effects after they are terminated. Second, psychotherapies and pharmacotherapies differ in terms of their applicability across drug classes. For example, while the same psychotherapy can often be applied, with only minor adaptation, across marijuana, cocaine, and heroin dependence, most available pharmacotherapies are applicable to only a single class of substance use (e.g., methadone produces cross-tolerance to heroin but typically does not directly affect cocaine use). Finally, these two major forms of treatment differ in their roles and focus of action. The roles of pharmacotherapies are typically detoxification, stabilization and maintenance, reduction of reinforcing properties of drugs, and treatment of coexisting psychiatric disorders. The roles and common tasks of most psychotherapies include fostering motivation, teaching coping skills, changing reinforcement contingencies, enhancing affect management, improving interpersonal functioning, and often, fostering compliance with pharmacotherapy (Carroll, 1997; Rounsaville & Carroll, 1992).

Each form of treatment also has its weaknesses. Psychosocial treatments for drug use disorders are beleaguered by problems associated with attrition, and no one form of psychosocial treatment has emerged as superior to others. Similarly, most pharmacotherapies are insufficient when delivered alone, that is, without concurrent psychosocial support. Furthermore, as noted above, most pharmacotherapies are narrow in their targets and affect only a single class of substance use; this is a marked disadvantage in the many cases where the individual abuses multiple substances concurrently (e.g., cocaine-heroin or alcohol-cocaine use).

Thus, as is highlighted throughout this review, combinations of psychotherapy and pharmacotherapy are generally seen as more effective than either type of treatment alone. This may be because with combination treatments, improvement is usually seen over a broader range of symptoms, each form of treatment may offset drawbacks of the other, and there is greater opportunity for patient–treatment matching (Carroll, 1997).

Treatments with High Levels of Empirical Support Are Not Those Most Widely Practiced

In the field of addictions treatment, and especially in the United States, there tends to be an inverse relationship between treatments with the highest level of empirical support and those most widely practiced. For example, many methadone programs continue to offer ineffective doses of methadone and inadequate psychosocial treatment (Ball & Ross, 1991; General Accounting Office, 1990). Opioid detoxification without follow-up care, which is associated with extremely high rates of relapse, remains a commonly used approach. Poorly defined psychosocial approaches and "alternative treatments" (e.g., acupuncture) with scant empirical support are widely available, whereas well-supported approaches, such as behavioral treatments, are rare in many clinical programs.

This chapter provides an overview of the current status of the treatment out-come literature for the major classes of drug dependence (opioids, cocaine, and marijuana). Based on the empirical literature and limited to randomized clinical trials of adult substance users that have evaluated drug abuse outcomes, this chapter focuses on what clinicians should know about the current status of treating drug users.

TREATMENT STRATEGIES FOR DRUG DEPENDENCE: WHAT RESEARCH REVEALS

OPIOIDS

Successful treatments for opiate dependence have generally involved some combination of psychotherapy and pharmacotherapy, most convincingly demonstrated by the disappointing results usually achieved when either modality is used alone. Purely pharmacologic approaches have generally yielded poor retention and limited outcomes, but marked improvements have been noted when a behavioral or psychotherapeutic component is added to pharmacologic interventions such as medication-assisted detoxification (e.g., Rawson, Mann, Tennant, & Clabough, 1983), narcotic antagonist programs (e.g., Meyer, Mirin, Altman, & McNamee, 1976), and methadone maintenance (e.g., McLellan, Arndt, Metzger, Woody, & O'Brien, 1993).

Conversely, while it has been almost impossible to engage opiate addicts in treatment with a purely psychotherapeutic approach (Rounsaville & Kleber, 1985), delivery of psychotherapy within methadone maintenance programs has enabled investigators to rigorously contrast different psychotherapeutic approaches and identify those addicts who benefit most from professional psychotherapy over standard drug counseling during methadone maintenance (e.g., Woody *et al.*, 1983). Thus, studies demonstrating efficacy of psychotherapy or behavioral treatments for opiate addicts have generally involved psychotherapy-pharmacotherapy combinations, in which initial stabilization of the patient (usually through methadone maintenance) is required before the patient can become available for psychotherapy.

Methadone Maintenance

The development of methadone maintenance in the 1960s revolutionized the treatment of opioid addiction as it displayed for the first time the ability to keep addicts in treatment and to reduce their illicit opioid use, outcomes with which nonpharmacologic treatments had fared comparatively poorly (O'Malley, Anderson, & Lazare, 1972). Beyond its ability to retain opioid addicts in treatment and attenuate opioid use, by substituting the longer-acting methadone for shorter-acting illicit opioids, methadone maintenance provides an important means of stabilization for many opioid addicts, and thus offers the opportunity to evaluate and treat concurrent medical, psychiatric, and psychosocial problems (Kreek, 1992; Lowinsohn, Marion, Joseph, & Dole, 1992; Ward, Mattick, & Hall, 1992). Methadone maintenance also reduces the risk of HIV infection and other serious medical morbidities associated with intravenous drug use (Ball, Lange, Myers, & Friedman,

1988; Kreek, 1992). Despite its many advantages, methadone maintenance treatment remains controversial (O'Brien, 1996). This is in large part because of the lengthy treatment episodes generally required to produce satisfactory outcomes; ongoing high rates of concurrent cocaine, alcohol, and benzodiazepine abuse seen in many programs; illicit diversion of take-home methadone doses; and the difficulties seen for most patients in detoxification from methadone and transition to a drug-free state.

Moreover, there is a great deal of variability in the effectiveness of different methadone maintenance programs, which is largely the result of variability in delivery of adequate dosing of methadone as well as variability in provision and quality of psychosocial services (Ball & Ross, 1991). The importance of psychosocial treatments in the context of methadone treatment was impressively demonstrated by McLellan and colleagues (1993). In this study, 92 opiate addicts were randomly assigned to receive either (1) methadone maintenance with doses of proven effectiveness, but without psychosocial services, (2) methadone maintenance with standard services, which included regular meetings with a counselor, or (3) enhanced methadone maintenance, which included regular counseling plus on-site medical and psychiatric services, employment counseling, and family therapy, in a 24-week trial. Although some patients did reasonably well in the methadone alone condition, 69% of this group had to be transferred out of this condition within 3 months of the study inception because their substance use did not improve or worsened to a level associated with unacceptable risks, or because they experienced significant medical or psychiatric problems that required a more intensive level of care. In terms of drug use and psychosocial outcomes, best outcomes were seen in the enhanced methadone maintenance condition, with intermediate outcomes for the standard methadone services condition, and poorest outcomes for the methadone alone condition. This study underlines that although methadone maintenance treatment has powerful effects in terms of keeping addicts in treatment and making them available for psychosocial interventions, a purely pharmacologic approach will not be sufficient for most patients and better outcomes are associated with higher levels of psychosocial treatments.

Psychotherapy in the Context of Methadone Maintenance. A study that established the value of psychotherapy in methadone maintenance treatment was conducted at the Philadelphia VA by Woody and colleagues (1983). This study is a landmark because it was the first in this area to include important design features such as random assignment to treatment conditions, specification of treatment in manuals, use of experienced and well-trained therapists, ongoing monitoring of therapy implementation, multidimensional ratings of outcome by independent raters, and adequate sample size.

One hundred ten opiate addicts entering a methadone maintenance program were randomly assigned to one of three treatments: drug counseling alone, drug counseling plus supportive-expressive psychotherapy (SE), or drug counseling plus cognitive-behavioral psychotherapy (CB). After a 6-month course of treatment, while the SE and CB groups did not differ significantly from each other on most measures of outcome, subjects who received either form of professional psychotherapy evidenced greater improvement in more outcome domains than the subjects who received drug counseling alone (Woody et al., 1983). Furthermore, gains made by the subjects who received professional psychotherapy were sustained over a 12-month follow-up, whereas subjects receiving drug counseling alone evidenced some attrition of gains (Woody, McLellan, Luborsky, O'Brien, 1987).

This study also demonstrated differential response to psychotherapy as a function of patient characteristics, which may point to the best use of psychotherapy (relative to drug counseling) when resources are scarce: While methadone-maintained opiate addicts with lower levels of psychopathology tended to improve regardless of whether they received professional psychotherapy or drug counseling, those with higher levels of psychopathology tended to improve only if they received psychotherapy. In addition, this study provides indications on differential response to psychotherapy by concurrent psychiatric disorder. For example, depressed addicts improved with psychotherapy, while addicts with antisocial personality disorder (ASP) tended to show little or no improvement unless they also had a depressive disorder (Woody, McLellan, Luborsky, & O'Brien, 1985). In a later analysis, Gerstley and colleagues (1989) expanded these findings and pointed out heterogeneity in treatment response among subjects with ASP. That is, response to psychotherapy for subjects with antisocial personality disorder who were able to form a positive working relationship with their therapist was better than for antisocials who did not. This suggests that there is variability in the treatment process and outcome even for the poor-prognosis group of substance abusers with antisocial personality disorder. Finally, a partial replication of this study in community drug abuse treatment settings (Woody, McLellan, Luborsky, & O'Brien, 1995) demonstrated better outcome across time for those treated with supportive-expressive therapy compared with drug counseling alone.

Despite sound empirical support in other types of substance use and intuitive appeal, few studies of motivational approaches have been completed with drug-dependent populations. Recently, however, Saunders, Wilkinson, and Phillips (1995) compared brief motivational counseling to an educational control condition for 122 subjects attending a methadone maintenance clinic. Subjects treated with motivational counseling had fewer opioid-related problems and greater commitment to abstinence; however, statistically significant differences were not seen on outcome variables including severity of opioid dependence.

Behavioral Treatments in the Context of Methadone Maintenance. A variety of behavioral approaches have been evaluated to reduce illicit substance use among methadone-maintained opiate addicts. Several features of standard methadone maintenance treatment (daily attendance, frequent urine monitoring, reinforcing properties of methadone) have offered researchers the opportunity to control reinforcers available to patients and hence to evaluate the effects of both positive and negative contingencies on outcome within methadone maintenance programs (Carroll & Rounsaville, 1995).

For example, methadone take-home privileges contingent on reduced drug use is an attractive approach, as it capitalizes on an inexpensive reinforcer which is potentially available in all methadone maintenance programs. Stitzer and her colleagues (Stitzer, Iguchi, Kidorf, & Bigelow, 1993) have done extensive work in evaluating methadone take-home privileges as a reward for decreased illicit drug use. In a series of well-controlled trials, this group of researchers has demonstrated (1) the relative benefits of positive over negative contingencies (Stitzer,

Bickel, Bigelow, & Liebson, 1986), (2) the attractiveness of take-home privileges over other incentives available within methadone maintenance clinics (Stitzer & Bigelow, 1978), (3) the effectiveness of targeting and rewarding drug-free urines over other, more distal behaviors such as group attendance (Iguchi et al., 1996), and (4) the benefits of using take-home privileges contingent on drug-free urines over noncontingent take-home privileges (Stitzer, Iguchi, & Felch, 1992).

Several studies have evaluated negative contingencies only (Dolan, Black, Penk, Rabinowitz, & DeFord, 1985; McCarthy & Borders, 1985; Saxon, Calsyn, Kivlahan, & Roszell, 1993). These have demonstrated that approximately 40% to 60% of subjects are able to reduce or stop illicit substance use under threat of methadone dose reduction or treatment termination. However, fully half the subjects in these studies do not reduce their substance use under these conditions and are forced to leave treatment. Often, patients who do not comply with behavioral requirements and are terminated are those with more frequent or severe polysubstance use (Dolan et al., 1985; Saxon et al., 1993). Thus, these studies demonstrate that while negative contingencies may reduce or stop illicit substance use in some methadone-maintenance patients, these somewhat draconian procedures may also have the undesirable effect of terminating treatment for those severely impaired patients who may need treatment most but who have difficulty complying (Stitzer et al., 1986). Moreover, continued drug-positive urines in a patient may indicate the need to raise, rather than lower, the dose of methadone (as well as to increase the intensity of psychosocial interventions).

The use of cue exposure procedures, aimed at extinguishing cues for conditioned craving for opiates by pairing exposure to specific conditioned cues with conditions incompatible with use (Childress, Ehrman, Rohsenow, Robbins, & O'Brien, 1992), does seem helpful in reducing craving but the efficacy of these procedures in influencing other outcomes, such as reduced illicit drug use, has not yet been convincingly demonstrated (McLellan, Childress, O'Brien, & Ehrman, 1986). Similar findings have also been reported for extinction procedures with cocaine patients (Childress, Ehrman, McLellan, & O'Brien, 1988), in whom extinction of craving to some cocaine cues has been demonstrated, but it is not yet clear whether extinction generalizes to other cues that are more difficult to control in laboratory or treatment settings, or whether extinction of craving has an appreciable effect on drug use (Childress et al., 1992).

Other Maintenance Therapies

A longer-acting opioid, LAAM (levo-alpha-acetylemethadol), was recently approved by the FDA, and appears comparable to methadone in reducing opioid use (American Psychiatric Association, 1995; O'Brien, 1996). Because of LAAM's longer halflife, a major advantage of LAAM compared with methadone is that dosing can occur three times a week, rather than daily, allowing for fewer clinic visits (Tennant, Rawson, Pumphrey, & Seecof, 1986), thus broadening its appeal to some patients. A partial opioid agonist, buprenorphine, is another new maintenance pharmacotherapy. A potential advantage of buprenorphine is that it may have a better safety profile and lower risk of overdose, as high doses do not produce respiratory depression and other agonist effects seen in methadone and LAAM (American Psychiatric Association, 1995; O'Brien, 1996). In addition, withdrawal symptoms after termination of low-dose buprenorphine treatment may be milder. Early studies have suggested that buprenorphine may be comparable to methadone in retention and reduction of opioid use; however, early reports that buprenorphine treatment was also associated with decreased cocaine use have not been widely supported (Strain, Stitzer, Liebson, & Bigelow, 1994). It is important to note that, like methadone, both LAAM and buprenorphine are unlikely to be effective without concurrent psychosocial treatment. Hence, a major unanswered question is the optimal type and level of psychosocial treatment to be delivered with these new maintenance approaches.

Opioid Antagonists

Naltrexone, an opioid antagonist, offers an important alternative to maintenance treatments. Naltrexone is nonaddicting and can be prescribed without concerns about diversion, has a benign side-effect profile, and may be less costly, in terms of demands on professional time and patient time, than the daily or nearly daily clinic visits required for maintenance treatment (Rounsaville, 1995). Most important are behavioral aspects of the treatment, as unreinforced opiate use allows extinction of relationships between cues and drug use. However, naltrexone has not, despite its many advantages, fulfilled its promise. Naltrexone treatment programs remain comparatively rare and underutilized in comparison with methadone maintenance programs. This is in large part due to problems with retention, particularly during the induction phase, in which on average 40% of patients drop out during the first month of treatment and 60% drop out by 3 months (Greenstein, Fudala, & O'Brien, 1992). However, the addition of behavioral and psychotherapeutic interventions targeted to address naltrexone's weaknesses consistently points to the value of these interventions in improving naltrexone compliance and outcome. Successful approaches have included contingency management (Grabowski *et al.*, 1979; Meyer *et al.*, 1976), behavioral therapies (Callahan *et al.*, 1980), and family therapy (Anton, Hogan, Jalali, Riordan, & Kleber, 1981).

COCAINE

While a wide variety of pharmacologic approaches have been evaluated (including tricyclic antidepressants such as desipramine, anticonvulsants such as carbamazepine, or selective serotonin reuptake inhibitors, such as fluoxetine), none, as yet, has consistently demonstrated its effectiveness relative to placebo in keeping cocaine abusers in treatment or reducing their cocaine use (American Psychiatric Association, 1995; Meyer, 1992; O'Brien, 1996).

However, several psychosocial strategies have emerged as effective treatments for cocaine dependence (Crits-Cristoph & Siqueland, 1996; General Accounting Office, 1996). Perhaps the most exciting findings pertaining to the effectiveness of psychosocial treatments for cocaine dependence have been the recent reports of Higgins and colleagues (Higgins & Budney, 1993; Higgins *et al.*, 1991) of the effectiveness of a program incorporating positive incentives for abstinence, reciprocal relationship counseling, and disulfiram into a community reinforcement approach (CRA; Sisson & Azrin, 1989). The Higgins strategy has four organizing features which are grounded in principles of behavioral pharmacology: (1) drug use and abstinence must be swiftly and accurately detected, (2) abstinence is positively reinforced, (3) drug use results in loss of reinforcement, and (4) emphasis is placed on the development of competing reinforcers to drug use (Higgins & Budney, 1993).

In this program, urine specimens are required three times weekly. Abstinence, assessed through drug-free urine screens, is reinforced through a voucher system in which patients receive points redeemable for items consistent with a drug-free lifestyle, such as movie tickets, sporting goods, and the like, but patients never receive money directly. To encourage longer periods of consecutive abstinence, the value of the points earned by the patients increases with each successive clean urine specimen, and the value of the points is reset back to its original level when the patient produces a drug-positive urine screen or the patient does not provide a urine specimen.

In a series of well-controlled clinical trials, Higgins has demonstrated (1) there was high acceptance, retention, and rates of abstinence for patients randomized to this approach (85% completing a 12-week course of treatment; 65% achieving 6 or more weeks of abstinence) relative to standard 12-step–oriented substance abuse counseling (Higgins & Budney, 1993; Higgins *et al.*, 1991); (2) rates of abstinence did not decline when less valuable incentives, such as lottery tickets, were substituted for the voucher system (Higgins, Budney, Bickel, & Hughes, 1993); (3) the value of the voucher system itself (as opposed to other program elements) in reducing cocaine use was assessed by comparing the behavioral system with and without the vouchers (Higgins *et al.*, 1994); (4) the durability of treatment effects after cessation of the voucher system (Higgins *et al.*, 1995) was high; and (5) this approach could be generalized to other populations and treatment settings, including methadone maintenance programs (Silverman *et al.*, 1996).

Cognitive-behavioral treatment (CBT) for cocaine dependence has also been widely studied and has a fair level of empirical support (American Psychiatric Association, 1995, Crits-Christoph & Siqueland, 1996; General Accounting Office, 1996). CBT usually incorporates skills training aimed at bringing about or maintaining early abstinence (e.g., coping with craving for cocaine, managing thoughts about drug use, monitoring high-risk situations for relapse) with in-session and extrasession practice of skills. While cognitive-behavioral treatments have not been consistently found to be significantly more effective than alternative, "active" treatments such as Interpersonal Psychotherapy or 12-step–oriented counseling (Carroll, Rounsaville, & Gawin, 1991; Wells, Peterson, Gainey, Hawkins, & Catalano, 1994), areas where CBT may emerge as particularly advantageous include durability of effects (Carroll, Rounsaville, Nich, *et al.*, 1994) and treatment of more severely dependent cocaine abusers (Carroll *et al.*, 1991; Carroll, Rounsaville, Gordon, *et al.*, 1994).

MARIJUANA

Treatment of marijuana abuse and dependence is a relatively understudied area to date, in part because comparatively few individuals with marijuana use disorders are present for treatment. As in the treatment of cocaine dependence, there are currently no effective pharmacotherapies for marijuana abuse or dependence and psychosocial approaches remain the backbone of treatment, but few controlled trials of psychosocial approaches have been completed. Stephens, Roffman, and Simpson (1994) evaluated a relapse prevention approach versus a social support group intervention for 212 individuals seeking treatment for marijuana use. No significant treatment effects for days of marijuana use or abstinence rates were found posttreatment or through the 1-year follow-up. More recently, this group (Stephens & Roffman, 1996) compared a delayed treatment control, a 2-session motivational approach, and the more intensive (14-session) relapse prevention approach and found better marijuana outcomes for the two active treatments compared with the delayed-treatment control group, but no significant differences between the brief and the more intensive treatment.

SUMMARY

Scientific advances in the past 10 years have greatly increased clinicians' repertoire of effective treatment approaches for drug use disorders. While a number of powerful pharmacotherapies have emerged that have greatly enhanced outcomes in the treatment of opioid dependence (including methadone, naltrexone, LAAM, and buprenorphine), no effective pharmacotherapies have yet been shown to be generally effective for most classes of drug abuse, including cocaine, marijuana, or benzodiazepene abuse. Moreover, even for those classes of substance abuse for which we have effective pharmacotherapies, these medications, when used without supportive psychosocial treatments, have been shown to be woefully ineffective in retaining drug abusers or reducing their drug use. Although psychosocial treatments remain the backbone of treatment for drug abuse (despite the perception that such treatments are too "weak" to retain or effectively treat drug abusers when used alone), a number of promising treatments with strong empirical support, particularly behavioral and cognitive therapies, are underutilized in clinical practice. Efforts to move empirically validated treatments into the clinical arena will require further research in areas of particular interest to clinicians, including (1) the types of patients for whom primarily psychotherapeutic approaches are sufficient, and the optimal type and intensity of psychosocial treatments when combined with available pharmacotherapies; (2) the value or contribution of different components of treatment to outcome; (3) the optimal intensity or duration of available treatment strategies; and (4) data evaluating contrasts and combinations of the most effective forms of treatment. Finally, across most areas of substance abuse, combinations of psychosocial and pharmacologic treatment appear to be particularly promising in addressing the myriad and complex nature of drug abusers' problems.

REFERENCES

American Psychiatric Association. (1994). *Diagnostic and statistical manual of mental disorders* (4th. ed.). Washington, DC: Author.

American Psychiatric Association, Work Group on Substance Use Disorders. (1995). Practice guidelines for the treatment of patients with substance use disorders: Alcohol, cocaine, opioids. *American Journal of Psychiatry, 152* (Suppl.), 2–59.

Anton, R. F., Hogan, I., Jalali, B., Riordan, C. E., & Kleber, H. D. (1981). Multiple family therapy and nal-trexone in the treatment of opiate dependence. *Drug and Alcohol Dependence, 8,* 157–168.

Ball, J., Lange, W. R., Myers, C. P., & Friedman, S. R. (1988). Reducing the risk of AIDS through methadone maintenance treatment. *Journal of Health and Social Behavior, 29,* 214–216.

Ball, J. C., & Ross, A. (1991). *The effectiveness of methadone maintenance treatment.* New York: Springer-Verlag.

Callahan, E. J., Rawson, R. A., McCleave, B., Aries, R., Glazer, M., Liberman, R. P. (1980). The treatment of heroin addiction: Naltrexone alone and with behavior therapy. *International Journal of the Ad-dictions, 15,* 795–807.

Carroll, K. M. (1997). Integrating psychotherapy and pharmacotherapy to improve drug abuse out-comes. *Journal of Addictive Behaviors, 22,* 233–245.

Carroll, K. M., & Rounsaville, B. J. (1990). Can a technology model be applied to psychotherapy re-search in cocaine abuse treatment? In L. S. Onken & J. D. Blaine (Eds.), *Psychotherapy and coun-seling in the treatment of drug abuse* (NIDA Research Monograph Series No. 104, pp. 91–104). Rockville, MD: National Institute on Drug Abuse.

Carroll, K. M., & Rounsaville, B. J. (1995). Psychosocial treatments for substance dependence. In J. M. Oldham & M. B. Riba (Eds.), *American Psychiatric Press review of psychiatry* (Vol. 14, pp. 127–149). Washington, DC: American Psychiatric Press.

Carroll, K. M., Rounsaville, B. J., & Gawin, F. H. (1991). A comparative trial of psychotherapies for am-bulatory cocaine abusers: Relapse prevention and interpersonal psychotherapy. *American Jour-nal of Drug and Alcohol Abuse, 17,* 229–247.

Carroll, K. M., Rounsaville, B. J., Gordon, L. T., Nich, C., Jatlow, P. M., Bisighini, R. M., & Gawin, F. H. (1994). Psychotherapy and pharmacotherapy for ambulatory cocaine abusers. *Archives of General Psychiatry, 51,* 177–187.

Carroll, K. M., Rounsaville, B. J., Nich, C., Gordon, L. T., Wirtz, P. W., & Gawin, F. H. (1994). One year follow-up of psychotherapy and pharmacotherapy for cocaine dependence: Delayed emergence of psychotherapy effects. *Archives of General Psychiatry, 51,* 989–997.

Childress, A. R., Ehrman, R. N., McLellan, A. T., & O'Brien, C. P. (1988). Conditioned craving and arousal in cocaine addiction: A preliminary report. In L. S. Harris (Ed.), *Problems of drug depen-dence, 1987* (NIDA Research Monograph Series No. 81, pp. 74–80). Rockville, MD: National Insti-tute on Drug Abuse.

Childress, A. R., Ehrman, R., Rohsenow, D. J., Robbins, S. J., & O'Brien, C. P. (1992). Classically condi-tioned factors in drug dependence. In J. H. Lowinsohn, P. Ruiz, & R. B. Millman (Eds.), *Compre-hensive textbook of substance abuse* (2nd ed., pp. 56–69). New York: Williams and Wilkins.

Crits-Christoph, P., & Siqueland, L. (1996). Psychosocial treatment for drug abuse: Selected review and recommendations for national health care. *Archives of General Psychiatry, 53,* 749–756.

Dolan, M. P., Black, J. L., Penk, W. E., Rabinowitz, R., & DeFord, H. A. (1985). Contracting for treatment termination to reduce illicit drug use among methadone maintenance treatment failures. *Journal of Consulting and Clinical Psychology, 53,* 549–551.

General Accounting Office. (1990). *Methadone maintenance: Some treatment programs are not effec-tive; greater federal oversight needed.* Washington, DC: Author.

General Accounting Office. (1996). *Cocaine treatment: Early results from various approaches.* Wash-ington, DC: Author.

Gerstley, L., McLellan, A. T., Alterman, A. I., Woody, G. E., Luborsky, L., & Prout, M. (1989). Ability to form an alliance with the therapist: A possible marker of prognosis for patients with antisocial per-sonality disorder. *American Journal of Psychiatry, 146,* 508–512.

Grabowski, J., O'Brien, C. P., Greenstein, R., Ternes, T., Long, M., & Steinberg-Donato, S. (1979). Effects of contingency payment on compliance with a naltrexone regimen. *American Journal of Drug and Alcohol Abuse, 6,* 355–365.

Greenstein, R. A., Fudala, P. J., & O'Brien, C. P. (1992). Alternative pharmacotherapies for opiate ad-diction. In J. H. Lowinsohn, P. Ruiz, & R. B. Millman (Eds.), *Comprehensive textbook of substance abuse* (2nd ed., pp. 562–573). New York: Williams and Wilkins.

Higgins, S. T., & Budney, A. J. (1993). Treatment of cocaine dependence through the principles of be-havior analysis and behavioral pharmacology. In L. S. Onken, J. D. Blaine, & J. J. Boren (Eds.), *Be-havioral treatments for drug and alcohol dependence* (NIDA Research Monograph Series No. 137, pp. 97–121). Rockville, MD: National Institute on Drug Abuse.

Higgins, S. T., Delaney, D. D., Budney, A. J., Bickel, W. K., Hughes, J. R., Foerg, F., & Fenwick, J. W. (1991). A behavioral approach to achieving initial cocaine abstinence. *American Journal of Psychiatry, 148,* 1218–1224.

Higgins, S. T., Budney, A. J., Bickel, W. K., & Hughes, J. R. (1993). Achieving cocaine abstinence with a behavioral approach. *American Journal of Psychiatry, 150,* 763–769.

Higgins, S. T., Budney, A. J., Bickel, W. K., Foerg, F. E., Donham, R., & Badger, G. J. (1994). Incentives improve outcome in outpatient behavioral treatment of cocaine dependence. *Archives of General Psychiatry, 51,* 568–576.

Higgins, S. T., Budney, A. J., Bickel, W. K., Badger, G. J., Foerg, F., & Ogden, D. (1995). Outpatient behavioral treatment for cocaine dependence: One-year outcome. *Experimental and Clinical Psychopharmacology, 3,* 205–212.

Iguchi, M. Y., Lamb, R. J., Belding, M. A., Platt, J. J., Husband, S. D., & Morral, A. R. (1996). Contingent reinforcement of group participation versus abstinence in a methadone maintenance program. *Experimental and Clinical Psychopharmacology, 4,* 17.

Kreek, M. J. (1992). Rationale for maintenance pharmacotherapy of opiate dependence. In C. P. O'Brien & J. H. Jaffe (Eds.), *Addictive behaviors* (pp. 205–230). New York: Raven.

Lowinsohn, J. H., Marion, I. J., Joseph, H., & Dole, V. P. (1992). Methadone maintenance. In J. H. Lowinsohn, P. Ruiz, & R. B. Millman (Eds.), *Comprehensive textbook of substance abuse* (2nd ed., pp. 550–561). New York: Williams and Wilkins.

McCarthy, J. J., & Borders, O. T. (1985). Limit setting on drug abuse in methadone maintenance treatment. *American Journal of Psychiatry, 142,* 1419–1423.

McLellan, A. T., Luborsky, L., Woody, G. E., O'Brien, C. P., & Kron, R. (1981). Are the addiction-related problems of substance abusers really related? *Journal of Nervous and Mental Disease, 169,* 232–239.

McLellan, A. T., Childress, A. R., O'Brien, C. P., & Ehrman, R. N. (1986). Extinguishing conditioned responses during treatment for opiate dependence: Turning laboratory findings into clinical procedures. *Journal of Substance Abuse Treatment, 3,* 33–40.

McLellan, A. T., Arndt, I. O., Metzger, D. S., Woody, G. E., & O'Brien, C. P. (1993). The effects of psychosocial services in substance abuse treatment. *Journal of the American Medical Association, 269,* 1953–1959.

McLellan, A. T., Alterman, A. I., Metzger, D. S., Grissom, G. R., Woody, G. E., Luborsky, L., & O'Brien, C. P. (1994). Similarity of outcome predictors across opiate, cocaine, and alcohol treatments: Role of treatment services. *Journal of Consulting and Clinical Psychology, 62,* 1141–1158.

Meyer, R. E. (1992). New pharmacotherapies for cocaine dependence . . . revisited. *Archives of General Psychiatry, 49,* 900–904.

Meyer, R. E., Mirin, S. M., Altman, J. L., & McNamee, B. (1976). A behavioral paradigm for the evaluation of narcotic antagonists. *Archives of General Psychiatry, 33,* 371–377.

O'Brien, C. P. (1996). Recent developments in the pharmacotherapy of substance abuse. *Journal of Consulting and Clinical Psychology, 64,* 677–686.

O'Malley, J. E., Anderson, W. H., & Lazare, A. (1972). Failure of outpatient treatment of drug abuse: I. Heroin. *American Journal of Psychiatry, 128,* 865–868.

Rawson, R. A., Mann, A. G., Tennant, F. S., & Clabough, D. (1983). Efficacy of psychotherapeutic counseling during 12-day ambulatory heroin detoxification. In L.S. Harris (Ed.), *Problems of drug dependence, 1982* (NIDA Research Monograph Series No. 43, pp. 310–314). Rockville, MD: National Institute on Drug Abuse.

Rounsaville, B. J. (1995). Can psychotherapy rescue naltrexone treatment of opioid addiction? In L. S. Onken & J. D. Blaine, *Potentiating the efficacy of medications: Integrating psychosocial therapies with pharmacotherapies in the treatment of drug dependence* (NIDA Research Monograph Series No. 105, pp. 37–52). Rockville, MD: National Institute on Drug Abuse.

Rounsaville, B. J., & Carroll, K. M. (1992). Individual psychotherapy for drug abusers. In J. H. Lowinsohn, P. Ruiz, & R. B. Millman (Eds.), *Comprehensive textbook of substance abuse* (2nd ed., pp. 496–508). New York: Williams and Wilkins.

Rounsaville, B. J., & Kleber, H. D. (1985). Psychotherapy/counseling for opiate addicts: Strategies for use in different treatment settings. *International Journal of the Addictions, 20,* 869–896.

Saunders, B., Wilkinson, C., & Phillips, M. (1995). The impact of a brief motivational intervention with opiate users attending a methadone programme. *Addiction, 90,* 415–424.

Saxon, A. J., Calsyn, D. A., Kivlahan, D. R., & Roszell, D. K. (1993). Outcome of contingency contracting for illicit drug use in a methadone maintenance program. *Drug and Alcohol Dependence, 31,* 205–214.

Silverman, K., Higgins, S. T., Brooner, R. K., Montoya, I. D., Cone, E. J., Schuster, C. R., & Preston, K. L. (1996). Sustained cocaine abstinence in methadone maintenance patients through voucher-based reinforcement therapy. *Archives of General Psychiatry, 53,* 409–415.

Sisson, R. W., & Azrin, N. H. (1989). The community reinforcement approach. In R. K. Hester & W. R. Miller (Eds), *Handbook of alcoholism treatment approaches* (pp. 242–258). New York: Pergamon.

Stephens, R. S., & Roffman, R. A. (1996, June 24). *Treating adult marijuana dependence.* Paper presented at the 58th annual meeting of the College on Problems of Drug Dependence, San Juan, Puerto Rico.

Stephens, R. S., Roffman, R. A., & Simpson, E. E. (1994). Treating adult marijuana dependence: A test of the relapse prevention model. *Journal of Consulting and Clinical Psychology, 62,* 92–99.

Stitzer, M. L., & Bigelow, G. E. (1978). Contingency management in a methadone maintenance program: Availability of reinforcers. *International Journal of the Addictions, 13,* 737–746.

Stitzer, M. L., Bickel, W. K., Bigelow, G. E, & Liebson, I. A. (1986). Effect of methadone dose contingencies on urinalysis test results of polydrug-abusing methadone maintenance patients. *Drug and Alcohol Dependence, 18,* 341–348.

Stitzer, M. L., Iguchi, M. Y., & Felch, L. J. (1992). Contingent take-home incentive: Effects on drug use of methadone maintenance patients. *Journal of Consulting and Clinical Psychology, 60,* 927–934.

Stitzer, M. L., Iguchi, M. Y., Kidorf, M., & Bigelow, G. E. (1993). Contingency management in methadone treatment: The case for positive incentives. In L. S. Onken, J. D. Blaine, & J. J. Boren (Eds.), *Behavioral treatments for drug abuse and dependence* (NIDA Research Monograph Series No. 137, pp. 19–36). Rockville, MD: National Institute on Drug Abuse.

Strain, E. C., Stitzer, M. L., Liebson, I. A., & Bigelow, G. E. (1994). Buprenorphine versus methadone in the treatment of opioid-dependent cocaine users. *Psychopharmacology (Berl), 116,* 401–406.

Tennant, F. S., Rawson, R. A., Pumphrey, E., & Seecof, R. (1986). Clinical experiences with 959 opioid-dependent patients treated with levo-alpha-acetylmethadol (LAAM). *Journal of Substance Abuse Treatment, 3,* 195–202.

Ward, J., Mattick, R., & Hall, W. (1992). *Key issues in methadone maintenance treatment.* Sydney, Australia: University of New South Wales Press.

Waskow, I. E. (1984). Specification of the technique variable in the NIMH treatment of depression collaborative research program. In J. B. W. Williams & R. L. Spitzer (Eds.), *Psychotherapy research: Where are we and where should we go* (pp. 150–159). New York: Guilford.

Wells, E. A., Peterson, P. L., Gainey, R. R., Hawkins, J. D., & Catalano, R. F. (1994). Outpatient treatment for cocaine abuse: A controlled comparison of relapse prevention and Twelve-Step approaches. *American Journal of Drug and Alcohol Abuse, 20,* 1–17.

Woody, G. E., Luborsky, L., McLellan, A. T., O'Brien, C. P., Beck, A. T., Blaine, J., Herman, I., & Hole, A. (1983). Psychotherapy for opiate addicts: Does it help? *Archives of General Psychiatry, 40,* 639–645.

Woody, G. E., McLellan, A. T., Luborsky, L., & O'Brien, C. P. (1985). Sociopathy and psychotherapy outcome. *Archives of General Psychiatry, 42,* 1081–1086.

Woody, G. E., McLellan, A. T., Luborsky, L., & O'Brien, C. P. (1987). Twelve-month follow-up of psychotherapy for opiate dependence. *American Journal of Psychiatry, 144,* 590–596.

Woody, G. E., McLellan, A. T., Luborsky, L., & O'Brien, C. P. (1995). Psychotherapy in community methadone programs: A validation study. *American Journal of Psychiatry, 152,* 1302–1308.

17

Treating Eating Disorders

KATHARINE L. LOEB AND G. TERENCE WILSON

INTRODUCTION

This chapter reviews the outcome literature pertinent to the treatment of eating disorders. The information provided is applicable to the individual prepared to relinquish what is often a long-standing pattern of disordered eating and associated symptomatology. However, the decision to seek treatment for an eating disorder commonly carries with it a degree of ambivalence about change, which varies depending on the particular eating disorder, its chronicity, and the individual characteristics of the patient. As is the case with other psychological disorders, the hesitancy that emerges as treatment begins derives from the fear that what one may have to give up in order to get better will be too great a sacrifice. In bulimia nervosa, for example, patients are often reluctant to abandon the hope that they will reach an (unrealistic) body weight goal; they want to continue engaging in dieting but forgo the ego dystonic features of the disorder, namely, binge eating and purging. These two aims are generally incompatible, given the documented contribution of dietary restriction in the development and maintenance of binge eating syndromes (Polivy & Herman, 1993). In anorexia nervosa, patients almost invariably fear the loss of identity and uniqueness that they believe will come with achieving a normal weight; individuals with this disorder usually present for treatment as a result of external pressure for change. The clinician must therefore be vigilant about the fluctuating and tenuous nature of readiness to change in these patient populations, and foster an acceptance of what can and cannot be changed (Wilson, 1996a; see Chapter 9, this volume).

KATHARINE L. LOEB   •   Eating Disorders Clinic, Rutgers University, Piscataway, New Jersey 08854.
G. TERENCE WILSON   •   Graduate School of Applied and Professional Psychology, Rutgers University, Piscataway, New Jersey 08855.

Treating Addictive Behaviors, 2nd ed., edited by Miller and Heather. Plenum Press, New York, 1998.

THE EATING DISORDERS

ANOREXIA NERVOSA

Anorexia nervosa is the eating disorder with the longest documented history. Its core diagnostic features (American Psychiatric Association, 1994) are as follows: a purposefully maintained, abnormally low body weight; an excessive fear of weight gain; body image disturbance; and, in postmenarcheal females, amenorrhea. Anorexia nervosa has two subtypes: binge eating/purging type, in which the patient engages in either or both of these behaviors, and restricting type, in which these behaviors are absent.

BULIMIA NERVOSA

Bulimia nervosa was first described in 1979 (Russell, 1979). This disorder is characterized by recurrent episodes of binge eating (defined as the consumption of excessively large amounts of food in a discrete period of time, along with a sense of loss of control) followed by regular inappropriate behaviors designed to compensate for the overeating. Individuals with bulimia nervosa place undue importance on body shape and weight as determinants of their self-evaluation. This disorder also has two subtypes based on the type of compensatory behavior employed by the patient: self-induced vomiting or laxative, diuretic, or enema misuse, or both define the purging type; excessive exercise, fasting, or both define the nonpurging type. In order to qualify for a diagnosis of bulimia nervosa, individuals must possess a normal or above normal body weight; underweight patients who engage in binge eating and purging should be considered for a diagnosis of anorexia nervosa.

BINGE EATING DISORDER

Binge eating disorder is currently under consideration for inclusion as a formal diagnostic category (American Psychiatric Association, 1994). The proposed criteria for the disorder include repeated binge eating in the absence of the inappropriate compensatory mechanisms seen in bulimia nervosa; clinically significant distress over the binge eating behavior; and the presence of behavioral and emotional correlates of binge eating.

Binge eating disorder is strongly associated with obesity; conversely, the majority of obese individuals presenting for treatment do not meet criteria for binge eating disorder (Spitzer et al., 1992; Spitzer et al., 1993). Obesity is considered a medical condition and is therefore not listed as a psychiatric diagnosis in DSM-IV (American Psychiatric Association, 1994). "Compulsive overeating," an overused catchall term, also does not represent a formal eating disorder, but probably encompasses a wide range of disordered eating behavior, including grazing and overeating at meals. It is theoretically possible, however, that established treatments for binge eating disorder may also be effective for other types of overeating patterns, although research has not yet been conducted to directly address this issue. For obesity, cognitive-behavioral, dietary, and certain pharmacological treatment programs have all been found to be effective in the short term, but safe, long-term solutions for this condition remain elusive (Brownell & Fairburn, 1995).

EATING DISORDERS AND ADDICTIONS

While the eating disorders, and binge eating behavior in particular, share many characteristics of the addictive disorders, their distinctions carry important therapeutic and theoretical implications (see Wilson, 1993 for a detailed analysis of this issue). For example, on the surface, binge eating and psychoactive substance abuse both seem to be phenomena of excess. The binge eater can, in a single episode of overeating, ingest over 5,000 kcal (Walsh, Hadigan, Kissileff, & LaChaussee, 1992); a claim frequently heard by clinicians is that cravings prompt the out-of-control consumption of sweet and salty binge foods. While this pattern appears to parallel reports of alcohol or drug dependence, their respective interventions should feature at least one fundamental difference. In the case of substance abuse, control or abstinence is the direct goal of many treatment approaches. Conversely, for binge eaters, it is the very avoidance of forbidden foods that leads to the physiological and psychological sense of deprivation implicated in the perpetuation of the binge eating cycle. Thus, the patient with bulimia nervosa who is restricting all day and binge eating all night would be encouraged to increase her food intake and decrease "control" (see the description of cognitive behavioral therapy on page 234).

Extreme dietary restriction can also play a role in the evolution of eating disorders for those patients whose binge eating episodes are superimposed on an overall pattern of overeating. Anecdotally, the majority of individuals with binge eating disorder participating in treatment programs at our clinic report that (1) historically, periods when they engaged in popular commercial diets were invariably followed by periods of increased binge eating, and (2) they are haunted by rules dictated in these diets even when they are not actively attempting to follow them. The cognitive behavioral therapy (CBT) employed with binge eating disorder promotes flexible, regular eating (Fairburn, 1995), and has been shown to be effective (see the following discussion). Thus, even for binge eaters who overeat in general, it is not necessary, and perhaps harmful, to promote abstinence and control as they are advocated in some treatment approaches for addictive disorders.

Another relevant issue is how to treat patients with comorbid psychoactive substance abuse and eating disorders. While there are no guiding empirical data on this matter, common clinical sense dictates that if the alcohol or drug problem is sufficiently severe to impair engagement in an eating disorder protocol, it should be made the priority of treatment (see Chapter 13, this volume). Concomitant intervention programs, however, have been developed and implemented (e.g., Mitchell, Specker, & Edmonson, 1997).

TREATMENT MODALITIES

This section describes the major approaches for the treatment of eating disorders; the next section will review the outcome literature pertaining to these treatments. Before discussing particular modalities, however, it is important to note that many interventions can be delivered at various levels of intensity. For instance, cognitive behavioral therapy (CBT) for bulimia nervosa can be administered via a self-help manual (Schmidt, Tiller, & Treasure, 1993; Treasure *et al.*,

1994), through nonprofessional or therapist-guided use of such a manual (Carter & Fairburn, 1997; Cooper, Coker, & Fleming, 1994, 1996; Huon, 1985; Loeb, Wilson, & Gilbert, 1998), in group treatment (e.g., Schneider & Agras, 1985), as individual psychological treatment (e.g., Walsh *et al.*, 1997), or in the context of day treatment (e.g., Kaplan & Olmsted, 1997) or inpatient programs. In addition, treatment can be assigned within a stepped-care model (Fairburn & Peveler, 1990; Garner & Needleman, 1996; Treasure *et al.*, 1996), beginning with the least intensive and most cost-effective intervention and moving upward depending on the patient's progress.

COGNITIVE BEHAVIORAL THERAPY

CBT for eating disorders was originally developed for the treatment of bulimia nervosa (Fairburn, 1981) and anorexia nervosa (Garner & Bemis, 1982), and has since been adapted for binge eating disorder (Fairburn, Marcus, & Wilson, 1993). CBT for bulimia nervosa is present-oriented and directly focused on symptom reduction. It consists of three stages, designed to be administered in weekly 50-minute sessions over the course of approximately 16 to 20 weeks. Stage 1 incorporates behavioral and psychoeducational components to achieve the following aims: (1) to orient the patient to the cognitive-behavioral model of the disorder, (2) to establish a regular pattern of eating (3 meals plus 2 to 3 snacks), as well as a weekly weighing regimen, (3) to convey the ineffectiveness and detrimental consequences of purging and extreme dietary restriction, and (4) to implement alternative activities to binge eating. Stage 2 teaches problem-solving skills, systematically reintroduces the patient to forbidden foods, and addresses shape and weight concerns using cognitive restructuring. Stage 3 focuses on relapse prevention.

CBT for binge eating disorder (Fairburn, Marcus, & Wilson, 1993) is based on CBT for bulimia nervosa, but reflects some fundamental differences between the two disorders. First, the majority of patients with binge eating disorder are obese, and their primary goal of treatment is weight loss. Therapy redirects patients' efforts to eliminating their binge eating first, with weight reduction being an important but secondary target of treatment. Second, obese binge eaters generally exhibit an overall chaotic eating pattern, which this intervention addresses by emphasizing stimulus control techniques, appropriate portion sizes, and sound nutrition. Third, the nature of shape and weight concerns among this population differs from that of individuals with bulimia nervosa; cognitive restructuring must acknowledge the difficulties of being overweight in a society that overvalues thinness. In addition, disabusing the patient of inaccurate notions about the nature of obesity is a key aim of the psychoeducational component of this treatment protocol.

CBT for anorexia nervosa has been described in the literature (e.g., Fairburn, Marcus, & Wilson, 1993; Garner, Vitousek, & Pike, 1997; Pike, Loeb, & Vitousek, 1996), but an empirically supported treatment protocol is not yet available. The commonalities between bulimia nervosa, for which an established CBT treatment exists, and anorexia nervosa suggest that the latter may also benefit from this approach.

INTERPERSONAL PSYCHOTHERAPY

Interpersonal psychotherapy (IPT) was originally developed for the treatment of depression (Klerman, Weissman, Rounsaville, & Chevron, 1984), and its adaptation to bulimia nervosa has produced encouraging results (Fairburn, Jones, Peveler, Hope, & O'Conner, 1993; Fairburn *et al.*, 1995). (See the following discussion; also see Chapter 16, this volume, for a discussion of IPT in the treatment of drug dependence.) In this treatment, the therapist takes an active but nondirective role in helping the patient identify and resolve interpersonal dysfunction that may be contributing to the eating disorder. However, eating disorder symptoms are not discussed beyond the initial phase of treatment. As with CBT, the focus is on the here-and-now and it is action-oriented. IPT has also been conducted in a group format for individuals with nonpurging bulimia nervosa (Wilfley *et al.*, 1993).

PHARMACOLOGICAL TREATMENTS

Many psychotropic agents have been tried with eating disorder patients, with the rationale ranging from the presence of associated symptomatology (such as depression) to targeting specific putative biological mechanisms of the disorders. Antidepressant medications, mood stabilizers, opiate antagonists, and fenfluramine have all been studied in bulimia nervosa; antipsychotic medications, antidepressants, anxiolytics, appetite-enhancing drugs, and prokinetic agents have been applied in the treatment of anorexia nervosa; and antidepressants and appetite suppressants have been given to obese binge eaters (see Garfinkel & Walsh, 1997 for an extensive review of the literature).

PSYCHODYNAMIC THERAPIES

Supportive-expressive therapy (Luborsky, 1984) and a more general supportive psychotherapy have been tested in controlled trials for bulimia nervosa (Garner *et al.*, 1993; Walsh *et al.*, 1997). These approaches are nondirective and are aimed at helping the patient uncover underlying dynamic processes that are being expressed as eating disorder symptoms.

OTHER APPROACHES

Additional treatment modalities have been applied to eating disorders. These include family therapy (e.g., Russell, Szmukler, Dare, & Eisler, 1987; Dodge, Hodes, Eisler, & Dare, 1995), feminist therapy (Fallon, Katzman, & Wooley, 1994), psychoeducation (Olmsted *et al.*, 1991; Davis, Olmsted, Rockert, Marques, & Dolhanty, 1997), and nutritional counseling (Laessle *et al.*, 1991). Overeaters Anonymous (OA; Yeary, 1987), one of the many 12-step offshoots of Alcoholics Anonymous, offers a valuable support system for many individuals. Some factions of OA promote abstinence from certain foods (e.g., sugar), to which overeaters are presumed to be addicted according to this approach. The addiction model's generalizability to eating disorders and obesity has, however, been criticized (Bemis, 1985; Wilson, 1993).

TREATMENT OUTCOME STUDIES

The following review focuses on controlled clinical trials in the treatment of eating disorders.

BULIMIA NERVOSA

CBT is the most extensively researched psychological intervention for bulimia nervosa. Studies of CBT for bulimia nervosa have attempted to answer three major questions: (1) Is CBT superior to a wait-list control? (2) how does CBT fare when compared to alternative interventions? and (3) is there any incremental value to combining CBT with antidepressant medication?

CBT has consistently been found to be superior to a wait-list control condition (e.g., Agras, Schneider, Arnow, Raeburn, & Telch, 1989; Wolf & Crowther, 1992). Five studies have examined CBT in relation to antidepressant medication (Agras et al., 1992; Fichter et al., 1991; Leitenberg et al., 1994; Mitchell et al., 1990; Walsh et al., 1997). Results of studies that employed a single agent indicate that CBT is more effective than medication, and that combining the two therapies may yield some modest incremental benefit (Agras et al., 1992; Walsh et al., 1997). Only one trial (Walsh et al., 1997) employed a two-stage medication intervention in which, if the first medication failed or produced intolerable side effects, a second agent was administered. This study compared the relative effectiveness of CBT or supportive psychotherapy in combination with medication or placebo; in addition, it compared medication alone with each psychotherapy-plus-medication group. CBT emerged as significantly superior to supportive psychotherapy in reducing the frequency of binge eating and purging as well as scores on a self-report measure of eating disorder symptoms (the Eating Attitudes Test [EAT; Garner, Olmsted, Bohr, & Garfinkel, 1982]). Active medication in combination with psychological treatment was superior to placebo plus psychotherapy in improving binge eating, depression, and EAT scores. Last, CBT plus medication was superior to medication alone in reducing vomiting and EAT scores; supportive psychotherapy, on the other hand, did not add any benefit to medication.

Other studies have compared CBT to alternative psychological interventions. Kirkley, Schneider, Agras, and Bachman (1985) examined the relative effectiveness of group CBT to a nondirective group therapy and found the former to be more effective in reducing the frequency of binge eating and vomiting, but not more effective in alleviating associated psychopathology (depression, anxiety, and dysfunctional thoughts). Fairburn, Kirk, O'Conner, and Cooper (1986) compared CBT to short-term focal psychotherapy, which overlapped to some extent with CBT (having included features such as self-monitoring and psychoeducation). Results showed that the two treatments yielded similar and significant improvement at the end of the acute phase of the study; however, at 8-month follow-up, the CBT group was vomiting less frequently. In addition, CBT had lower levels of general psychopathology and depression throughout follow-up. The authors note that the lack of group differences at posttreatment may be attributable to the shared elements of the two treatments. Garner and colleagues (1993) compared CBT with supportive-expressive therapy and found both to be equally effective in reducing the frequency of binge eating; however, CBT was superior in reducing purging, dietary restraint, shape and weight concerns, and depressive symptoms, and in increasing self-esteem.

Fairburn and colleagues (Fairburn *et al.,* 1991) studied the relative effects of CBT, behavior therapy (a dismantled version of CBT, minus its focus on shape and weight concerns), and IPT, and found CBT to be the best of the three interventions in reducing the entire package of the core features of bulimia nervosa. In a 12-month follow-up study (Fairburn, Jones, *et al.,* 1993), however, IPT was found to have "caught up" to CBT, suggesting that IPT's effects may be as strong but delayed in comparison to the time course of CBT. Overall, behavior therapy alone produced the least impressive results. A similar pattern was seen at 6-year follow-up (Fairburn *et al.,* 1995). Other trials have found CBT to be equal to behavior therapy after an acute phase of treatment but superior at follow-up (Cooper & Steere, 1995; Thackwray, Smith, Bodfish, & Meyers, 1993). Freeman, Barry, Dunkeld-Turnball, and Henderson (1988) found no differences between CBT and behavior therapy in a comparison of these treatments and "supportive and educational" group therapy and a wait-list control condition; however, no follow-up data were provided.

Taken as a whole, research results suggest the following about the treatment of bulimia nervosa. First, CBT is clearly the most empirically supported psychological intervention for bulimia nervosa. While long-term results of IPT appear promising, CBT has been studied more extensively and produces more rapid improvement, and thus should be employed as the first-line strategy in combating this disorder. Results from the most methodologically sound studies show that CBT produces a mean reduction in binge eating ranging from 73% to 93% and a mean reduction in purging ranging from 77% to 94%; remission (abstinence for at least 1 week) rates range from 51% to 71% for binge eating and 36% to 56% for purging (Wilson, Fairburn, & Agras, 1997). Second, while pharmacological trials in the treatment of bulimia nervosa have consistently demonstrated that medication is superior to placebo (Garfinkel & Walsh, 1997), it is inferior to CBT. The available evidence suggests that, at best, combining antidepressant medication with CBT results in only a modest incremental benefit compared with CBT alone (Agras *et al.,* 1992). However, the combination might be more effective than CBT alone in reducing depressive symptoms (Walsh *et al.,* 1997).

ANOREXIA NERVOSA

Few well-controlled clinical trials have been conducted in the treatment of anorexia nervosa; resistance to treatment and the relative rarity of the disorder are among the reasons for the paucity of good outcome research in this area. A study comparing CBT, behavioral treatment, and a weight-restoration–oriented control condition (all outpatient interventions) found improvement in, but no differences between the three groups (Channon, De Silva, Helmsley, & Perkins, 1989). However, this trial was compromised by methodological limitations, including a small sample size and nonindependent assessments. Hall and Crisp (1987) compared two posthospitalization treatments, dietary advice, and a combination of individual and family psychotherapy; results showed significant weight gain in the dietary advice group and a significant increase in social adjustment in the psychotherapy condition. Again, research design shortcomings, such as a small sample and overlap in the two interventions, limit the conclusions that can be drawn

from this study. A third study (Crisp *et al.,* 1991) randomized patients to (1) inpatient treatment followed by individual outpatient psychotherapy, (2) outpatient
individual and family therapy, (3) outpatient group therapy conducted separately
for patients and parents, or (4) no treatment. The treatment approach was primarily psychodynamic. All three active conditions exhibited significant improvement
(in terms of weight gain and social and sexual functioning) at 1 year; interestingly,
outpatient treatment fared as well as more intensive hospitalization. A 2-year follow-up study of group 2 compared to the control group indicated that the observed improvement was maintained in this condition (Gowers, Norton, Halek, &
Crisp, 1994). However, methodological problems, such as the lack of a clearly defined treatment protocol, temper the generalizability of these findings. The most
salient result from the outcome literature on anorexia nervosa is that family therapy may fare better than individual supportive therapy for patients 18 years old or
younger who have been ill for less than 3 years (Russell *et al.,* 1987); in this well-
controlled study, patients not fitting this profile did poorly in both conditions. A
more recent randomized, controlled trial (Robin, Siegel, & Moye, 1995), comparing behavioral family systems therapy to ego-oriented individual therapy for adolescents with a recent onset of anorexia nervosa, also yielded results in favor of
family therapy.

Although CBT has not been well studied in this population, there are strong
theoretical and practical bases for applying this approach to patients with
anorexia nervosa (Pike *et al.,* 1996), and relevant trials are under way (Halmi,
1997; Pike, 1997). Generally, treatment needs to begin in an inpatient setting in order to execute weight restoration in a controlled environment, using behavioral
techniques (Bemis, 1987). Once a patient has reached a medically safe weight, intensive outpatient psychotherapy, such as the CBT program described earlier, is
appropriate. This sequenced format of treatment may be beneficial in three re-
spects: (1) in allowing patients to generalize gains made in a hospital setting to
their natural environment, within the supportive context of therapy, (2) in fostering continued improvement, and (3) in preventing relapse. Pharmacotherapy for
anorexia nervosa has met with little success (Walsh, 1992).

BINGE EATING DISORDER

Psychological interventions, particularly CBT (Smith, Marcus, & Kaye, 1992;
Telch, Agras, Rossiter, Wilfley, & Kenardy, 1990), have shown promise for the
treatment of binge eating disorder. Wilfley and colleagues (1993) compared group
CBT, group IPT, and a wait-list control condition for obese binge eaters; the two active treatments yielded a significant reduction in binge eating frequency, whereas
the control did not. Agras and colleagues (1994) used an additive design to study
the effectiveness of three conditions: 9 months of weight loss treatment, 3 months
of CBT followed by 6 months of weight loss treatment, and 3 months of CBT followed by 6 months of both weight loss treatment and desipramine. At the end of
3 months, the CBT groups had reduced binge eating more than the weight loss
only group, but the weight loss only group had lost more weight at this time point.
At the end of 9 months, however, these differences disappeared. It is particularly
interesting that weight loss treatment improved binge eating as much as CBT; follow-up would be needed to determine whether there would be a rebound in binge

eating in the diet-only condition. Results from another study (Telch & Agras, 1993) suggest that dieting may maintain but not exacerbate binge eating in obese binge eaters. A 1-year follow-up (Agras, Telch, Arnow, Eldredge, & Marnell, 1997) of patients from the above study and two others (Agras et al., 1994; Agras et al., 1995; Eldredge et al., 1997), all of whom received CBT plus weight loss treatment, found that this treatment sequence yields improvements in binge eating that are fairly well maintained.

Marcus, Wing, and Fairburn (1995) compared CBT, a behavioral weight loss treatment, and a delayed treatment control condition for binge eating disorder. Results showed no difference between the two active conditions on the reduction of binge eating, but found the weight loss condition to be superior in reducing weight. Levine, Marcus, and Moulton (1996) demonstrated the effectiveness of an exercise intervention for obese women with binge eating disorder. A seventh study (Agras et al., 1995) found that a course of IPT was not beneficial to patients who did not improve with CBT, but an eighth showed that extending a course of CBT was helpful (Eldredge et al., 1997). Overall, pharmacological treatment alone appears to be a less viable option than CBT or IPT given the limited success of antidepressants in placebo-controlled trials (Agras et al., 1994; Alger, Schwalberg, Bigaouette, Michalek, & Howard, 1991; de Zwaan, Nutzinger, & Schoenbeck, 1992; Marcus et al., 1990; McCann & Agras, 1990), the potential side effects of appetite suppressants, and the likely relapse after stopping these agents (Devlin, 1996).

CONCLUSIONS

Effective treatments exist for anorexia nervosa, bulimia nervosa, and binge eating disorder (Wilson & Fairburn, 1998). CBT, the first-line treatment of choice for binge eating, can be applied with the knowledge that it is equally if not more effective than alternative interventions for bulimia nervosa and binge eating disorder. Nevertheless, CBT has its limitations. For example, only about half of the patients receiving CBT for bulimia nervosa cease binge eating and purging by the end of treatment, highlighting the need for developing strategies for nonresponders (Wilson, 1996b). In addition, more research is needed on the treatment of anorexia nervosa, pertaining to controlled outcome studies and to techniques for enhancing motivation for change in this difficult population (Vitousek, Watson, & Wilson, in press). The field would also benefit from a focus, in the next generation of research, on effective treatment approaches for patients with concomitant diagnoses.

REFERENCES

Agras, W. S., Schneider, J. A., Arnow, B., Raeburn, S. D., & Telch, C. F. (1989). Cognitive behavioral and response prevention treatments for bulimia nervosa. *Journal of Consulting and Clinical Psychology, 57,* 215–221.

Agras, W. S., Rossiter, E. M., Arnow, B., Schneider, J. A., Telch, C. F., Raeburn, S. D., Bruce, B., Perls, M., & Koran, L. M. (1992). Pharmacologic and cognitive-behavioral treatment for bulimia nervosa: A controlled comparison. *American Journal of Psychiatry, 149,* 82–87.

Agras, W. S., Telch, C. F., Arnow, B., Eldredge, K., Wilfley, D. E., Raeburn, S. D., Henderson, J., & Marnell, M. (1994). Weight loss, cognitive-behavioral, and desipramine treatments in binge eating disorder: An additive design. *Behavior Therapy, 25,* 225–238.

Agras, W. S., Telch, C. F., Arnow, B., Eldredge, K., Detzer, M. J., Henderson, J., & Marnell, M. (1995). Does interpersonal therapy help patients with binge eating disorder who fail to respond to cognitive-behavioral therapy? *Journal of Consulting and Clinical Psychology, 63,* 356–360.

Agras, W. S., Telch, C. F., Arnow, B., Eldredge, K., & Marnell, M. (1997). One-year follow-up of cognitive-behavioral therapy for obese individuals with binge eating disorder. *Journal of Consulting and Clinical Psychology, 65,* 343–347.

Alger, S. A., Schwalberg, M. D., Bigaouette, J. M., Michalek, A. V., & Howard, L. J. (1991). Effect of tricyclic antidepressants and opiate agonist on binge-eating behavior in normoweight bulimic and obese, binge-eating subjects. *American Journal of Clinical Nutrition, 53,* 865–871.

American Psychiatric Association. (1994). *Diagnostic and statistical manual of mental disorders* (4th ed.). Washington, DC: Author.

Bemis, K. M. (1985). Abstinence and nonabstinence models for the treatment of bulimia. *International Journal of Eating Disorders, 4,* 407–437.

Bemis, K. (1987). The present status of operant conditioning for the treatment of anorexia nervosa. *Behavior Modification, 11,* 432–463.

Brownell, K. D., & Fairburn, C. G. (1995). *Eating disorders and obesity: A comprehensive handbook.* New York: Guilford.

Carter, J. C., & Fairburn, C. G. (1997). *Cognitive behavioural self-help for binge eating disorder: A controlled effectiveness study.* Manuscript submitted for publication.

Channon, S., De Silva, P., Helmsley, D., & Perkins, R. (1989). A controlled trial of cognitive-behavioural and behavioural treatment of anorexia nervosa. *Behaviour Research and Therapy, 27,* 529–535.

Cooper, P. J., & Steere, J. (1995). A comparison of two psychological treatments for bulimia nervosa: Implications for models of maintenance. *Behaviour Research and Therapy, 33,* 875–886.

Cooper, P. J., Coker, S., & Fleming, C. (1994). Self-help for bulimia nervosa: A preliminary report. *International Journal of Eating Disorders, 16,* 401–404.

Cooper, P. J., Coker, S., & Fleming, C. (1996). An evaluation of the efficacy of supervised cognitive behavioral self-help for bulimia nervosa. *Journal of Psychosomatic Research, 40,* 281–287.

Crisp, A. H., Norton, K., Gowers, S., Halek, C., Bowyer, C., Yeldham, D., Levett, G., & Bhatt, A. (1991). A controlled study of the effect of therapies aimed at adolescent and family psychopathology in anorexia nervosa. *British Journal of Psychiatry, 159,* 325–333.

Davis, R., Olmsted, M., Rockert, W., Marques, T., & Dolhanty, J. (1997). Group psychoeducation for bulimia nervosa with and without additional psychotherapy process sessions. *International Journal of Eating Disorders, 22,* 25–34.

Devlin, M. J. (1996). Assessment and treatment of binge eating disorder. *Psychiatric Clinics of North America, 19,* 761–772.

de Zwaan, M., Nutzinger, D. O., & Schoenbeck, G. (1992). Binge eating in overweight women. *Comprehensive Psychiatry, 33,* 256–261.

Dodge, E., Hodes, M., Eisler, I., & Dare, C. (1995). Family therapy for bulimia nervosa in adolescents: An exploratory study. *Journal of Family Therapy, 17,* 59–78.

Eldredge, K. L., Agras, W. S., Arnow, B., Telch, C. F., Bell, S., Castonguay, L., & Marnell, M. (1997). The effects of extending cognitive-behavioral therapy for binge eating disorder among initial treatment nonresponders. *International Journal of Eating Disorders, 21,* 347–352.

Fairburn, C. G. (1981). A cognitive behavioural approach to the treatment of bulimia. *Psychological Medicine, 11,* 707–711.

Fairburn, C. G. (1995). *Overcoming binge eating.* New York: Guilford.

Fairburn, C. G., & Peveler, R. C. (1990). Bulimia nervosa and a stepped care approach to management. *Gut, 31,* 1220–1222.

Fairburn, C. G., Kirk, J., O'Conner, M., & Cooper, P. J. (1986). A comparison of two psychological treatments for bulimia nervosa. *Behaviour Research and Therapy, 24,* 629–643.

Fairburn, C. G., Jones, R., Peveler, R. C., Carr, S. J., Solomon, R. A., O'Conner, M. E., Burton, J., & Hope, R. A. (1991). Three psychological treatments for bulimia nervosa. *Archives of General Psychiatry, 48,* 463–469.

Fairburn, C. G., Jones, R., Peveler, R. C., Hope, R. A., & O'Conner, M. (1993). Psychotherapy and bulimia nervosa: The longer-term effects of interpersonal psychotherapy, behavior therapy and cognitive behavior therapy. *Archives of General Psychiatry, 50,* 419–428.

Fairburn, C. G., Marcus, M., & Wilson, G. T. (1993). Cognitive behavioral treatment for binge eating and bulimia nervosa: A comprehensive treatment manual. In C. G. Fairburn & G. T. Wilson (Eds.), *Binge eating: Nature, assessment, and treatment* (pp. 361–404). New York: Guilford.

Fairburn, C. G., Norman, P. A., Welch, S. L., O'Conner, M. E., Doll, H. A., & Peveler, R. C. (1995). A prospective study of outcome in bulimia nervosa and the long-term effects of three psychological treatments. *Archives of General Psychiatry, 52,* 304–312.

Fallon, P., Katzman, M. A., & Wooley, S. C. (Eds.). (1994). *Feminist perspectives on eating disorders.* New York: Guilford.

Fichter, M. M., Leibl, K., Rief, W., Brunner, E., Schmidt-Auberger, S., & Engel, R. R. (1991). Fluoxetine versus placebo: A double-blind study with bulimic inpatients undergoing intensive psychotherapy. *Pharmacopsychiatry, 24,* 1–7.

Freeman, C. P. L., Barry, F., Dunkeld-Turnball, J., & Henderson, A. (1988). Controlled trial of psychotherapy for bulimia nervosa. *British Medical Journal, 296,* 521–525.

Garfinkel, P. E., & Walsh, B. T. (1997). Drug therapies. In D. M. Garner & P. E. Garfinkel (Eds.), *Handbook of treatment for eating disorders* (2nd ed., pp. 372–380). New York: Guilford.

Garner, D. M., & Bemis, K. M. (1982). A cognitive-behavioral approach to anorexia nervosa. *Cognitive Therapy and Research, 6,* 123–150.

Garner, D. M., & Needleman, L. D. (1996). Stepped-care and decision-tree models for treating eating disorders. In J. K. Thompson (Ed.), *Body image, eating disorders, and obesity: An integrative guide for assessment and treatment* (pp. 225–252). Washington, DC: American Psychological Association.

Garner, D. M., Olmsted, M. P., Bohr, Y., & Garfinkel, P. E. (1982). The eating attitudes test: Psychometric features and clinical correlates. *Psychological Medicine, 12,* 871–878.

Garner, D. M., Rockert, W., Davis, R., Garner, M. V., Olmsted, M. P., & Eagle, M. (1993). Comparison between cognitive-behavioral and supportive-expressive therapy for bulimia nervosa. *American Journal of Psychiatry, 150,* 37–46.

Garner, D. M., Vitousek, K. M., & Pike, K. M. (1997). Cognitive-behavioral therapy for anorexia nervosa. In D. M. Garner & P. E. Garfinkel (Eds.), *Handbook of treatment for eating disorders* (2nd ed., pp. 94–144). New York: Guilford.

Gowers, S., Norton, K., Halek, C., & Crisp, A. (1994). Outcome of outpatient psychotherapy in a random allocation treatment study of anorexia nervosa. *International Journal of Eating Disorders, 15,* 165–177.

Hall, A., & Crisp, A. H. (1987). Brief psychotherapy in the treatment of anorexia nervosa: Outcome at one year. *British Journal of Psychiatry, 151,* 185–191.

Halmi, K. A. (1997). Personal communication.

Huon, G. F. (1985). An initial validation of a self-help program for bulimia. *International Journal of Eating Disorders, 4,* 573–588.

Kaplan, A. S., & Olmsted, M. P. (1997). Partial hospitalization. In D. M. Garner & P. E. Garfinkel (Eds.), *Handbook of treatment for eating disorders* (2nd ed., pp. 354–360). New York: Guilford.

Kirkley, B. G., Schneider, J. A., Agras, W. S., & Bachman, J. A. (1985). Comparison of two group treatments for bulimia nervosa. *Journal of Consulting and Clinical Psychology, 53,* 43–48.

Klerman, G. L., Weissman, M. M., Rounsaville, B. J., & Chevron, E. S. (1984). *Interpersonal psychotherapy of depression.* New York: Basic Books.

Laessle, P. J., Beumont, P. J. V., Butow, P., Lennerts, W., O'Conner, M., Pirke, K. M., Touyz, S. W., & Waadt, S. (1991). A comparison of nutritional management with stress management in the treatment of bulimia nervosa. *British Journal of Psychiatry, 159,* 250–261.

Leitenberg, H., Rosen, J. C., Wolf, J., Vara, L. S., Detzer, M. J., & Srebnik, D. (1994). Comparison of cognitive-behavior therapy and desipramine in the treatment of bulimia nervosa. *Behaviour Research and Therapy, 32,* 37–45.

Levine, M. D., Marcus, M. D., & Moulton, P. (1996). Exercise in the treatment of binge eating disorder. *International Journal of Eating Disorders, 19,* 171–177.

Loeb, K. L., Wilson, G. T., & Gilbert, J. (1998). *A comparison of supervised and unsupervised self-help for binge eating.* Paper presented at the Eighth International Conference on Eating Disorders, New York.

Luborsky, L. (1984). *Principles of psychodynamic psychotherapy: A manual for supportive-expressive treatment.* New York: Basic Books.

Marcus, M. D., Wing, R. R., Ewing, L., Kern, E., Gooding, W., & McDermott, M. (1990). A double-blind, placebo-controlled trial of fluoxetine plus behavior modification in the treatment of obese binge eaters and non-binge eaters. *American Journal of Psychiatry, 147,* 876–881.

Marcus, M. D., Wing, R. R., & Fairburn, C. G. (1995). Cognitive treatment of binge eating versus behavioral weight control in the treatment of binge eating disorder. *Annals of Behavioral Medicine, 17,* S090.

McCann, U. D., & Agras, W. S. (1990). Successful treatment of nonpurging bulimia nervosa with desipramine: A double-blind, placebo-controlled study. *American Journal of Psychiatry, 147,* 1509–1513.

Mitchell, J. E., Pyle, R. L., Eckert, E. D., Hatsukami, D., Pomeroy, C., & Zimmerman, R. (1990). A comparison study of antidepressants and intensive group psychotherapy in the treatment of bulimia nervosa. *Archives of General Psychiatry, 47,* 149–157.

Mitchell, J. E., Specker, S., & Edmonson, K. (1997). Management of substance abuse and dependence. In D. M. Garner & P. E. Garfinkel (Eds.), *Handbook of treatment for eating disorders* (2nd ed., pp. 415–423). New York: Guilford.

Olmsted, M. P., Davis, R., Rockert, W., Irvine, M. J., Eagle, M., & Garner, D. M. (1991). Efficacy of a brief group psychoeducational intervention for bulimia nervosa. *Behaviour Research and Therapy, 29,* 71–83.

Pike, K. M. (1997). *Relapse prevention in anorexia nervosa.* Paper presented at the International Conference on Eating Disorders, London.

Pike, K. M., Loeb, K., & Vitousek, K. (1996). Cognitive-behavioral therapy for anorexia nervosa and bulimia nervosa. In J. K. Thompson (Ed.), *Body image, eating disorders, and obesity: An integrative guide for assessment and treatment* (pp. 253–302). Washington, DC: American Psychological Association.

Polivy, J., & Herman, C. P. (1993). Etiology of binge eating: Psychological mechanisms. In C. G. Fairburn & G. T. Wilson (Eds.), *Binge eating: Nature, assessment, and treatment* (pp. 173–205). New York: Guilford.

Robin, A. L., Siegel, P. T., & Moye, A. (1995). Family versus individual therapy for anorexia: Impact on family conflict. *International Journal of Eating Disorders, 17,* 313–312.

Russell, G. (1979). Bulimia nervosa: An ominous variant of anorexia nervosa. *Psychological Medicine, 9,* 429–448.

Russell, G. F. M., Szmukler, G. I., Dare, C., & Eisler, I. (1987). An evaluation of family therapy in anorexia nervosa and bulimia nervosa. *Archives of General Psychiatry, 44,* 1047–1056.

Schmidt, U., Tiller, J., & Treasure, J. (1993). Self-treatment of bulimia nervosa: A pilot study. *International Journal of Eating Disorders, 13,* 273–277.

Schneider, J. A., & Agras, W. S. (1985). A cognitive behavioral group treatment of bulimia. *British Journal of Psychiatry, 146,* 66–69.

Smith, D. E., Marcus, M. D., & Kaye, W. (1992). Cognitive-behavioral treatment of obese binge eaters. *International Journal of Eating Disorders, 12,* 257–262.

Spitzer, R. L., Devlin, M., Walsh, B. T., Hasin, D., Wing, R., Marcus, M., Stunkard, A., Wadden, T., Yanovksi, S., Agras, S., Mitchell, J., & Nonas, C. (1992). Binge eating disorder: A multisite field trial of the diagnostic criteria. *International Journal of Eating Disorders, 11,* 191–203.

Spitzer, R. L., Yanovksi, S., Wadden, T., Wing, R., Marcus, M., Stunkard, A., Devlin, M., Mitchell, J., Hasin, D., & Horne, R. L. (1993). Binge eating disorder: Its further validation in a multisite study. *International Journal of Eating Disorders, 13,* 137–153.

Telch, C. F., & Agras, W. S. (1993). The effects of a very low calorie diet on binge eating. *Behavior Therapy, 24,* 177–193.

Telch, C. F., Agras, W. S., Rossiter, E. M., Wilfley, D., & Kenardy, J. (1990). Group cognitive-behavioral treatment for the nonpurging bulimic: An initial evaluation. *Journal of Consulting and Clinical Psychology, 58,* 629–635.

Thackwray, D. E., Smith, M. C., Bodfish, J. W., & Meyers, A. W. (1993). A comparison of behavioral and cognitive-behavioral interventions for bulimia nervosa. *Journal of Consulting and Clinical Psychology, 61,* 639–645.

Treasure, J., Schmidt, U., Troop, N., Tiller, J., Todd, G., Keilen, M., & Dodge, E. (1994). First step in managing bulimia nervosa: Controlled trial of therapeutic manual. *British Medical Journal, 308,* 686–689.

Treasure, J., Schmidt, U., Troop, N., Tiller, J., Todd, G., & Turnball, S. (1996). Sequential treatment for bulimia nervosa incorporating a self-care manual. *British Journal of Psychiatry, 168,* 94–98.

Vitousek, K., Watson, S., & Wilson, G. T. (in press). Enhancing motivation for change in treatment-resistant eating disorders. *Clinical Psychology Review.*

Walsh, B. T. (1992). Pharmacological treatment of eating disorders. In K. Halmi (Ed.), *The psychobiology and treatment of anorexia nervosa and bulimia nervosa* (pp. 329–340). Washington, DC: American Psychiatric Press.

Walsh, B. T., Hadigan, C. M., Kissileff, H. R., & LaChaussee, J. L. (1992). Bulimia nervosa: A syndrome of feast and famine. In G. H. Anderson & S. H. Kennedy (Eds.), *The biology of feast and famine* (pp. 3–20). New York: Academic Press.

Walsh, B. T., Wilson, G. T., Loeb, K. L., Devlin, M. J., Pike, K. M., Fleiss, J. L., & Wanternaux, C. (1997). Psychological and pharmacological treatment of bulimia nervosa. *American Journal of Psychiatry, 154,* 523–531.

Wilfley, D. E., Agras, W. S., Telch, C. S., Rossiter, E. M., Schneider, J. A., Cole, A. G., Sifford, L., & Raeburn, S. D. (1993). Group cognitive-behavioral therapy and group interpersonal psychotherapy for the nonpurging bulimic individual: A controlled comparison. *Journal of Consulting and Clinical Psychology, 61,* 296–305.

Wilson, G. T. (1993). Binge eating and addictive disorders. In C. G. Fairburn & G. T. Wilson (Eds.), *Binge eating: Nature, assessment, and treatment* (pp. 97–120). New York: Guilford.

Wilson, G. T. (1996a). Acceptance and change in the treatment of eating disorders and obesity. *Behavior Therapy, 27,* 417–439.

Wilson, G. T. (1996b). Treatment of bulimia nervosa: When CBT fails. *Behaviour Research and Therapy, 34,* 197–212.

Wilson, G. T., & Fairburn, C. G. (1998). Treatments for eating disorders. In P. E. Nathan & J. M. Gorman (Eds.), *Treatments that work* (pp. 501–530). New York: Oxford University Press.

Wilson, G. T., Fairburn, C. G., & Agras, W. S. (1997). Cognitive-behavioral therapy for bulimia nervosa. In D. M. Garner & P. E. Garfinkel (Eds.), *Handbook of treatment for eating disorders* (2nd ed., pp. 67–93). New York: Guilford.

Wolf, E. M., & Crowther, J. H. (1992). An evaluation of behavioral and cognitive-behavioral group interventions for the treatment of bulimia nervosa in women. *International Journal of Eating Disorders, 11,* 3–15.

Yeary, J. (1987). The use of Overeaters Anonymous in the treatment of eating disorders. *Journal of Psychoactive Drugs, 19,* 303–309.

18

Strategies for Tobacco Cessation

DAVID A. F. HAAGA AND LINDSEY KIRK

INTRODUCTION

Cigarette smoking is considered the leading preventable cause of death in the United States (USDHHS, 1990). Cigarette smoking has been implicated in lung, oral, and other cancers, as well as cardiovascular disease, pulmonary disease, fetal complications, and other disorders (Peto, Lopez, Boreham, Thun, & Heath, 1992). Smoking cessation substantially reduces the risks of various diseases, and eventually returns former smokers to the same risk levels as nonsmokers (USDHHS, 1990). Despite these well-publicized risks of smoking and benefits of smoking cessation, about one-fourth of the adult population in the United States currently smokes cigarettes (American Psychiatric Association, 1996). Moreover, whereas the majority of smokers express a desire to quit, and about one third try to quit smoking in a given year (American Psychiatric Association, 1994), on any given attempt to quit, only 4% to 5% of smokers trying to quit on their own succeed, as defined by a full year of continuous abstinence after smoking cessation (Cohen *et al.*, 1989).

Cigarette smoking is thus a highly prevalent, addictive behavior with severe negative consequences, and smoking cessation affords clinically significant health benefits but is quite difficult to achieve on one's own. Identification of effective strategies for helping patients quit smoking should therefore be a very high priority for health professionals. The purpose of this chapter is to describe briefly some smoking cessation methods supported by research. Our focus is on relatively intensive strategies for helping smokers. One important component of the overall antismoking effort is brief advice from health care professionals, which has tremendous potential for making an impact at the population level and is reviewed in this volume by Heather (Chapter 10).

DAVID A. F. HAAGA AND LINDSEY KIRK • Department of Psychology, American University, Washington, D.C. 20016.

Treating Addictive Behaviors, 2nd ed., edited by Miller and Heather. Plenum Press, New York, 1998.

ENHANCING MOTIVATION TO QUIT SMOKING

The general problem of motivating addicts to contemplate and then to attempt behavior change is taken up by Miller in Chapter 9 of this volume. Nevertheless, it is common to encounter residual ambivalence on the part of participants in smoking cessation programs. That is, motivation is not all-or-none, and even those who have progressed far enough to initiate a formal attempt to quit smoking sometimes leave considerable room for motivational enhancement.

WHEN IS THE RIGHT TIME TO QUIT SMOKING?

In a word, now. Smoking cessation should not be on the back burner awaiting the (hypothetical) time when there will be few other time commitments, no forthcoming visits from difficult guests, little pressure at work or school, unfailingly cooperative children, and so on.

Therapists as well as patients sometimes question the wisdom of quitting smoking right away, particularly when the patient also abuses alcohol or other drugs. Given that the prevalence of cigarette smoking is very high among alcohol-dependent people (e.g., 90%, Bobo, 1992), this is an important practical issue in treatment planning. Some studies show smokers with a history of alcohol or other drug problems to be less successful than other smokers in trying to quit (Hughes, 1993b), though researchers are only beginning to target this subgroup specifically for smoking cessation programs (Martin et al., 1997). Of importance is the fact that no studies have found quitting smoking to worsen alcohol or other drug problems. To the contrary, if anything, successful smoking cessation is associated positively with the likelihood of success in addressing other addictions (for a review, see Shiffman & Balabanis, 1995). There is therefore no reason automatically to delay smoking cessation efforts simply because patients have other drug problems (Sees, Clark, & Westly, 1993).

PERSONALIZING HEALTH RISKS

Assuming that therapists are convinced of the wisdom of proceeding with efforts to motivate smokers to quit, the next question faced is what to do. One frequently used motivational strategy is to try to help patients personalize the risks of continued smoking and the benefits of quitting (Ockene & Kristeller, 1994). The premise of such an approach is that general knowledge of the pros and cons of smoking and smoking cessation is insufficient unless the smoker applies these concepts to her or his own situation. Some studies have achieved very high rates of cessation with postcoronary patients (Burling, Singleton, Bigelow, Baile, & Gottlieb, 1984), and the more severe the coronary heart disease the higher the cessation rate (for a review, see Ockene & Zapka, 1997). These results are a testament to the power of the principle of taking the consequences of smoking personally, but of course it would be ideal not to have to wait until someone has suffered a myocardial infarction to focus their attention on the importance of smoking cessation.

A new technological development relevant to the goal of personalizing health risks is the availability of screening tests for genetic susceptibility to certain forms of cancer. It is possible that results indicative of enhanced cancer risk would serve to motivate current smokers to view smoking cessation as a more urgent priority. In one self-help smoking cessation experiment, smokers randomly assigned to receive feedback on the basis of a blood test as to their genetic susceptibility to lung cancer reported increased fear, increased perceived risk of lung cancer, and increased perceived health benefits of quitting smoking (Lerman *et al.,* 1997). There was no significant effect of genetic susceptibility feedback on smoking cessation rate, however. One-year follow-up confirmed the motivational effect of genetic testing in that participants given this feedback were more likely to try to quit smoking, but they were no more likely than controls to achieve abstinence (Audrain *et al.,* 1997).

From the perspective of social cognitive theory (Bandura, 1986), it is important to remember that "motivation" is not fueled solely by the perception that quitting smoking would be a good idea. Rather, the smoker must also perceive himself or herself as capable of quitting smoking. That is, self-efficacy (I can learn these coping skills and abstain from smoking) *and* response-outcome expectations (if I abstain, I will improve my breathing, save money, reduce cancer risk . . .) must be positive for a serious attempt to be initiated. Contemplation of quitting smoking is associated specifically with enhanced expectation of benefits to be derived from quitting, but translating such contemplation into effective action and maintenance of smoking cessation seems to entail enhanced self-efficacy as well (Dijkstra, DeVries, & Bakker, 1996).

DEBRIEFING PAST RELAPSES

One impediment to motivation for some long-term smokers enrolling in smoking cessation programs is pessimism bred of having tried and failed to quit smoking in the past. For such smokers it may be helpful to point out that number of previous (failed) attempts to quit is not strongly, if at all, correlated with success on the current attempt (Cohen *et al.,* 1989). This finding is subject to multiple interpretations (e.g., the subgroup still around having to keep trying after 10 or more attempts are particularly tough cases, and this may be offset by the educational value of past relapses for guiding current strategies) but at a minimum implies that there is no basis for those who have relapsed many times before to conclude that their addictions are beyond the reach of treatment.

Another tack, borrowed from the applied science of marketing, is to bill the techniques to be used in the current smoking cessation attempt as somehow new and different, with the implication that past failures are no longer applicable to the current situation. This may account in part for the tremendous, immediate commercial success of the nicotine patch (Fiore, Jorenby, Baker, & Kenford, 1992).

PREPARING FOR QUIT DAY

Assuming that the smoker is well motivated for a cessation attempt, the further question arises as to how she or he should go about cutting down on smoking prior to quitting altogether.

RAPID-PACED AVERSIVE SMOKING

Behavior therapy approaches developed in the 1960s and 1970s included an array of creative means of trying to make smoking aversive so as to discourage further smoking. These included contingent mild electric shock, holding the smoky air in longer than is typical before exhaling ("smokeholding"), drastically increasing the rate of smoking (satiation), and blowing warm, stale smoke into smokers' faces as they smoked (Schwartz, 1987). The most widely studied approach was rapid-paced aversive smoking (Lichtenstein, Harris, Birchler, Wahl, & Schmahl, 1973), which involves puffing more frequently than is typical (e.g., every 6 seconds). Although a number of studies supported the efficacy of rapid smoking, it is not recommended for routine practice. First, safety concerns were raised about its use, especially for smokers with coronary heart disease (Hauser, 1974). Subsequent research actually found promising results in terms of the safety of the procedure, but the recommendation remained that "[p]ersons with cardiac disease should be treated with rapid smoking only if medical backup is available" (Schwartz, 1987, p. 78). Second, a metanalysis (Law & Tang, 1995) found that the small subset of rapid-smoking studies featuring biochemical corroboration of self-reported abstinence did not support its long-term efficacy.

NICOTINE FADING AND SELF-MONITORING

A nonaversive alternative to rapid smoking is nicotine fading (also called "brand switching"). In this 3-week procedure, participants switch brands of cigarettes on a weekly basis to a lower-nicotine brand. Typically, the progression is from a brand 30% lower in nicotine than the smoker's usual brand (week 1) to one 60% lower (week 2) to one 90% lower (week 3), followed by quitting smoking altogether (Foxx & Brown, 1979). There is no requirement to decrease the number of cigarettes smoked while progressing through the nicotine fading procedure. In principle one could achieve the same aim of reducing blood nicotine levels gradually, and thereby ease the discomfort of withdrawal symptoms after smoking cessation, by cutting down on the number of cigarettes rather than the nicotine content of each one. Nicotine fading is preferred, though, for two reasons. First, if one were to smoke fewer cigarettes but stick to the same brand, the contrast between (declining) plasma nicotine level and the nicotine level of the cigarette being smoked is increasing over time, perhaps inadvertently making each cigarette more salient and more reinforcing (Berecz, 1984). Second, a tortuous process of number fading before getting to zero can have the effect of making each remaining cigarette seem more of a precious reward, not the ideal frame for preparing to quit smoking.

Nicotine fading is usually implemented along with self-monitoring procedures, such as keeping a record of the time, place, and circumstance (any relevant stressors, thoughts, and emotions) of each cigarette smoked. This is intended to help smokers become more aware of their smoking patterns and to guide the selection of personally useful coping skills that might serve the same psychological functions (e.g., relaxation, stimulation, something to do, a ritual, a break from tasks) after smoking cessation as cigarettes are currently serving for the smoker. The combination of nicotine fading and self-monitoring played an important role in an effective, widely disseminated, broad-spectrum behavior therapy approach to smoking cessation developed by Lando (1977; McGovern & Lando, 1991). Coping skills training is dissociable from nicotine fading as a means of preparing to quit, though, and is reviewed separately on page 250.

SCHEDULED REDUCED SMOKING

A concern about nicotine fading is that it enables smokers to retain high-preference cigarettes, and to continue to smoke in conjunction with personally relevant external smoking cues. A scheduled smoking procedure was developed to break well-established associations between environmental cues, mood, and smoking. This procedure involves having people smoke according to a preset schedule, based on gradually increasing intercigarette intervals. An initial study by Cinciripini and colleagues (1994) found that a multicomponent treatment incorporating scheduled smoking led to higher 1-year abstinence rates (41%) than did a minimal-contact self-help control condition (6%). A follow-up study confirmed experimentally the importance of scheduling smoking rather than allowing it to be ad lib (Cinciripini *et al.*, 1995). Scheduled reduced smoking yielded a higher abstinence rate at 1-year follow-up (44%) than did nonscheduled reduced smoking (18%), or nonscheduled, nonreduced smoking (i.e., abrupt quitting) (22%). Scheduled reduced smoking did not differ significantly from scheduled, nonreduced smoking (32%). All groups in this study received cognitive-behavioral relapse prevention training as discussed on page 251. Scheduled reduced smoking was also associated with improved adaptation to nonsmoking, as indicated by reduced tension, fatigue, withdrawal, and urges to smoke.

The scheduled reduced smoking program consists of 1 week of baseline, 4 weeks of reducing, and 4 weeks of maintenance and relapse prevention. During the baseline week participants smoke as usual while noting time of day and environmental cues. After 3 days, they bring a 3-week supply of cigarettes (based on their baseline rate of daily consumption) to the clinic. During weeks 2 and 3, smoking intervals are set by dividing two thirds (week 2) and one third (week 3) of the participant's average baseline smoking rate by the average number of waking hours in their day. For example, someone who typically smokes 24 cigarettes in a 16-waking-hour day would be assigned during week 2 to smoke 1 cigarette each hour (two thirds of 24 = 16 cigarettes per day, and 16 cigarettes spread evenly across 16 waking hours = 1 per hour). In week 3 this participant would smoke once every 2 hours ($^1/_3$ × 24 = 8 cigarettes per day, scheduled evenly across 16 waking hours = 1 every 2 hours). In week 4, intervals are lengthened again, reducing consumption by one third of the rate for week 2 every day until the person reaches 2 to 4 cigarettes per day (which should be within 1 to 2 days of the target quit date). Independent replication of the efficacy findings is needed, and research is needed to determine the mechanisms of action, but scheduled reduced smoking appears to be a very promising method of preparing for the actual cessation of cigarette smoking (Cinciripini, Wetter, & McClure, 1997).

PSYCHOLOGICAL METHODS OF COPING WITH ABSTINENCE

Regardless of the means used to prepare for quit day, sustaining abstinence after smoking cessation is challenging. In this section we describe psychological techniques of possible use in meeting this challenge.

General Coping Skills Training

In addition to planning a method to reduce or eliminate smoking, clinicians can teach new coping skills to regulate emotions and deal with stress and other negative experiences. Behavioral coping skills include leaving the situation, using substitute behaviors, or self-management skills (such as assertiveness, time management, etc.). Cognitive coping skills include identifying maladaptive thoughts, then challenging and critically evaluating them. Descriptive research suggests that no one coping tactic is across the board more effective than others but that use of both behavioral and cognitive coping tactics is preferable to either alone or to the failure to make any explicit coping effort (Shiffman, 1984). Accordingly, some treatment programs have taught a great many specific coping techniques, in the hope that more smokers will find some tactics that are valuable for them (Stevens & Hollis, 1989).

Specific Coping Tactics

Clearly it is somewhat inefficient to teach dozens of coping techniques in the hope that a few will "take" with a given smoker and prove useful in managing urges and maintaining abstinence. Moreover, there may be a danger of overloading people with a panoply of techniques, such that none really is taught well and practiced thoroughly. Two directions for attempting to improve on this state of affairs are discernible in current research.

First, we can try to test experimentally the value of specific coping tactics in achieving particular outcomes. For example, continuing regular smokers prevented from smoking for a period of about 3 hours in the laboratory (most of the time being spent watching a movie) reported significantly less craving for a cigarette if they were given access to chewing gum during this time (Cohen, Collins, & Britt, 1997). This finding does not speak to the relevance of the tactic of chewing gum for those who are trying to quit smoking altogether for any length of time, but it does support the common clinical impression that chewing gum can be a useful alternative response for smokers to employ when experiencing craving.

Second, we can try to improve our ability to identify individual differences in smoking patterns and motives and thereby our ability to tailor coping-skills training to the individual smoker (see Chapter 13, this volume). Traditionally, smoking patterns and motives have been evaluated with generalized, traitlike self-report inventories. However, evidence for the validity of such scales is not strong (Shiffman, 1993a), and the assumption of traitlike consistency in the situations that are challenging for a particular smoker may be somewhat overgeneralized. It is possible that in vivo, computer-assisted self-monitoring methods such as the "ecological momentary assessment" techniques developed by Stone and Shiffman (1994) will provide more precise situational data useful for individualized treatment planning.

REFRAMING LAPSES

Identification of high-risk situations, and coping skills training oriented toward managing them, is incorporated in some treatment programs in a more general relapse prevention model (Marlatt & Gordon, 1985).

A unique feature of the relapse prevention model is the hypothesis that an abstinence violation effect (AVE) increases the probability that an initial lapse after smoking cessation will result in relapse to regular smoking. The AVE consists of feeling guilty about the initial lapse and attributing it to internal, stable, and global causes. Thus, a recent ex-smoker who smokes one cigarette after eating dinner with still-smoking friends could conclude "I blew it; I guess I'm really addicted and just don't have the willpower to quit smoking." Such a reaction would increase the probability of resuming regular smoking relative to viewing the same event as an indication that one needs to come up with better means of coping with (or at least temporarily avoiding) the indirect social pressure to smoke associated with socializing with these friends.

Studies of the utility of the relapse prevention model, and in particular its unique focus on differentiating lapses from relapses and trying to reduce the AVE by helping smokers reframe lapses, have yielded mixed results. Minneker-Hugel, Unland, and Buchkremer (1992), for example, found that relapse prevention strategies did not provide a significant increase in the effectiveness of smoking cessation therapy.

In contrast, Davis and Glaros (1986) found that smokers who learn relapse prevention skills maintain cessation longer and smoke fewer cigarettes if they do relapse than controls who did not receive the training. Carroll (1996) reviewed 12 studies that evaluated relapse prevention treatment for smoking and found strong evidence for its effectiveness, when compared with no-treatment controls. However, the results showed inconsistent support for relapse prevention compared with other active treatments (Carroll, 1996).

Several explanations for these mixed results are possible, and at this point there are insufficient data to choose among them. First, relapse prevention may in fact be better than nothing, but not better than other plausible treatments and therefore not uniquely effective (Carroll, 1996). Second, the descriptive model may be accurate, but the technology for implementing it to improve smoking cessation programs underdeveloped. Shiffman (1993b) suggests, for instance, that the main procedure utilized in most smoking cessation clinics to take into account the AVE is simply teaching patients the nature of the effect. It may prove useful to borrow from the technical tool bag of cognitive therapy of depression, which appears to work at least in part by changing similar attributional patterns as they relate to negative life events (DeRubeis et al., 1990). Third, we need to consider the possibility that disputing the AVE and otherwise trying to help patients learn to limit and recover from lapses is not extremely effective because the basic model is incorrect. Many of the supportive data linking attributions and guilt feelings to the lapse–relapse transition come from retrospective studies.

The AVE may reflect after-the-fact interpretations of relapses on the part of smokers. Haaga (1989) investigated recent ex-smokers' thoughts in high-risk situations through an articulated thoughts during simulated situations paradigm (Davison, Robins, & Johnson, 1983) and found that cognitions associated with the AVE did not distinguish between people who would later recover from an initial lapse and those who would fall into a full-blown relapse. Shiffman and colleagues (1996) assessed indicators of the AVE by using handheld computers to record people's real-time reactions to an initial lapse. They found that evidence of an AVE response to the initial lapse failed to predict progression into full relapse. These studies suggest that having an initial reaction to a lapse consistent with the AVE may not lead to relapse as previously thought. Perhaps in previous studies, AVE seemed to be related to eventual relapse because people were reporting their reactions to the initial lapse retrospectively, and were influenced by the knowledge that they eventually did relapse (Haaga, 1989; Shiffman *et. al.,* 1996).

NICOTINE REPLACEMENT

Numerous pharmacological approaches to smoking cessation have been proposed and are being studied actively, including antidepressant medications, but only nicotine replacement strategies have been clearly documented as bolstering long-term abstinence (Hajek, 1996).

Two types of nicotine replacement—nicotine gum and transdermal nicotine patches—are available over the counter in the United States ("Nicotine Patches Available OTC," 1996). These products deliver nicotine to the body in order to minimize the withdrawal symptoms associated with smoking cessation. It is thought that minimizing physical withdrawal might make it easier for the patient to break the smoking habit and then gradually withdraw from the nicotine after a period of successful abstinence from smoking.

Nicotine Gum

Nicotine gum is available in 2 mg and 4 mg strengths, with 4 mg recommended for highly nicotine-dependent patients and those who have failed with a 2 mg trial. Gum is usually prescribed for the first few months of quitting, but can be continued. It can be prescribed for use as needed, or for scheduled dosing, for a typical period of 3 months. Recent work suggests that scheduling gum use works better.

A metanalysis of nicotine chewing gum by Cepeda-Benito (1993) reviewed 33 studies comparing nicotine chewing gum to a control (placebo or no gum) with random assignment and double-blind procedures. Effect sizes were calculated at short (0–8 weeks after completion of treatment) and long term (10–14 months after completion of treatment) follow-up, and considered whether nicotine gum was used in the context of intensive treatment (a comprehensive smoking cessation program with a minimum of 3 hours of therapy within a 4-week period) or brief treatment (when the other criteria were not met). Over all conditions, the nicotine gum performed significantly better than controls. Nicotine gum was superior to both placebo and no-gum controls at both short and long term for the intensive treatments. However, the gum was only superior to placebo and no gum at the short-term assessment for the brief strategies. This suggests that nicotine gum does not have an effect on long-term abstinence when used outside the context of intensive therapy, which has clear implications for the likely utility of nicotine gum for patients who are buying it over the counter and using it without adjunctive treatment.

Several studies have investigated the hypothesis that pretreatment levels of nicotine dependence would predict differential responses to nicotine gum treatment. In one such trial, 173 smokers were classified as high or low on nicotine dependence using the Fagerstrom Tolerance Questionnaire and were randomly assigned to nicotine gum (2 mg, chewed ad libitum), or no gum (Niaura, Goldstein, & Abrams, 1994). All smokers received a 5-week treatment program concurrently; this consisted of four counseling sessions and a self-help manual. Smokers with high levels of nicotine dependence were more likely to quit with the gum (32%) than without it (12%). Low-nicotine smokers were slightly less likely to quit with the gum (14%) than without it (20%), though this difference was not significant. The relative differences in outcome persisted at 1-year follow-up, but were statistically nonsignificant.

These results and those from similar studies (for a review, see Hughes, 1993a) support the possible utility of a patient–treatment matching scheme in which only smokers high in nicotine dependence would receive nicotine gum. However, while it is reliably found that low-dependence smokers receive less benefit from nicotine gum than do high-dependence smokers, findings are inconsistent with respect to whether they derive any benefit. Accordingly, it may well make sense for even low-dependence smokers to try nicotine gum (AHCPR, 1996).

NICOTINE PATCH

The transdermal nicotine patch is easier to use than nicotine gum, with once per day dosing and steadier nicotine replacement. The nicotine patch is available for 16-hour or 24-hour use, with starting doses of 22 mg and 15 mg of nicotine, respectively. The patch may have advantages over nicotine gum in terms of ease of use and reduced compliance problems. However, pregnant women and cardiac patients need special consideration of the risks and benefits before deciding to use the nicotine patch.

A metanalysis of 17 double-blind, placebo-controlled nicotine patch studies of 4 weeks or longer, with random assignment and biochemical verification of abstinence, found average abstinence rates for the patch to be 22% at 6-month follow-up, compared to 9% for placebo patches (Fiore, Smith, Jorenby, & Baker, 1994). There did not appear to be a difference in the effectiveness of the 16- and 24-hour patch, and treatment duration beyond 8 weeks did not enhance effectiveness. Gradual weaning from the patch did not improve outcome. The nicotine patch significantly increased cessation rates when added either to intensive counseling or minimal adjunctive therapy. This suggests that when nicotine replacement therapy is used in the absence of intensive therapy, the patch may be more effective than nicotine gum. Differences between nicotine and placebo patches have been clearest in studies measuring outcome as continuous abstinence rather than point prevalence; the latter measure allows for the possibility that someone is abstinent at the time of follow-up but has relapsed one or more times since smoking cessation (Richmond, 1997).

Overall the transdermal nicotine patch is an effective aid to smoking cessation, much more so than placebo, but still not by any means a universal cure. No consistent indicators of differential response to the patch have been found that could guide rational patient–treatment matching; notably, several studies have failed to show differential response to transdermal nicotine on the basis of pretreatment nicotine dependence (e.g., Kenford *et al.*, 1994; Stapleton *et al.*, 1995).

COMBINING NICOTINE PATCH AND NICOTINE GUM

Both nicotine gum and the nicotine patch have thus been shown to result in significantly higher abstinence rates than placebos in smoking cessation trials. Does combining the two methods yield still better results? In a within-subject experiment on this question (Fagerstrom, Schneider, & Lunell, 1993), 28 smokers were exposed for 3 days each to four conditions (with 4-day smoking intervals to return to baseline levels of withdrawal symptoms): (1) double active = active gum (2 mg) + active patch (16-hour), (2) gum only active = active gum + placebo patch, (3) patch active = placebo gum + active patch, and (4) double placebo = placebo gum + placebo patch. Withdrawal symptoms were lowest during the "double active" condition, intermediate for the two conditions in which one form of nicotine replacement was active and the other placebo, and highest for double placebo. These results indicate that the combined group was significantly more effective than either single-active condition at reducing withdrawal. Consistent with this finding, the addition of 2 mg nicotine gum ad-lib to a patch appears to increase smoking cessation rates (Fagerstrom, 1994).

OTHER DELIVERY SYSTEMS FOR NICOTINE REPLACEMENT

Nicotine gum and nicotine patch are the most extensively studied nicotine replacement procedures, but others are available as well. Nicotine nasal spray was developed as a new form of nicotine replacement therapy because it is faster acting than the nicotine patch, and easier to use than nicotine gum. A randomized clinical trial assigned 255 smokers to nicotine nasal spray or a piperine placebo, using 8 to 32 doses per day for 6 months (Schneider *et al.*, 1995). Nicotine nasal spray significantly enhanced abstinence rates over placebo. Active versus placebo abstinence rates were 25% versus 10% (6 months) and 18% versus 8% (1 year). It was concluded that nicotine nasal spray is a safe, effective alternative for nicotine replacement in smoking cessation.

Finally, a smokeless nicotine inhaler, permitting smokers to suck nicotine through a plastic tube that resembles a fat cigarette, was recently made available. The inhaler delivers a much lower dose of nicotine than does a puff of a cigarette, and none of the tar. Ostensible advantages of this delivery system for nicotine replacement are that it sustains the ritual of bringing hand to mouth and replicates the sensation in the back of one's throat typical of smoking a cigarette. Results to date suggest that the inhaler may be expected to work approximately as well as other nicotine replacement methods ("FDA Approves First Smokeless Nicotine Inhaler," 1997)

COMBINING NICOTINE REPLACEMENT WITH
PSYCHOLOGICAL METHODS

There is nothing incompatible about nicotine replacement strategies and the psychological strategies noted earlier in this chapter. Indeed, it makes sense conceptually that a combination treatment would be particularly useful to the extent that nicotine replacement works by alleviating withdrawal symptoms whereas behavioral and cognitive techniques work by disrupting stimulus–response connections (e.g., scheduled reduced smoking) and providing alternative coping techniques for managing negative affect and high-risk situations. Combined behavior therapy and nicotine replacement therapy may work better than either alone (Klesges, Ward, & DeBon, 1996).

SPECIAL POPULATIONS

A large number of smokers may also suffer from psychiatric disorders, notably mood disorders, anxiety disorders, and schizophrenia (American Psychiatric Association, 1996). It is estimated that between 50% and 90% of people with mental disorders smoke (American Psychiatric Association, 1994). These comorbid disorders can make it more difficult to stop smoking. One such area of overlap that has received empirical attention is between depression and smoking. An increase in negative mood after quitting smoking is likely to predict relapse, and such increases in negative mood appear to be more common in people with a history of major depressive disorder (Hall *et. al.*, 1996). Hall, Muñoz, and Reus (1994) tested the utility of a 5-weekly session group cognitive-behavioral therapy (CBT), adapted from CBT for depression and including pleasant-events scheduling and cognitive restructuring. This "mood-management" treatment significantly enhanced the efficacy of nicotine gum plus an initial five sessions of group support and education about the consequences of smoking; the beneficial effect of CBT was obtained only for the smokers with a history of major depressive disorder. In a follow-up study controlling for length of treatment between the CBT and educational interventions, the history-of-depression X treatment condition interaction was not significant, though the trend was again for higher long-term abstinence among the depression-history-positive smokers if they were in the CBT condition (Hall *et. al.*, 1996).

CONCLUSIONS

Space constraints preclude an exhaustive review or a detailed methodological critique of research in this area. Additional details and documentation can be obtained from the practice guidelines published by the American Psychiatric Association (1996), the Agency for Health Care Policy and Research (1996), or the Quality Assurance Review (Mattick *et al.*, 1994).

Consistent with the overall perspective of this book, we view quitting smoking as a process, not a single event. Many smokers need multiple attempts before they can quit smoking indefinitely, and even a given attempt has multiple phases. To summarize the implications of the work reviewed in this chapter, we can follow the timeline of a single attempt to quit smoking:

(a) *Go/No-Go decision:* There is no need routinely to wait until other addictions have been successfully treated in order to attempt smoking cessation. Help bolster smokers' motivation to quit by personalizing the costs of smoking and the benefits of cessation. Increase self-efficacy, perhaps by promoting the novelty of the treatment method and by debriefing past relapses.

(b) *The month or so before complete abstinence:* Help smokers choose and implement one of two empirically supported nonaversive methods of cutting down on smoking prior to quitting altogether: nicotine fading or scheduled reduced smoking. Initiate coping skills training.

(c) *First two months after quit date:* Recommend nicotine replacement (transdermal patch or gum). Continue training in, and practice of, multiple cognitive and behavioral coping techniques for managing personally relevant high-risk situations.

By making smoking cessation a high priority in clinical practice, encouraging all smokers to quit, and adopting empirically supported methods, we can make a substantial positive impact on the length and quality of patients' lives.

REFERENCES

Agency for Health Care Policy and Research (AHCPR). (1996). Smoking cessation clinical practice guideline. *Journal of the American Medical Association, 275,* 1270–1280.

American Psychiatric Association. (1994). *Diagnostic and statistical manual of mental disorders* (4th ed.). Washington, DC: Author.

American Psychiatric Association. (1996). Practice guidelines for the treatment of patients with nicotine dependence. *American Journal of Psychiatry, 153,* 1–31.

Audrain, J., Boyd, N. R., Roth, J., Main, D., Caporaso, N. E., & Lerman, C. (1997). Genetic susceptibility testing in smoking cessation treatment: One-year outcomes of a randomized trial. *Addictive Behaviors, 22,* 741–751.

Bandura, A. (1986). *Social foundations of thought and action: A social cognitive theory.* Englewood Cliffs, NJ: Prentice Hall.

Berecz, J. M. (1984). Superiority of a low-contrast smoking cessation method. *Addictive Behaviors, 9,* 273–278.

Bobo, J. K. (1992). Nicotine dependence and alcoholism epidemiology and treatment. *Journal of Psychoactive Drugs, 24,* 123–129.

Burling, T. A., Singleton, G. E., Bigelow, G. E., Baile, W. F., & Gottlieb, S. H. (1984). Smoking following myocardial infarction: A critical review of the literature. *Health Psychology, 3,* 83–96.

Carroll, K. M. (1996). Relapse prevention as a psychosocial treatment: A review of controlled clinical trials. *Experimental and Clinical Psychopharmacology, 4,* 46–54.

Cepeda-Benito, A. (1993). Meta-analytical review of the efficacy of nicotine chewing gum in smoking treatment programs. *Journal of Consulting and Clinical Psychology, 61,* 822–830.

Cinciripini, P. M., Lapitsky, L. G., Wallfisch, A., Mace, R., Nezami, E., & Van Vunakis, H. (1994). An evaluation of a multicomponent treatment program involving scheduled smoking and relapse prevention procedures: Initial findings. *Addictive Behaviors, 19,* 13–22.

Cinciripini, P. M., Lapitsky, L., Seay, S., Wallfisch, A., Kitchens, K., & Vunakis, H. V. (1995). The effects of smoking schedules on cessation outcome: Can we improve on common methods of gradual and abrupt nicotine withdrawal? *Journal of Consulting and Clinical Psychology, 63,* 388–399.

Cinciripini, P. M., Wetter, D. W., & McClure, J. B. (1997). Scheduled reduced smoking: Effects on smoking abstinence and potential mechanisms of action. *Addictive Behaviors, 22,* 759–767.

Cohen, L. M., Collins, F. L., Jr., & Britt, D. M. (1997). The effect of chewing gum on tobacco withdrawal. *Addictive Behaviors, 22,* 769–773.

Cohen, S., Lichtenstein, E., Prochaska, J. O., Rossi, J. S., Gritz, E. R., Carr, C. R., Orleans, C. T., Schoenbach, V. J., Biener, L., Abrams, D., DiClemente, C., Curry, S., Marlatt, G. A., Cummings, K. M., Emont, S. L., Giovino, G., & Ossip-Klein, D. (1989). Debunking myths about self-quitting. *American Psychologist, 44,* 1355–1365.

Davis, J., & Glaros, A. (1986). Relapse prevention and smoking cessation. *Addictive Behaviors, 11,* 105–114.

Davison, G. C., Robins, C., & Johnson, M. K. (1983). Articulated thoughts during simulated situations: A paradigm for studying cognition in emotion and behavior. *Cognitive Therapy and Research, 7,* 17–40.

DeRubeis, R. J.,, Evans, M. D., Hollon, S. D., Garvey, M. J., Grove, W. M., & Tuason, V. B. (1990). How does cognitive therapy work: Cognitive change and symptom change in cognitive therapy and pharmacotherapy for depression. *Journal of Consulting and Clinical Psychology, 58,* 862–869.

Dijkstra, A., DeVries, H., & Bakker, M. (1996). Pros and cons of quitting, self-efficacy, and the stages of change in smoking cessation. *Journal of Consulting and Clinical Psychology, 64,* 758–763.

Fagerstrom, K. (1994). Combined use of nicotine replacement products. *Health Values, 18,* 15–20.

Fagerstrom, K. O., Schneider, N. G., & Lunell, E. (1993). Effectiveness of nicotine patch and nicotine gum as individual versus combined treatments for tobacco withdrawal symptoms. *Psychopharmacology, 111,* 271–277.

FDA approves first smokeless nicotine inhaler. (1997, May 6). *Washington Post,* p. A9.

Fiore, M. C., Jorenby, D. E., Baker, T. B., & Kenford, S. L. (1992). Tobacco dependence and the nicotine patch: Clinical guidelines for effective use. *Journal of the American Medical Association, 268,* 2687–2694.

Fiore, M. C., Smith, S. S., Jorenby, D. E., & Baker, T. B. (1994). The effectiveness of the nicotine patch for smoking cessation: A meta-analysis. *Journal of the American Medical Association, 271,* 1940–1947.

Foxx, R. M., & Brown, R. A. (1979). Nicotine fading and self-monitoring for cigarette abstinence or controlled smoking. *Journal of Applied Behavior Analysis, 12,* 111–125.

Haaga, D. A. F. (1989). Articulated thoughts and endorsement procedures for cognitive assessment in the prediction of smoking relapse. *Psychological Assessment, 1,* 112–117.

Hajek, P. (1996). Current issues in behavioral and pharmacological approaches to smoking cessation. *Addictive Behaviors, 21,* 699–707.

Hall, S. M., Muñoz, R. F., & Reus, V. I. (1994). Cognitive-behavioral intervention increases abstinence rates for depressive-history smokers. *Journal of Consulting and Clinical Psychology, 62,* 141–146.

Hall, S. M., Muñoz, R. F., Reus, V. I., Sees, K. L., Duncan, C., Humfleet, G. L., & Hartz, D. T. (1996). Mood management and nicotine gum in smoking treatment: A therapeutic contact and placebo-controlled study. *Journal of Consulting and Clinical Psychology, 64,* 1003–1009.

Hauser, R. (1974). Rapid smoking as a technique of behavior modification: Caution in selection of subjects. *Journal of Consulting and Clinical Psychology, 42,* 625.

Hughes, J. R. (1993a). Pharmacotherapy for smoking cessation: Unvalidated assumptions, anomalies, and suggestions for future research. *Journal of Consulting and Clinical Psychology, 61,* 751–760.

Hughes, J. R. (1993b). Treatment of smoking cessation in smokers with past alcohol/drug problems. *Journal of Substance Abuse Treatment, 10,* 181–187.

Kenford, S. L., Fiore, M. C., Jorenby, D. E., Smith, S. S., Wetter, D., & Baker, T. B. (1994). Predicting smoking cessation: Who will quit with and without the nicotine patch? *Journal of the American Medical Association, 271,* 589–594.

Klesges, R. C., Ward, K. D., & DeBon, M. (1996). Smoking cessation: A successful behavioral/pharmacologic interface. *Clinical Psychology Review, 16,* 479–496.

Lando, H. A. (1977). Successful treatment of smokers with a broad-spectrum behavioral approach. *Journal of Consulting and Clinical Psychology, 45,* 361–366.

Law, M., & Tang, J. L. (1995). An analysis of the effectiveness of interventions intended to help people stop smoking. *Archives of Internal Medicine, 155,* 1933–1941.

Lerman, C., Gold, K., Audrain, J., Lin, T. H., Boyd, N. R., Orleans, C. T., Wilfond, B., Louben, G., & Caporaso, N. (1997). Incorporating biomarkers of exposure and genetic susceptibility into smoking cessation treatment: Effects on smoking-related cognitions, emotions, and behavior change. *Health Psychology, 16,* 87–99.

Lichtenstein, E., Harris, D. E., Birchler, G. R., Wahl, J. M., & Schmahl, D. P. (1973). Comparison of rapid smoking, warm, smoky air, and attention placebo in the modification of smoking behavior. *Journal of Consulting and Clinical Psychology, 40,* 92–98.

Marlatt, G. A., & Gordon, J. R. (Eds.). (1985). *Relapse prevention.* New York: Guilford.

Martin, J. E., Calfas, K. J., Patten, C. A., Polarek, M., Hofstetter, C. R., Noto, J., & Beach, D. (1997). Prospective evaluation of three smoking interventions in 205 recovering alcoholics: One-year results of Project SCRAP-Tobacco. *Journal of Consulting and Clinical Psychology, 65,* 190–194.

Mattick, R. P., Baillie, A., Digiusto, E., Gourlay, S., Richmond, R., & Stanton, H. J. (1994). A summary of the recommendations for smoking cessation interventions: The quality assurance in the treatment of drug dependence project. *Drug and Alcohol Review, 13,* 171–177.

McGovern, P. G., & Lando, H. A. (1991). Reduced nicotine exposure and abstinence outcome in two nicotine fading methods. *Addictive Behaviors, 16,* 11–20.

Minneker-Hugel, E., Unland, H., & Buchkremer, G. (1992). Behavioral relapse prevention strategies in smoking cessation. *International Journal of the Addictions, 27,* 627–634.

Niaura, R., Goldstein, M. G., & Abrams, D. B. (1994). Matching high- and low-dependence treatment with or without nicotine replacement. *Preventive Medicine, 23,* 70–77.

Nicotine patches available OTC. (1996, October). *FDA Consumer,* pp. 2–3.

Ockene, J. K., & Kristeller, J. L. (1994). Tobacco. In M. Galanter & H. D. Kleber (Eds.), *The American Psychiatric Press textbook of substance abuse treatment* (pp. 157–177). Washington, DC: American Psychiatric Press.

Ockene, J. K., & Zapka, J. G. (1997). Physician-based smoking intervention: A rededication to a five-step strategy to smoking research. *Addictive Behaviors, 22,* 835–848.

Peto, R., Lopez, A. D., Boreham, J., Thun, M., & Heath, C., Jr. (1992). Mortality from tobacco in developed countries: Indirect estimation from national vital statistics. *Lancet, 339,* 1268–1278.

Richmond, R. L. (1997). A comparison of measures used to assess effectiveness of the transdermal nicotine patch at one year. *Addictive Behaviors, 22,* 753–757.

Schneider, N. G., Olmstead, R., Mody, F. V., Doan, K., Franzon, M., Jarvik, M. E., & Steinberg, C. (1995). Efficacy of a nicotine nasal spray in smoking cessation: A placebo-controlled, double-blind trial. *Addiction, 90,* 1671–1682.

Schwartz, J. L. (1987). *Review and evaluation of smoking cessation methods: The United States and Canada, 1978–1985* (NIH Publication No. 87-2940). Washington, DC: U.S. Department of Health and Human Services.

Sees, K. L., Clark, H., & Westly, H. (1993). When to begin smoking cessation in substance abusers. *Journal of Substance Abuse Treatment, 10,* 189–195.

Shiffman, S. (1984). Coping with temptations to smoke. *Journal of Consulting and Clinical Psychology, 52,* 261–267.

Shiffman, S. (1993a). Assessing smoking patterns and motives. *Journal of Consulting and Clinical Psychology, 61,* 732–742.

Shiffman, S. (1993b). Smoking cessation treatment: Any progress? *Journal of Consulting and Clinical Psychology, 61,* 718–722.

Shiffman, S., & Balabanis, M. (1995). Associations between alcohol and tobacco. In J. B. Fertig & J. P. Allen (Eds.), *Alcohol and tobacco: From basic science to clinical practice* (Research Monograph No. 30, pp. 17–36). Bethesda, MD: National Institutes of Health.

Shiffman, S., Hickcox, M., Paty, J. A., Gnys, M., Kassel, J. D., & Richards, T. J. (1996). Progression from a smoking lapse to relapse: Prediction from abstinence violation effects, nicotine dependence, and lapse characteristics. *Journal of Consulting and Clinical Psychology, 64,* 993–1002.

Stapleton, J. A., Russell, M. A. H., Feyerabend, C., Wiseman, S. M., Gustavsson, G., Sawe, U., & Wiseman, D. (1995). Dose effects and predictors of outcome in a randomized trial of transdermal nicotine patches in general practice. *Addiction, 90,* 31–42.

Stevens, V. J., & Hollis, J. F. (1989). Preventing smoking relapse, using an individually tailored skills-training technique. *Journal of Consulting and Clinical Psychology, 57,* 420–424.

Stone, A. A., & Shiffman, S. (1994). Ecological momentary assessment (EMA) in behavioral medicine. *Annals of Behavioral Medicine, 16,* 199–202.

U.S. Department of Health and Human Services (USDHHS). (1990). *The health consequences of smoking cessation: A report of the US Surgeon General.* Washington, DC: U.S. Government Printing Office.

19

Treating Pathological Gambling

VANESSA C. LÓPEZ VIETS

INTRODUCTION

Pathological gambling is a disorder that is currently receiving widespread attention around the world. It certainly warrants much notice, because as reviewed here, the prevalence of pathological gambling is growing in many countries. The seriousness of this disorder is multiplied when considering its co-occurrence with other disorders and problems. The treatment picture is not bleak, however, because there are several techniques that treatment providers can use to help individuals with a gambling disorder. This chapter focuses on treatment approaches that have been documented to be helpful for pathological gamblers who are at the readiness stage of the transtheoretical model. Using Custer and Milt's (1985) "chart of compulsive gambling and recovery," one could view the "critical phase" (e.g., honest desire for help) as the start of the gambler's readiness for change. The therapies described in this chapter may provide practitioners with a background on how best to treat clients who are motivated to seek help for their gambling addiction.

DEFINING PATHOLOGICAL GAMBLING

The U.S. mental health care community formally recognized pathological gambling in 1980 (American Psychiatric Association, 1980) as a "disorder of impulse control not elsewhere classified." Current diagnostic criteria for pathological gambling (American Psychiatric Association, 1994) specify that "persistent and recurrent" gambling is evidenced by at least five of the following behaviors:

VANESSA C. LÓPEZ VIETS • Department of Psychology, University of New Mexico, Albuquerque, New Mexico 87131.

Treating Addictive Behaviors, 2nd ed., edited by Miller and Heather. Plenum Press, New York, 1998.

- Preoccupation with gambling
- Gambling with larger amounts of money to achieve excitement
- Repeated efforts to reduce or stop gambling
- Restlessness or irritability when reducing or stopping gambling
- Gambling to escape problems or relieve negative moods
- Placing more and/or larger bets to compensate for losses ("chasing" losses)
- Lying to significant others to conceal level of involvement with gambling
- Committing crimes to pay for gambling activities
- Loss of significant relationship or career opportunity because of gambling
- Dependence on others for money to pay for debts caused by gambling

Some confusion has arisen as to the proper terminology for individuals with gambling problems. Common terms used to refer to these individuals include compulsive, pathological, and problem gamblers. These words are often used interchangeably. Recently, however, some distinctions between these terms have been noted. Some researchers have argued that *compulsive* is an inappropriate descriptor of most gamblers, because it refers to individuals who desire to resist an impulse (Allcock, 1986). Most gamblers enjoy gambling and do not want to quit, thereby showing little resistance during the early stages of the disorder (Lesieur & Rosenthal, 1991). *Pathological* refers to people who are at the severe and extreme end of a gambling continuum. It is the term used in *DSM-IV* (American Psychiatric Association, 1994). Finally, *problem* gambling includes all gambling activity that has a negative impact on any of the gambler's life domains (e.g., interpersonal, financial, legal; Lesieur & Rosenthal, 1991). It is an umbrella term that includes both compulsive and pathological gambling (Lesieur & Rosenthal, 1991).

There is also some ambiguity as to what activities constitute gambling. Gambling can encompass a variety of behaviors (e.g., buying a lottery ticket, buying aggressive stocks, purchasing a raffle ticket for a good cause, risk taking). Vague definitional borders of gambling can make it difficult to establish specific criteria for treatment outcomes such as "abstinence," "controlled gambling," and "relapse." López Viets and Miller (1997) recommended calendar-based timeline follow-back procedures to obtain more precise and comprehensive information about various gambling behaviors.

There is less disagreement that pathological gambling qualifies as an addiction. Pathological gamblers report gambling to achieve a state of arousal that is comparable to a drug-induced "high" (Lesieur & Rosenthal, 1991). Furthermore, like many substance abusers, pathological gamblers engage in their activity to escape the daily hassles and problems of life (Lesieur & Blume, 1991b). Both groups of individuals also have been found to experience many of the same symptoms as a result of their problem behaviors. Evidence of cravings, tolerance (i.e., gambling increasing amounts of money to achieve excitement), and withdrawal symptoms (e.g., irritability) among pathological gamblers has been documented in the literature (Lesieur & Rosenthal, 1991; Wray & Dickerson, 1981). In fact, diagnostic measures for pathological gambling were developed from psychoactive substance dependence criteria (Lesieur & Rosenthal, 1991).

There is also striking clinical overlap between pathological gambling and substance abuse. As is reviewed here, gamblers abuse more substances and drug abusers experience more gambling problems than the general population. In addition, similar psychological profiles between pathological gamblers and substance abusers have been shown. For example, elevated scores on the psychopathic deviance and depression scales of the MMPI have been noted consistently in both pathological gamblers and substance abusers (Moravec & Munley, 1983). Other measures including the Eysenck Personality Questionnaire and the California Personality Inventory have shown few distinctions between gamblers and substance abusers, and significant differences between these two groups and controls (Blaszczynski, Buhrich, & McConaghy, 1985; McCormick, Taber, Kruedelbach, & Russo, 1987).

Despite the apparent parallels between pathological gambling and substance abuse, there are also clinically relevant differences. Walker (1989) emphasized the distinction between physiological and psychological dependence, arguing that an addiction results from the physiological dependence on substances, and is maintained to ward off withdrawal symptoms. In contrast, pathological gambling is an activity that fosters psychological dependence resulting from partial reinforcement schedules (Walker, 1989). In addition, Lesieur (1994) observed practices such as "chasing" (betting more money to try to recover losses) which appear to be uniquely characteristic of pathological gambling. Furthermore, he argued that gamblers can more easily conceal their problem than alcohol and drug addicts, because there are fewer physical signs (Lesieur, 1994). Another notable difference between pathological gamblers and substance users may be reflected in the content and format of their 12-step meetings. According to Lesieur (1994), Gamblers Anonymous (GA) does not emphasize spirituality, consists of fewer but longer "step" meetings, and uses "pressure relief" sessions to help the gambler formulate a financial plan. Given some of these issues, Lesieur (1994) cautioned treatment professionals to be sensitive to the distinct experiences that pathological gamblers encounter.

PREVALENCE OF PATHOLOGICAL GAMBLING

Opportunities to gamble are expanding. According to Lesieur (1996), gambling has been legalized in 48 out of 50 states and in more than 90 nations around the world. As the availability and accessibility of gambling expand, the prevalence of pathological gambling increases. In 1974, 0.77% of the U.S. population was estimated to be involved in "probable compulsive gambling" (cited in Lesieur & Rosenthal, 1991). More recent estimates of probable pathological gambling range from 0.1% to 5.0% ("New Mexico Survey of Gambling Behavior," 1996; Sommers, 1988; Volberg, 1993; Volberg & Steadman, 1988). The variability in incidence rates seems to arise from differences in the local availability of legalized gambling. For example, Iowa has fewer gambling opportunities, and its residents gamble about half as much than those in other states (Lesieur, 1992).

Researchers from other nations have found prevalence estimates that are similar to those of the United States. Many prevalence studies have been conducted in different parts of Canada. For example, 6-month prevalence rates in Edmonton have been estimated to be 0.23% (Bland, Newman, Orn, & Stebelsky, 1993). Others have found higher prevalence estimates in other parts of Canada (e.g., Ladouceur,

1991). Although fewer prevalence studies have been completed in Spain, estimates indicate that up to 1.7% of adults are pathological gamblers and an additional 3.0% are at risk (Echeburúa, Báez, & Fernández-Montalvo, 1994). Niewijk and Remmers (1995) reported that in the Netherlands and on the Dutch island of Curaçao, prevalence rates of problem gambling ranged from 3.0% to 5.0%. In an examination of international prevalence studies, Walker and Dickerson (1996) found that the percentage of people scoring 5 or higher on the South Oaks Gambling Screen (SOGS), a widely used gambling measure, ranged from 1.2% in Canada to 7.1% in Australia.

Several of these prevalence studies have also found particular demographic variables that are typically associated with pathological gamblers. In general, more males than females tend to be problem or pathological gamblers (Bland et al., 1993; Volberg & Steadman, 1988), but a recent New Mexico survey found that men and women had gambled about equally in the past month, and more females than males were classified as problem gamblers ("New Mexico Survey of Gambling Behavior," 1996). Age is not a consistent correlate of pathological gambling. Some surveys have reported that individuals under the age of 30 tend to engage in pathological gambling more than the general population (Volberg, 1993), while others have not supported these findings (Volberg & Steadman, 1989). A more consistent observation is that individuals who began gambling at a young age demonstrate more gambling-related problems than those with a later onset (Reno, 1994). This suggests the importance of focusing on gambling in adolescents. In addition, some ethnic minorities have reported higher rates of problem gambling (Lesieur & Rosenthal, 1991; "New Mexico Survey of Gambling Behavior," 1996). Finally, low education and low income were found to be positively related to pathological gambling in some surveys (e.g., Volberg & Steadman, 1988). In spite of these findings, treatment studies to date have seldom included females, minorities, adolescents, and individuals from low income and educational backgrounds in their samples of gamblers. In any event, the need for treatment of problem gambling is likely to increase.

COMORBIDITY OF PATHOLOGICAL GAMBLING AND OTHER PSYCHOLOGICAL DISORDERS

Pathological gamblers have demonstrated higher rates of certain psychological disorders than individuals from the general population. Substance abuse disorders, in particular, have been consistently documented to co-occur with pathological gambling. Ramirez, McCormick, Russo, and Taber (1983) found that 39% of their inpatient sample met criteria for alcohol or drug abuse within a year of hospital admission, and 47% met lifetime criteria. Similarly, Lesieur and Blume (1991b) revealed that 48% of female GA members met criteria for substance abuse and dependence, a significantly higher rate than that of the general adult female population. In another study, 80% of pathological gamblers indicated that their primary problem was substance abuse only or a combination of substance abuse and gambling (Lesieur & Blume, 1992). Conversely, studies of substance abusers in treatment have shown a high incidence of problem and pathological gambling (Daghestani, Elenz, & Crayton, 1996; Feigelman, Kleinman, Lesieur, Millman, & Lesser, 1995; Lesieur, Blume, & Zoppa, 1986). Of particular interest, Lesieur and

Heineman (1988) found that 14% of substance-abusing youth in a therapeutic community were probable pathological gamblers.

Affective disorders have also been frequently observed in treatment samples of pathological gamblers. McCormick, Russo, Ramirez, and Taber (1984) found that 76% and 38% of inpatients were diagnosed with major depressive and hypomanic disorders, respectively. Within GA, 26% of women reported having suffered from serious depression, and 12% of respondents had attempted suicide before the onset of gambling problems (Lesieur & Blume, 1991b). Linden, Pope, and Jonas (1986) also reported high rates of major depression in their sample of male GA members. They found that 72% of gamblers had experienced a major depressive episode while 28% suffered from recurrent major depression. Moreover, these researchers observed a high prevalence of bipolar and panic disorders and agoraphobia in their study sample. Of further importance, pathological gamblers with substance abuse problems have reported more symptoms of negative affectivity than their nonabusing counterparts (McCormick, 1993).

Generalized impulsivity and disinhibition are also associated with problem gambling. Pathological gamblers have displayed more attention problems and reported more childhood behaviors that are consistent with attention deficit disorder than matched controls (Carlton et al., 1987; Rugle & Melamed, 1993). More disinhibition of aggressive impulses has also been reported by severe gamblers compared to moderate gamblers (McCormick, 1993). In addition, 15.5% of pathological gamblers have met criteria for antisocial personality disorder (Blaszczynski, Steel, & McConaghy, 1997), consistent with elevated scores on scale 4 (psychopathic deviance) of the MMPI (Moravec & Munley, 1983). In light of these findings on comorbidity, it appears that a comprehensive psychological assessment is warranted when treating pathological gamblers.

TREATMENT APPROACHES

The approaches described in this chapter were selected because of their documented effectiveness in the treatment of pathological gambling. These chosen treatment methods have often been used in group and case studies, and less often have been tested under the rigors of controlled trials. Gamblers Anonymous was also included because of its reputation as a common source of support for people with gambling problems. This paper is not meant to be an exhaustive review of the treatment literature. For more comprehensive reviews of treatment techniques, refer to Blaszczynski and Silove (1995) or López Viets and Miller (1997).

BEHAVIORAL THERAPY

The basic premise behind behavioral treatment approaches is that pathological gambling is "a learned maladaptive behavior that can be unlearned" (Blaszczynski & Silove, 1995). Behavioral studies have provided some of the most extensive and encouraging treatment literature on pathological gambling.

Initial promise was found in the earliest case studies using aversive techniques to treat problem gamblers (Barker & Miller, 1966; Goorney, 1968; Seager, Pokorny, & Black; 1966). With a larger sample, Seager (1970) demonstrated that almost half of his clients had ceased to gamble following the use of electrical aversion therapy. Koller (1972) found that approximately two thirds of his sample had either substantially reduced or abstained from gambling.

Aversion therapy has fallen out of clinical usage, however, and other behavioral strategies have proven at least as effective. The combination of behavioral strategies in the management of pathological gambling also began with case studies. Cotler (1971) used behavioral monitoring, contingency management, aversion therapy, covert sensitization, and marital counseling to treat a pathological gambler. His client abstained from gambling for 5 months after treatment, but then relapsed. Using imaginal desensitization and progressive muscle relaxation, McConaghy (1991) noted a lengthy period of abstinence in a female problem gambler, followed by a relapse but significantly reduced gambling levels. Greenberg and Rankin (1982) treated 26 gamblers using behavioral analysis, urge control techniques, and in some cases, exposure and covert sensitization. Five of their clients displayed control over their gambling when followed up between 9 and 54 months; none of their clients completely abstained from gambling. In a larger study, Blaszczynski, McConaghy, and Frankova (1991) used one of four techniques to treat 120 gamblers: imaginal desensitization, aversion therapy, imaginal relaxation, or in vivo exposure. They followed up 63 clients for a mean follow-up period of 66 months and reported abstinence in 18 clients and controlled gambling in 25 individuals. The other 20 reported uncontrolled gambling.

Behavioral procedures have also been applied with the specific aim of reducing or controlling gambling. Dickerson and Weeks (1979) found that contingency contracting and spousal interventions limited the frequency of betting and the amount of money gambled by the client. In addition, Rankin (1982) showed that a weekly wagering limit greatly reduced their client's gambling activity. Moreover, both studies found additional benefits of therapy including improved marital relationships, stable occupations, and the cessation of criminal activity.

One team of investigators in Australia has conducted controlled research comparing the effectiveness of different behavioral techniques. McConaghy, Armstrong, Blaszczynski, and Allcock (1983) randomized 20 gamblers to receive either aversion therapy (AT) or imaginal desensitization (ID). The ID group demonstrated greater reductions in gambling behaviors and urges and less anxiety than the AT group. In a subsequent study, the same researchers (McConaghy, Armstrong, Blaszczynski, & Allcock, 1988) compared imaginal desensitization (ID) and imaginal relaxation (IR) and found that both treatments reduced anxiety. In addition, gamblers who reported a decrease in anxiety cut back on their gambling behaviors. The investigators recommended the use of imaginal relaxation in the treatment of pathological gamblers because of its relatively low cost.

COGNITIVE AND COGNITIVE-BEHAVIORAL THERAPIES

Cognitive and cognitive-behavioral therapies emphasize the impact of people's thoughts on their behavior. These treatment orientations target and challenge the maladaptive cognitions that contribute to and maintain the problem behavior. Hence, in treating pathological gamblers, distorted beliefs about gambling are modified to reduce or eliminate the wagering behavior (Gaboury & Ladouceur, 1989). Some types of irrational beliefs include thinking one has influence over gambling outcomes, making predictions, and using superstitious practices (Sylvain & Ladouceur, 1992). The following treatment approaches have either relied exclusively on cognitive restructuring techniques or have used them in combination with other procedures.

One of the earliest studies to utilize cognitive-behavioral techniques was conducted by Bannister (1977), who used rational emotive therapy and covert sensitization to treat a gambler. As a side note, Valium was given to the client during his inpatient treatment. After a lengthy period of time, the gambler was assessed, and he and his wife reported that he had abstained from gambling.

Toneatto and Sobell (1990) targeted a gambler's misperceptions about gambling by helping him evaluate the evidence behind his beliefs. At the end of treatment, the client became aware of the substantial amount of money he had lost over several years and the ineffectiveness of his gambling strategies, and his gambling diminished in frequency.

Sylvain and Ladouceur (1992) utilized education, cognitive restructuring, and relapse prevention to treat 3 pathological gamblers. Clients were taught to question the validity of their control over gambling activities and to replace these thoughts with more accurate ones. All of the clients increased their ability to identify their cognitive distortions and substitute more appropriate verbalizations for the distortions. Moreover, one client discontinued gambling while another greatly reduced it.

Sharpe and Tarrier (1992) used relaxation, exposure, and cognitive restructuring techniques to treat a problem gambler. They found that both his gambling urges and behaviors had dramatically decreased. In addition, he reported improvements in his level of depression.

One of the few outcome studies to treat adolescent gamblers provided them with information sessions, cognitive restructuring, problem-solving training, social-skills training, and relapse prevention (Ladouceur, Boisvert, & Dumont, 1994). Following the termination of therapy, all 4 clients had more accurate perceptions about gambling and lowered problem severity scores. They also reported having completely refrained from gambling activities at the 3- and 6-month follow-up sessions.

At least one study has compared the efficacy of different cognitive and behavioral procedures. Echeburúa and colleagues (1994), a Spanish team of researchers, randomly allocated 64 clients to one of the following treatments: (1) individual stimulus control and in vivo exposure with response prevention, (2) group cognitive restructuring, (3) a combination of the first two treatments, or (4) a wait-list control. The researchers found that individual behavior therapy was more beneficial to the clients than the other treatments, including the combined approach. Specifically, gamblers in this group quit or showed significant reductions in gambling compared to other group members. In addition, they had fewer relapses than their counterparts in the other treatment approaches. Clients in all experimental groups reported less depression than individuals in the control group.

MULTIMODAL APPROACHES

The use of a broad range of techniques is not uncommon in the treatment of pathological gamblers. Studies using several procedures to treat problem gambling frequently have been conducted in inpatient units that were often associated with U.S. Veterans' Administration hospitals.

Combined gambling and substance abuse treatment units often use multiple approaches to treat a diverse clientele. For example, 60 veteran gamblers were provided with group therapy, education, and GA meetings in an inpatient facility specifically designed for alcohol abusers (Russo, Taber, McCormick, & Ramirez, 1984). A little over half of the gambling clients had abstained from gambling for a year. Furthermore, the abstinent clients reported improved social, financial, and psychological functioning. The same program was evaluated again in a prospective study following the progress of a group of clients (Taber, McCormick, Russo, Adkins, & Ramirez, 1987). Similar levels of improvement were found with regard to abstinence as in the former study. Also, clients reported significant decreases in alcohol abuse.

In a study of another combined inpatient program, gamblers received treatment consisting of psychotherapy (individual and group), education, psychodrama, family counseling, and GA (Lesieur & Blume, 1991a). Approximately two thirds of the clients had abstained from gambling since treatment. Moreover, a modified version of the Addiction Severity Index indicated notable reductions across problem domains (e.g., legal). About half of the clients reported the group psychotherapy to be the most helpful component of the program.

A multimodal approach comprised of individual, group, and family therapy was administered on an outpatient basis to a group of pathological gamblers (Blackman, Simone, Thoms, & Blackman, 1989). It is also important to note that some attended GA and others were given medications. Significant reductions in weekly amount wagered and in gambling frequency were noted.

GAMBLERS ANONYMOUS

GA was established in 1957 and has become one of the most well-known sources of help for problem gambling. Despite the widespread popularity of GA, there is little empirical support for its effectiveness with pathological gamblers. The largest study to examine the impact of GA found that meeting attendance was associated with gambling abstinence in a small percentage of gamblers in Scotland (Brown, 1985). More specifically, after 1 and 2 years of involvement in GA, approximately 7.0% of attendees remained abstinent. Although there is a need for more controlled outcome studies for pathological gambling in general, there is great need for such investigations to be conducted with a program as prevalent as GA, which may require designs other than randomized trials.

COMBINING APPROACHES

How might one design a treatment program based on the current treatment outcome literature? This was the question that faced us as pathological gamblers began to present for treatment at the University of New Mexico Center on Alcoholism, Substance Abuse, and Addictions (CASAA). Given that cognitive and behavioral approaches currently appear to be the most promising in helping this population reduce or stop gambling, we incorporated the techniques of these therapies into a program called Better Future. To enhance cost-effectiveness, the program was designed as an open group cycling through 8 weeks of 1-hour sessions. Prior to group therapy, clients are screened for substance abuse and mood disorders, and are seen individually to complete a comprehensive gambling profile assessing gambling behavior, problems, and motivation for change. At the conclusion of this assessment clients are given self-monitoring forms to begin using prior to their first treatment session. The content for the group includes the following: (1) high-risk situations and practical coping strategies, (2) cognitive restructuring, (3) decreasing arousal, (4) coping with urges and lapses, (5) alternative coping skills, (6) social support, (7) problem-solving and refusal skills, and (8) increasing pleasant activities. Each session provides in-session exercises as well as homework assignments.

CONCLUSION

Overall, the treatment of pathological gambling appears encouraging. To date, behavioral, cognitive, and combined cognitive-behavioral therapies appear to be most effective at treating gambling problems. Outcome data for these treatment approaches indicate that often up to two thirds of clients show significant reductions in or abstain from gambling.

Multimodal methods seem helpful in treating inpatient and outpatient samples of pathological gamblers, but it is not clear what specific treatment components are most therapeutic. It is interesting to note that attendance at GA meetings is a common part of treatment in settings that use multiple techniques. Nevertheless, GA's individual effectiveness remains largely untested. More evaluations with clearer outcome data will help better assess these approaches.

In addition to gambling outcomes, many of the treatment studies reviewed in this chapter have found secondary gains in other life domains. The treatment literature indicates that clients often report an improvement in psychosocial functioning. It is not uncommon to find that treated clients report a reduction in depression, anxiety, and other psychological afflictions. As was reviewed here, pathological gambling and other psychological disorders are highly associated with one another. What is less clear is the extent to which clients are able to maintain treatment gains in their level of psychological functioning. These findings point to the need to make gambling treatment broad-spectrum. It is recommended that treatment providers recognize and treat concomitant psychosocial problems, as well as the gambling, so that a client's overall prognosis improves.

In sum, pathological gamblers seem to respond well to cognitive-behavioral techniques. Nevertheless, more clinical research in this area is still needed, especially with regard to other treatment approaches. Explicit outcome data assessing gambling and psychosocial functioning at follow-up points of at least 1 year are strongly recommended. Although current approaches are promising, more work is needed to advance effective treatment for this unique client population.

REFERENCES

Allcock, C. C. (1986). Pathological gambling. *Australian and New Zealand Journal of Psychiatry, 20,* 259–265.
American Psychiatric Association. (1980). *Diagnostic and statistical manual of mental disorders* (3rd ed., rev.). Washington, DC: Author.

American Psychiatric Association. (1994). *Diagnostic and statistical manual of mental disorders* (4th ed.). Washington, DC: Author.

Bannister, G., Jr. (1977). Cognitive and behavior therapy in a case of compulsive gambling. *Cognitive Therapy and Research, 1,* 223–227.

Barker, J. C., & Miller, M. (1966). Aversion therapy for compulsive gambling. *Lancet, 1,* 491–492.

Blackman, S., Simone, R. V., Thoms, D. R., & Blackman, S. (1989). The Gamblers Treatment Clinic of St. Vincent's North Richmond Community Mental Health Center: Characteristics of the clients and outcome of treatment. *International Journal of the Addictions, 24,* 29–37.

Bland, R. C., Newman, S. C., Orn, H., & Stebelsky, G. (1993). Epidemiology of pathological gambling in Edmonton. *Canadian Journal of Psychiatry, 38,* 108–112.

Blaszczynski, A., & Silove, D. (1995). Cognitive and behavioral therapies for pathological gambling. *Journal of Gambling Studies, 11,* 195–220.

Blaszczynski, A., Steel, Z., & McConaghy, N. (1997). Impulsivity in pathological gambling: The antisocial impulsivist. *Addiction, 92,* 75–87.

Blaszczynski, A., Buhrich, N., & McConaghy, N. (1985). Pathological gamblers, heroin addicts and controls compared on the E.P.Q. "addiction scale." *British Journal of Addiction, 80,* 315–319.

Blaszczynski, A., McConaghy, N., & Frankova, A. (1991). Control versus abstinence in the treatment of pathological gambling: A two to nine year follow-up. *British Journal of Addiction, 86,* 299–306.

Brown, R. I. F. (1985). The effectiveness of Gamblers Anonymous. In W. R. Eadington (Ed.), *The gambling studies: Proceedings of the sixth national conference on gambling and risk taking* (pp. 259–284). Reno, NV: Bureau of Business and Economic Research, University of Nevada, Reno.

Carlton, P. L., Manowitz, P., McBride, H., Nora, R., Swatzburg, M., & Goldstein, L. (1987). Attention deficit disorder and pathological gambling. *Journal of Clinical Psychiatry, 48,* 487–488.

Cotler, S. B. (1971). The use of different behavioral techniques in treating a case of compulsive gambling. *Behavior Therapy, 2,* 579–584.

Custer, R., & Milt, H. (1985). *When luck runs out: Help for compulsive gamblers and their families.* New York: Warner.

Daghestani, A. N., Elenz, E., & Crayton, J. W. (1996). Pathological gambling in hospitalized substance abusing veterans. *Journal of Clinical Psychiatry, 57,* 360–363.

Dickerson, M. G., & Weeks, D. (1979). Controlled gambling as a therapeutic technique for compulsive gamblers. *Journal of Behavior Therapy and Experimental Psychiatry, 10,* 139–141.

Echeburúa, E., Báez, C., & Fernández-Montalvo, J. (1994). Efectividad diferencial de diversas modalidades terapéuticas en el tratamiento psicológico del juego patológico: Un estudio experimental. *Análisis y Modificación de Conducta, 20,* 617–643.

Feigelman, W., Kleinman, P. H., Lesieur, H. R., Millman, R. B., & Lesser, M. L. (1995). Pathological gambling among methadone patients. *Drug and Alcohol Dependence, 39,* 75–81.

Gaboury, A., & Ladouceur, R. (1989). Erroneous perceptions and gambling. *Journal of Social Behavior and Personality, 4,* 411–420.

Goorney, A. B. (1968). Treatment of a compulsive horse race gambler by aversion therapy. *British Journal of Psychiatry, 114,* 329–333.

Greenberg, D., & Rankin, H. (1982). Compulsive gamblers in treatment. *British Journal of Psychiatry, 140,* 364–366.

Koller, K. M. (1972). Treatment of poker-machine addicts by aversion therapy. *Medical Journal of Australia, 1,* 742–745.

Ladouceur, R. (1991). Prevalence estimates of pathological gambling in Quebec. *Canadian Journal of Psychiatry, 36,* 732–734.

Ladouceur, R., Boisvert, J. M., & Dumont, J. (1994). Cognitive-behavioral treatment for adolescent pathological gamblers. *Behavior Modification, 18,* 230–242.

Lesieur, H. R. (1992). Compulsive gambling. *Society, 29,* 43–50.

Lesieur, H. R. (1994). Pathological gambling and chemical dependency: Differences. *Bettor Times, 3,* 1–4.

Lesieur, H. R. (1996, February). Gaming addictions workshop, Albuquerque, New Mexico.

Lesieur, H. R., & Blume, S. B. (1991a). Evaluation of patients treated for pathological gambling in a combined alcohol, substance abuse, and pathological gambling treatment unit using the Addiction Severity Index. *British Journal of Addiction, 86,* 1017–1028.

Lesieur, H. R., & Blume, S. B. (1991b). When lady luck loses: Women and compulsive gambling. In N. Van Den Bergh (Ed.), *Feminist perspectives on addictions* (pp. 181–197). New York: Springer.

Lesieur, H. R., & Blume, S. B. (1992). Modifying the Addiction Severity Index for use with pathological gamblers. *American Journal on Addictions, 1,* 240–247.

Lesieur, H. R., & Heineman, M. (1988). Pathological gambling among youthful multiple substance abusers in a therapeutic community. *British Journal of Addiction, 83,* 765–771.

Lesieur, H. R., & Rosenthal, R. J. (1991). Pathological gambling: A review of the literature (Prepared for the American Psychiatric Association Task Force on DSM-IV Committee on Disorders of Impulse Control Not Elsewhere Classified). *Journal of Gambling Studies, 7,* 5–39.

Lesieur, H. R., Blume, S. B., & Zoppa, R. M. (1986). Alcoholism, drug abuse, and gambling. *Alcoholism: Clinical and Experimental Research, 10,* 33–38.

Linden, R. D., Pope, H. G., Jr., & Jonas, J. M. (1986). Pathological gambling and major affective disorder: Preliminary findings. *Journal of Clinical Psychiatry, 47,* 201–203.

López Viets, V. C., & Miller, W. R. (1997). Treatment approaches for pathological gamblers. *Clinical Psychology Review, 17,* 689–702.

McConaghy, N. (1991). A pathological or a compulsive gambler? *Journal of Gambling Studies, 7,* 55–64.

McConaghy, N., Armstrong, M. S., Blaszczynski, A., & Allcock, C. (1983). Controlled comparison of aversive therapy and imaginal desensitization in compulsive gambling. *British Journal of Psychiatry, 142,* 366–372.

McConaghy, N., Armstrong, M. S., Blaszczynski, A., & Allcock, C. (1988). Behavior completion versus stimulus control in compulsive gambling: Implications for behavioral assessment. *Behavior Modification, 12,* 371–384.

McCormick, R. A. (1993). Disinhibition and negative affectivity in substance abusers with and without a gambling problem. *Addictive Behaviors, 18,* 331–336.

McCormick, R. A., Russo, A. M., Ramirez, L. F., & Taber, J. I. (1984). Affective disorders among pathological gamblers seeking treatment. *American Journal of Psychiatry, 141,* 215–218.

McCormick, R. A., Taber, J. I., Kruedelbach, N., & Russo, A. (1987). Personality profiles of hospitalized pathological gamblers: The California Personality Inventory. *Journal of Clinical Psychiatry, 43,* 521–527.

Moravec, J. D., & Munley, P. H. (1983). Psychological test findings on pathological gamblers in treatment. *International Journal of the Addictions, 18,* 1003–1009.

New Mexico survey of gambling behavior. (1996). Albuquerque: New Mexico Department of Health and University of New Mexico.

Niewijk, A., & Remmers, P. (1995). Study on gambling problems in Curaçao. *Jellinek Quarterly, 2,* 10–11.

Ramirez, L. F., McCormick, R. A., Russo, A. M., & Taber, J. I. (1983). Patterns of substance abuse in pathological gamblers undergoing treatment. *Addictive Behaviors, 8,* 425–428.

Rankin, H. (1982). Case histories and shorter communications. *Behavior Research and Therapy, 20,* 185–187.

Reno, R. A. (1994, October). *Empty dreams: The social significance of gambling. Focus on the Family.* Colorado Springs, CO: Public Policy Research Department.

Rugle, L., & Melamed, L. (1993). Neuropsychological assessment of attention problems in pathological gamblers. *Journal of Nervous and Mental Disease, 181,* 107–112.

Russo, A. M., Taber, J. I., McCormick, R. A., & Ramirez, L. F. (1984). An outcome study of an inpatient treatment program for pathological gamblers. *Hospital and Community Psychiatry, 35,* 823–827.

Seager, C. P. (1970). Treatment of compulsive gamblers by electrical aversion. *British Journal of Psychiatry, 117,* 545–553.

Seager, C. P., Pokorny, M. R., & Black, D. (1966). Aversion therapy for compulsive gambling. *Lancet, 1,* 546.

Sharpe, L., & Tarrier, N. (1992). A cognitive-behavioral treatment approach for problem gambling. *Journal of Cognitive Psychotherapy: An International Quarterly, 6,* 193–203.

Sommers, I. (1988). Pathological gambling: Estimating prevalence and group characteristics. *International Journal of the Addictions, 23,* 477–490.

Sylvain, C., & Ladouceur, R. (1992). Correction cognitive et habitudes de jeu chez les joueurs de poker vidéo. *Revue Canadienne des Sciences du Comportement, 24,* 479–489.

Taber, J. I., McCormick, R. A., Russo, A. M., Adkins, B. J., & Ramirez, L. F. (1987). Follow-up of pathological gamblers after treatment. *American Journal of Psychiatry, 144,* 757–761.

Toneatto, T., & Sobell, L. C. (1990). Pathological gambling treated with cognitive behavior therapy: A case report. *Addictive Behaviors, 15,* 497–501.

Volberg, R. A. (1993, January). *The prevalence of problem and pathological gambling.* Paper prepared for the 1st statewide conference of the Florida Council on Compulsive Gambling.

Volberg, R. A., & Steadman, H. J. (1988). Refining prevalence estimates of pathological gambling. *American Journal of Psychiatry, 145,* 502–505.

Volberg, R. A., & Steadman, H. J. (1989). Prevalence estimates of pathological gambling in New Jersey and Maryland. *American Journal of Psychiatry, 146,* 1618–1619.

Walker, M. B. (1989). Some problems with the concept of "gambling addiction": Should theories of addiction be generalized to include excessive gambling? *Journal of Gambling Behavior, 5,* 179.

Walker, M. B., & Dickerson, M. G. (1996). The prevalence of problem and pathological gambling: A critical analysis. *Journal of Gambling Studies, 12,* 233–249.

Wray, I., & Dickerson, M. (1981). Cessation of high frequency gambling and "withdrawal" symptoms. *British Journal of Addiction, 76,* 401–405.

20

Treating the Family

HOLLY BARRETT WALDRON AND NATASHA SLESNICK

INTRODUCTION

Theorists and researchers have long recognized the family as a major source of influence in the development and maintenance of substance use problems (cf. Hawkins, Catalano, & Miller, 1992; Kaufman & Kaufmann, 1992). A variety of family factors have been associated with substance abuse, including parental and sibling use, family members' attitudes toward use, poor family management practices, particular patterns of family interaction, and generally disturbed marital and family relationship functioning (Brook, Whiteman, Gordon, & Brook, 1988; Hops, Tildesley, Lichtenstein, Ary, & Sherman, 1990; Jacob & Leonard, 1988). Such factors represent genetic and environmental influences that are likely to be interdependent and bidirectional. For example, Dishion, Patterson, and Reid (1988) examined substance use among adolescents and found that parental drug use had both a direct effect, presumably resulting from modeling and opportunities for use, and an indirect effect, resulting from impaired parental control when parents were under the influence of drugs or alcohol. The presence of stressors, relationship conflict, negative affect, lack of openness, and poor cohesion in families, as well as seeking support in relationships outside the family, also may be variables having reciprocal influence with addictive behaviors.

Similarly, the family can play a major role in the process of change (Brown, Myers, Mott, & Vik, 1994; McCrady, 1986). Marital and family treatment approaches for addictive behaviors have been widely embraced in community mental health agencies and other clinical settings and have received considerable attention in outcome research evaluating the effectiveness of treatments for alcohol and drug use problems. Several reviewers examining controlled clinical trials

HOLLY BARRETT WALDRON AND NATASHA SLESNICK • Department of Psychology, University of New Mexico, Albuquerque, New Mexico 87131.

Treating Addictive Behaviors, 2nd ed., edited by Miller and Heather. Plenum Press, New York, 1998.

of family-based interventions have concluded that family therapy is an effective treatment for both adults and adolescents with problem substance use. Family therapy has been associated with higher rates of treatment engagement and retention, significant reductions in substance use from pre- to posttreatment, and improved functioning in other behavioral domains (Liddle & Dakof, 1995; O'Farrell, 1995; Stanton & Shadish, 1997; Waldron, 1997).

Family therapies have traditionally been derived primarily from theory and clinical experience, with research serving more to clarify and justify treatment models than to develop new models prospectively (Alexander, Holtzworth-Munroe, & Jameson, 1994). Family therapies for addictive behaviors have been developed on the basis of a variety of theoretical perspectives, including psycho-dynamic, disease-based, family systems, and cognitive and behavioral models (cf. Kaufman & Kaufmann, 1992). This chapter is intended to provide an overview of family therapy for treating addictive behaviors, addressing the theoretical underpinnings and practical application of each approach and the empirical foundations for the effectiveness of the interventions. The chapter focuses primarily on the three general approaches studied most extensively and engendering the bulk of empirical evidence: behavioral models, family systems models, and ecological and/or integrative models. Although marital and family therapies for addictive behaviors share similarities, the focus of intervention, specific techniques and strategies employed, and special problems encountered in therapy for couples and families are distinct. The emphasis in this chapter is on family-based interventions, rather than on couples (cf. McCrady, 1986; O'Farrell, 1995) or spouse-involved treatments (Chapter 11, this volume).

TREATMENT APPROACHES

Behavioral Family Models

Behavioral family therapy models have relied primarily on operant and social learning theories to understand the behavior of an individual in the context of the family. Behaviors such as substance use are viewed as a pattern of responses learned in the context of social interactions (e.g., observing parents, sibling, peers, or models in the media) and established as a result of family-related and other contingencies in the environment (Akers, Krohn, Lanza Kaduce, & Radosevich, 1979).

According to McCrady (1989), three components of family interactions can increase the likelihood of substance use. First, family members' behaviors can serve as stimulus cues or play a role in triggering substance use through interaction behaviors (e.g., making demands, criticizing, withdrawal of attention). Second, the organismic responses, such as internal emotional reactions and physiological responses, experienced by the individual that are often associated with problem use can be influenced by family members. Third, family members' responses to drinking or drug use can serve to reinforce use or punish sobriety, increasing the probability of future use and decreasing the probability of abstinence. Integrating social learning principles within an operant perspective, the individual's observations of the coping function of substance use reinforcing drinking or drug use for others in the social environment (e.g., drinking to relieve stress) could also influence the development and maintenance of substance use. From a behavioral family perspective, then, substance abuse is determined by factors in the environment, many of which involve the family-related consequences of substance use behavior and the antecedents that indicate the consequences that are in effect (Bry, 1988).

For treatment, many behavioral family models emphasize skill building and contingency management aimed to increase prosocial behavior (e.g., reinforcing behaviors incompatible with substance use, such as involvement in recreational or community activities) and to reduce substance use and related negative behaviors (e.g., loss of privileges as a punishment for curfew violation). Techniques include stimulus control strategies such as increasing parental monitoring to limit exposure to high-risk situations, and problem-solving or other coping skills training, implemented to provide families with a behavioral repertoire that will allow them to resolve problems independently (Fleischman, Horne, & Arthur, 1983). The increased positive interactions they experience when putting such skills to use, combined with homework assignments to increase desired behaviors outside the therapy setting, are presumed to reinforce the likelihood that the new behaviors will become established patterns in the natural environment.

FAMILY SYSTEMS MODELS

Family systems perspectives view the family as a basic unit or system subject to the same properties as other systems (e.g., homeostasis, hierarchical organization, reciprocal influence). The family system is characterized by the mutual interdependence of the members of the family together with the processes (e.g., rules for behaving, roles, repeated sequences of behaviors, communication interactions) in which they engage. Alcohol and substance abuse are conceptualized as maladaptive behaviors expressed by one or more family members, but reflecting dysfunction in the system as a whole (Stanton, Todd et al., 1982). Thus, drinking or drug use problems persist primarily as an aspect of current, ongoing interactions between the user and his or her intimates.

Some systems therapists assume that behaviors associated with substance use serve a function for families to cope with internal or external stressors or maintain other processes that have become established in the organization of the system (Stanton, Todd et al., 1982; Steinglass, Bennett, Wolin, & Reiss, 1987). For example, the attention required to cope with substance abuse in one family member may allow the family to avoid conflict in the marital dyad that could threaten the integrity of the family or could reflect the family's inability to cope with the transition of the abuser from childhood into adolescence. Others view substance use as occurring within the family social context, but do not ascribe functional properties to the behavior (Berg & Miller, 1992; Beutler et al., 1993). These differences notwithstanding, the essential core and distinguishing feature of systems models is that the locus of the problem transcends the individual and the focus of treatment should be relational.

Treatment is aimed at restructuring the interactional patterns associated with the abuse, theoretically making the abuse unnecessary to the maintenance of system functioning. Techniques include (1) forming a therapeutic relationship (i.e., joining) in which the therapist can elicit the recurring behavioral sequences (i.e., enactment), interrupting and destabilizing the dysfunctional behavioral exchanges; (2) helping family members understand the interrelatedness of their behaviors and see the symptomatic behavior in a way consistent with family change (e.g., reframing); and (3) restructuring or shifting family interaction patterns and establishing new behaviors [e.g., manipulating seating arrangements to fortify a weak parental dyad, establishing rules of communicating and solving problems that preclude triangulation or conflict avoidance (cf. Stanton, Todd *et al.*, 1982; Szapocznik & Kurtines, 1989)].

ECOLOGICAL AND INTEGRATIVE MODELS

Multisystemic or social ecological family therapy models view substance use and other related problem behaviors as the result of many sources of influence and occurring in the context of multiple systems (Henggeler *et al.*, 1991; Liddle, Dakof, & Diamond, 1991). Sessions may involve whole families, parts of the family system, and individual sessions. Therapists draw upon a variety of intervention strategies developed from cognitive, behavioral, and family systems models to facilitate the adolescent's decision making, emotion regulation, or other intrapersonal factors which may be influencing substance use, to modify behavioral exchanges in the family, and to implement interventions at the broader system levels such as the schools or legal system (Henggeler *et al.*, 1991; Liddle, Dakof, & Diamond, 1991).

Functional family therapy (FFT; Alexander & Parsons, 1982; Waldron & Slesnick, 1997) conceptually links behavioral and cognitive intervention strategies to the ecological theories of the family disturbance. As in other family systems models, problems with alcohol and drugs are viewed as behaviors which occur in the context of and have meaning for family relationships. The model is integrative, however, in that the relational formulation of the problem behavior is used to guide the implementation of behavior change strategies, drawn broadly from behavioral and other models of psychotherapy. The early part of therapy focuses on readiness to change and involves creating the context in which behavior change can occur, through treatment engagement, motivation enhancement, and a functional assessment of family relationships. The second phase focuses on establishing and maintaining behavior change both at the individual level and for the family as a whole. The Purdue brief family therapy model (Lewis, Piercy, Sprenkle, & Trepper, 1990) is similar to the FFT model, integrating elements of structural, strategic, functional, and behavioral family therapies and focusing on decreasing the family's initial resistance to change, assessing the relationship function of substance use behavior, disrupting maladaptive behavioral sequences, and reestablishing parental control.

TREATMENT EFFECTIVENESS: EMPIRICAL FINDINGS

EARLY FAMILY THERAPY RESEARCH

Much of the impetus for family therapy outcome research can be attributed to a small cadre of researchers evaluating the effectiveness of family systems interventions for adult and adolescent substance abusers more than two decades ago.

Stanton, Todd, and colleagues (1982) refined a structural-strategic family therapy approach for adults using heroin and other drugs. At a 12-month posttreatment assessment, the families who received family therapy showed dramatically less drug use compared to a matched group of clients in the methadone–individual counseling program. Similarly, other early studies with adult substance abusers also showed that a family systems approach may be more effective than individual therapy in reducing recidivism (Kaufman & Kaufmann, 1992) and maintaining abstinence from drugs and alcohol (Ziegler-Driscoll, 1977).

Examining treatment for substance-abusing adolescents and their families, Scopetta, King, Szapocznik, and Tillman (1979) investigated whether family interventions need to be ecologically focused, involving multiple systems, or whether intervention within the conjoint family context is sufficient. Both groups showed improved outcomes following treatment, although no differences were found between the two interventions. Szapocznik and his colleagues then evaluated two variations of structural family systems therapy, conjoint family therapy and one-person family therapy, for substance-abusing adolescents and their families (Szapocznik, Kurtines, Foote, Perez-Vidal, & Hervis, 1983, 1986). Families in both intervention conditions showed significant improvement at the end of therapy. Moreover, compared with conjoint therapy, one-person family therapy led to slightly greater improvement for some outcome measures.

The improved outcomes for substance abusers participating in treatment with their families that were observed in these early studies were promising and led to the initiation of more than a dozen controlled clinical trials evaluating the effectiveness of family therapy. These formal evaluations of family therapy for substance abuse were designed to improve on the early studies which were sometimes limited by small sample sizes and other methodological problems. Although the studies have varied considerably with respect to design and implementation (e.g., models examined, selection of comparison groups, severity of substance use, outcome measures employed, follow-up intervals), the body of work provides strong support for family-based interventions for addictive behaviors (cf. Stanton & Shadish, 1997; Waldron, 1997).

TREATMENT OUTCOME FOR ADOLESCENT SUBSTANCE ABUSE

A sizable number of controlled family therapy outcome studies evaluating the effectiveness of a variety of family therapy approaches for adolescent substance abuse have been completed, with encouraging results. Two studies of behavioral family therapy—Azrin, Donohue, Besalel, Kogan, and Acierno (1994) and Bry and Krinsley (1992)—found that family therapy produced greater reductions in substance use than other, nonfamily-based interventions. Similarly, Joanning, Thomas, Quinn, and Mullen (1992) compared a systems family therapy intervention with two comparison conditions, a family drug education intervention and adolescent group therapy. The results at posttreatment revealed that family therapy was most effective in decreasing problem behaviors and drug use, with 54% of youth in family therapy abstinent, compared to 29% in the family education condition and 17% in the group therapy condition. Ecological and integrative family interventions for adolescent substance abuse have also been effective. Henggeler and colleagues (1991) conducted two studies, comparing multisystemic family therapy with individual therapy in the first study and with a treatment-as-usual juvenile probation supervision intervention in the second. As they had found for delinquent adolescents and their families, multisystemic family therapy produced significantly better substance use outcomes at posttest. Liddle and colleagues (1993) compared a multisystemic, multidimensional family therapy to two alternative treatments: adolescent group therapy and a family education group. All three conditions were associated with reduced substance use, with greatest and most consistent improvement in the family therapy condition.

Studies of the FFT model have demonstrated treatment effectiveness for adolescents with a wide range of behavioral disturbances including substance use problems across a variety of sites and settings (Alexander, Pugh, & Parsons, in press; Barton, Alexander, Waldron, Turner, & Warburton, 1985). Moreover, evidence has been found for the preventive effects of FFT for siblings of problem youth and for the long-term effectiveness of the intervention (Gordon, Graves, & Arbuthnot, 1995; Klein, Alexander, & Parsons, 1977). Friedman (1989) compared FFT with a parenting skills group intervention and found significant improvement from pre- to posttreatment for both intervention conditions, with 93% treatment engagement for families in family therapy compared to only 67% of the parenting group families. Moreover, in a reanalysis of these data that included treatment dropouts as failures, a significant difference between the two family-based interventions emerged revealing the greater effectiveness of FFT (Stanton & Shadish, 1997). The Purdue brief family therapy model (Lewis et al., 1990), integrating elements of FFT, was compared to a didactic, family-oriented parenting skills intervention, again with both interventions associated with significant reductions in adolescent drug use at posttreatment. Moreover, a greater percentage of youth receiving family therapy decreased their use, compared with the parenting group intervention. Currently, another randomized clinical trial, funded by the National Institute on Drug Abuse, is underway to compare the effectiveness of FFT with other nonfamily-based interventions (i.e., cognitive-behavioral and group education interventions) for substance-abusing adolescents and their families (Waldron, 1994a). Preliminary data analysis of 14 families completing 3-month follow-up has indicated a high rate of treatment engagement (96%) for FFT, similar to Friedman (1989). With respect to substance use outcome, FFT was also associated with a 45% reduction in number of days of drug use (Waldron & Slesnick, 1997). Although promising, these findings must be interpreted with caution until the full study has been completed.

TREATMENT OUTCOME FOR ADULT SUBSTANCE ABUSE

Research examining the effectiveness of treatments for adult problem drinkers has provided considerable evidence that the involvement of spouses and significant others in treatment, especially in behavioral couples therapy, is associated with improved treatment engagement and reduced drinking behavior (cf. O'Farrell, 1995). Family-based interventions implemented unilaterally with parents, spouses, and other concerned individuals have also been shown to improve treatment engagement for adult drug abusers (cf. Chapter 11, this volume). By contrast, relatively little attention has been given to evaluating the effectiveness of conjoint family therapy approaches for adult substance abusers. In a study of behavioral couples therapy, Fals-Stewart, Birchler, and O'Farrell (1996) added a couples intervention for male substance abusers to a cognitive-behavioral treatment-as-usual package, involving individual and group therapy modalities, and found significantly reduced substance use for the couples intervention. In studies examining family systems approaches, Stanton, Todd, and associates (1982) and McLellan, Arndt, Metzger, Woody, and O'Brien (1993) found that the addition of a family intervention component to individual counseling and methadone maintenance led to improved outcomes for adult heroin addicts. Similarly, Kosten, Jalali, Hogan, and Kleber (1983) found that treating multiple families together in a group setting, multiple family therapy combined with standard care, was superior to standard care alone in promoting abstinence from drug use. Bernal and colleagues (1997) also found significant pre- to posttreatment reductions in substance use for adult clients and their families using contextual family therapy, an intergenerational approach based on psychodynamic and systems theories, but differences found for family therapy and a family education approach were small. Although these findings are encouraging, other studies have not found the expected results (Liddle & Dakof, 1995).

EVIDENCE FOR DIFFERENTIAL EFFECTIVENESS

Although only a few studies have directly compared family therapy models, making any conclusions premature, there is little evidence to support the superiority of one approach over another. The lack of meaningful differences in outcomes thus far could reflect the limited variation in theoretical orientation across models (Stanton & Shadish, 1997). For example, the vast majority of family-based interventions for substance abuse problems focus on present-oriented and directive approaches that include family interaction patterns and parenting behaviors as major targets of change. Alternatively, the similarities in outcomes across approaches may suggest that systemic change can be achieved in a variety of ways. The following section describes the practice of family therapy, using the anatomy of intervention model (AIM; Alexander, Barton, Waldron, & Mas, 1983) to depict family therapy process. The AIM model describes five generic phases common across most family therapy models, regardless of theoretical orientation: initial introduction and impression formation, motivation, assessment, behavior change, and generalization. Although the sequencing of and emphasis on each of the five phases may vary across models, AIM provides a useful structure for describing the tasks of family therapy and common techniques and strategies employed for each of the distinct phases.

FAMILY THERAPY PRACTICE

INITIAL INTRODUCTION PHASE

The family's initial impressions of treatment, while representing only a brief, transitory phase of family therapy, can have a significant influence on treatment engagement and retention (Alexander & Parsons, 1982; Stanton, Todd et al., 1982; Szapocznik et al., 1988). A host of interrelated factors can affect this early stage of treatment, including family beliefs and attitudes, aspects of the service delivery system (e.g., reputation, location), and a wide range of therapist characteristics and behaviors such as gender, cultural sensitivity, interpersonal warmth, and empathic listening (Alexander & Parsons, 1982). These factors generally relate to the families' perceptions of therapist credibility and the potential for development of the therapeutic alliance. The therapist's rationale for treatment, relationship-building skills, nondefensive response to direct challenges to therapist credibility (e.g., "Do you have children?"), and the ability to normalize problems and convey confidence in potential for change are also important in developing families' positive expectations for change.

ASSESSMENT

Assessment procedures vary considerably across theoretical models, and may include very structured assessments conducted prior to the beginning of treatment, as in behavioral models, or ongoing assessment that occurs in conjunction with other phases of therapy. Despite theoretical, methodological, and sequencing differences, however, family therapy models generally conduct assessment with respect to three primary targets of change: substance use, family relationship functioning, and the substance abuser's use of time (Stanton, Todd et al., 1982). In addition, the FFT model and other models integrating FFT constructs (e.g., PBFT model, Lewis et al., 1990) assess the relational functions served by the substance use and other behaviors in order to guide the process of behavior change (cf. Alexander & Parsons, 1982).

MOTIVATING FAMILIES: CREATING A CONTEXT FOR CHANGE

Many family therapy models acknowledge that engaging entire families in treatment is a significant challenge. Families with substance-abusing members frequently enter treatment with an established pattern of conflicted exchanges characterized by intense negativity (Hops et al., 1990) and marked resistance to the treatment process (Alexander & Parsons, 1982; Stanton, Todd et al., 1982; Szapocznik et al., 1988). The lack of motivation for change among individuals referred for substance-abuse treatment is widely recognized (Miller & Rollnick, 1991). This resistance is often compounded when family members, holding the view that only the referred substance abuser needs to change and blaming the substance abuser, refuse to attend family therapy. If the therapist accepts the resistance and agrees to meet with only one or two members of the family, he or she may reinforce the maladaptive patterns of interaction in the family that may contribute to the maintenance of problems instead of challenging them (Szapocznik & Kurtines, 1989).

The motivation phase is designed to effect a cognitive change that predisposes families to systemic change by offering them alternative, less negative, relationship-based definitions of the problem and engaging rationales for their participation in treatment. Behavioral models have emphasized building positive expectancies for treatment through the creation of the collaborative set and by providing theoretical and empirical rationales for treatment (Jacobson & Margolin, 1979). Family systems models have emphasized relabeling or reframing problem behavior to effect a shift in the family's perspective about their problems (Alexander & Parsons, 1982; Lewis *et al.*, 1990; Liddle *et al.*, 1992; Stanton, Todd *et al.*, 1982). Relabeling changes the meaning and value of a negative behavior by casting it in a more benign, or even benevolent, light. Morris, Alexander, and Waldron (1988) proposed that relabels may operate by (1) suspending the automatic negative thinking and response patterns in families, (2) requiring them to search for new explanations of family behavior, and (3) offering a cognitive perspective that opens the door to more effective communication and expression of feelings and reconnects families with their underlying love and caring for one another. If family members can be helped to consider that their own and others' behaviors are motivated and maintained by variables other than individual malevolence (e.g., anger reflects underlying hurt or worry), they are more likely to see change as possible and to be more motivated. In a related way, members of disturbed families often are unaware of how their behavior contributes to their current difficulties in a contingent or interdependent fashion. Another aspect of motivating families to change is helping family members recognize the relational interdependency of each family member's behavior with every other member (Alexander & Parsons, 1982).

Several structured interventions for motivating families have been developed focusing on getting resistant substance abusers and their families into treatment. Szapocznik and his colleagues (1988) proposed a structural analysis of the resistance in families, with different theoretically based interventions applied depending on the type of resistance encountered (e.g., ambivalent mother, strongly allied mothers and sons). Garrett and his colleagues have proposed the ARISE method that provides a three-step strategy to engage families and substance abusers in treatment, including intervening with the concerned family member making the initial contact, mobilizing the social network to engage the substance abuser, and working with the family to conduct an adapted Johnson Institute intervention (Garrett, Landau-Stanton, Stanton, Stellato-Kabat, & Stellato-Kabat, 1997). Both of these models view structured telephone interventions with families before "treatment" has begun as the appropriate points to begin the motivational process. (See Chapter 11, this volume, for a review of other unilateral family interventions to engage resistant substance abusers in treatment.) Other researchers are examining an intervention to provide feedback and develop discrepancies in families' views of their current functioning, in order to enhance families' motivation for change (Dishion & Kavanagh, in press). This unique approach involves the application of motivational interviewing principles and procedures (Miller & Rollnick, 1991) to family interventions aimed at enhancing engagement and motivation of resistant families.

STRATEGIES FOR LONG-TERM BEHAVIOR CHANGE

Family therapy models overlap considerably in their focus on certain strategies designed to help families change dysfunctional patterns of interaction. Communication and problem-solving skills training, strategies to increase rewarding family activities, contingency management practices, and other strategies to restructure family patterns and change behaviors are among the most common interventions implemented (Bry, 1988; Fleishmann *et al.*, 1983; Liddle *et al.*, 1992). The FFT model uses a menu approach to the behavior change phase. Therapists working with adolescent substance abusers and their families draw from a menu of treatment strategies and behavior change techniques (Waldron, 1994b). In addition to the commonly used skills training and pleasant shared activities modules, optional modules can also implemented, depending on the families' particular needs, such as affect regulation (i.e., anger management, depressed mood), relaxation training, self-esteem building, assertiveness training, drug refusal skills, contingency contracting, or methods of self-control. Stanton, Todd, and colleagues (1982) also note that after the referred family member's substance use has decreased and family interactions have improved, other family problems such as marital discord or parental drinking may need to be addressed.

Families with addictive behavior problems also often have limited access to community resources that reduce the risk for alcohol abuse. Multisystemic family therapy models emphasize the importance of enhancing extrafamilial resources that can be developed to support the treatment gains made in therapy. Many extrafamilial factors are more difficult to change, such as neighborhood crime or institutional racism. However, other factors may be modifiable for a family, such as responsiveness of school personnel or employers. The therapist can work with families to help them interact more effectively with legal and educational systems or may interact with staff directly on behalf of the adolescent and family (Alexander et al., in press; Henggeler et al., 1991; Liddle et al., 1992; Scopetta et al., 1979).

GENERALIZATION OF CHANGE AND RELAPSE PREVENTION

As behavioral changes are established in the family, the focus of sessions shifts toward maintenance of change and establishing the family's independence from the therapist (Alexander & Parsons, 1982; Henggeler et al., 1991). To develop independence, the therapist gradually takes a less active role in intrafamily process. As family members experience short-term changes, they are helped to consider alternative ways to continue positive change. Gradually, the family is encouraged to develop techniques that might work for them on their own and the interval between sessions is extended. In addition, the therapist may help the family anticipate stressors and problems, exploring solutions to those future difficulties. Relapse prevention strategies may also be implemented in family therapy sessions to help the family support the substance abuser in recognizing and avoiding triggers or high-risk events that may trigger a lapse and establish an emergency plan to deal with a lapse (Waldron, 1994b).

Therapy moves toward termination when (1) drug and alcohol use and other problem behaviors are reduced or eliminated, (2) adaptive interaction patterns and problem-solving styles have been developed and are occurring independent of the therapist's monitoring and prompting, and (3) the family appears to have the necessary motivation, skills, and resources to maintain a positive clinical trajectory without the support of ongoing services.

REFERENCES

Akers, R. L., Krohn, M. D., Lanza Kaduce, L., & Radosevich, M. (1979). Social learning and deviant behavior: A specific test of a general theory. *American Sociology Review, 44,* 636–655.

Alexander, J. F., & Parsons, B. V. (1982). *Functional family therapy.* Monterey, CA: Brooks/Cole.

Alexander, J. F., Barton, C., Waldron, H., & Mas, C. H. (1983). Beyond the technology of family therapy: The anatomy of intervention model. In K. D. Craig & R. H. McMahon (Eds.), *Advances in clinical behavior therapy* (pp. 48–73). New York: Brunner/Mazel.

Alexander, J. F., Holtzworth-Munroe, A., & Jameson, P. (1994). The process and outcome of marital and family therapy: Research review and evaluation. In S. L. Garfield & A. E. Bergin (Eds.), *Handbook of psychotherapy and behavior change* (4th ed., pp. 595–630). New York: Wiley.

Alexander, J. F., Pugh, C., & Parsons, B. V. (in press). Functional family therapy. In D. S. Elliott (Ed.), *Blueprints for violence prevention.* Boulder, CO: Center for the Study of Prevention and Violence, Institute of Behavioral Science, University of Colorado.

Azrin, N. H., Donohue, B., Besalel, V. A., Kogan, E. S., & Acierno, R. (1994). Youth drug abuse treatment: A controlled outcome study. *Journal of Child and Adolescent Substance Abuse, 3,* 1–16.

Barton, C., Alexander, J. F., Waldron, H., Turner, C. W., & Warburton, J. (1985). Generalizing treatment effects of Functional Family Therapy: Three replications. *Journal of Marriage and Family Therapy, 13,* 16–26.

Berg, I. K., & Miller, S. D. (1992). *Working with the problem drinker: A solution-focused approach.* New York: Norton.

Bernal, G., Flores-Ortiz, Y., Sorenson, J. L., Miranda, J., Diamond, G., & Bonilla, J. (1997). *Intergenerational family therapy with methadone maintenance patients and family members: Findings of a clinical outcome study.* Manuscript submitted for publication.

Beutler, L. E., McCray-Patterson, K., Jacob, T., Shoham, V., Yost, E., & Rohrbaugh, M. (1993). Matching treatment to alcoholism subtypes. *Psychotherapy, 30,* 463–472.

Brook, J. S., Whiteman, M., Gordon, A. S., & Brook, D. W. (1988). The role of older brothers in younger brothers' drug use viewed in the context of parent and peer influences. *Journal of Genetic Psychology, 151,* 59–75.

Brown, S. A., Myers, M. B., Mott, M. A., & Vik, P. (1994). Correlates of success following treatment for adolescent substance abuse. *Applied and Preventive Psychology, 3,* 61–73.

Bry, B. H. (1988). Family-based approaches to reducing adolescent substance use: Theories, techniques and findings. In E. R. Rahdert & J. Grabowski (Eds.), *Adolescent drug abuse: Analyses of treatment research* (National Institute on Drug Abuse Research Monograph No. 77, pp. 39–68). Rockville, MD: U.S. Department of Health and Human Services.

Bry, B. H., & Krinsley, K. E. (1992). Booster sessions and long-term effects of behavioral family therapy on adolescent substance use and school performance. *Journal of Behavioral Therapy and Experimental Psychiatry, 23,* 183–189.

Dishion, T. J., Patterson, G. R., & Reid, J. R. (1988). Parent and peer factors associated with drug sampling in early adolescence: Implications for treatment. In E. R. Rahdert & J. Grabowski (Eds.), *Adolescent drug abuse: Analyses of treatment research* (National Institute on Drug Abuse Research Monograph No. 77, pp. 69–93). Rockville, MD: U.S. Department of Health and Human Services.

Dishion, T., & Kavanagh, K. (in press). *Adolescent problem behavior: A family-centered assessment and intervention sourcebook.* New York: Guilford.

Fals-Stewart, W., Birchler, G. R., & O'Farrell, T. J. (1996). Behavioral couples therapy for male substance-abusing patients: Effects on relationship adjustment and drug-using behavior. *Journal of Consulting and Clinical Psychology, 64,* 959–972.

Fleischman, M. J., Horne, A. M., & Arthur, J. L. (1983). *Troubled families: A treatment program.* Champaign, IL: Research Press.

Friedman, A. S. (1989). Family therapy vs. parent groups: Effects on adolescent drug abusers. *American Journal of Family Therapy, 17,* 335–347.

Garrett, J., Landau-Stanton, J., Stanton, M. D., Stellato-Kabat, J., & Stellato-Kabat, D. (1997). ARISE: A method for engaging reluctant alcohol- and drug-dependent individuals in treatment. *Journal of Substance Abuse Treatments, 14,* 235–248.

Gordon, D. A., Graves, K., & Arbuthnot, J. (1995). The effect of Functional Family Therapy for delinquents on adult criminal behavior. *Criminal Justice and Behavior, 22,* 60–73.

Hawkins, J. D., Catalano, R. F., & Miller, J. Y. (1992). Risk and protective factors for alcohol and other drug problems in adolescence and early adulthood: Implications for substance abuse prevention. *Psychological Bulletin, 112,* 64–105.

Henggeler, S. W., Borduin, C. M., Melton, G. B., Mann, B. J., Smith, L. A., Hall, J. A., Cone, L., & Fucci, B. R. (1991). Effects of multisystemic therapy on drug use and abuse in serious juvenile offenders: A progress report from two outcome studies. *Family Dynamics of Addiction Quarterly, 1,* 40–51.

Hops, H., Tildesley, E., Lichtenstein, E., Ary, D., & Sherman, L. (1990). Parent–adolescent problem-solving interactions and drug use. *American Journal of Drug and Alcohol Abuse, 16,* 239–258.

Jacob, T., & Leonard, K. E. (1988). Alcoholic–spouse interaction as a function of alcoholism subtype and alcohol consumption interaction. *Journal of Abnormal Psychology, 97,* 231–237.

Jacobson, N. S., & Margolin, G. (1979). *Marital therapy.* New York: Brunner/Mazel.

Joanning, H., Thomas, F., Quinn, W., & Mullen, R. (1992). Treating adolescent drug abuse: A comparison of family systems therapy, group therapy, and family drug education. *Journal of Marital and Family Therapy, 18,* 345–356.

Johnson, V. E. (1986). *Intervention: How to help those who don't want help.* Minneapolis, MN: Johnson Institute.

Kaufman, E., & Kaufmann, P. (1992). *Family therapy of drug and alcohol abuse* (2nd ed.). Needham Heights, MA: Allyn & Bacon.

Klein, N. C., Alexander, J. F., & Parsons, B. V. (1977). Impact of family systems intervention on recidivism and sibling delinquency: A model of primary prevention and program evaluation. *Journal of Consulting and Clinical Psychology, 45,* 469–474.

Kosten, T. R., Jalali, B. Hogan, I., & Kleber, H. D. (1983). Family denial as a prognostic factor in opiate addict treatment outcome. *Journal of Nervous and Mental Disease, 171,* 611–616.

Lewis, R. A., Piercy, F. P., Sprenkle, D. H., & Trepper, T. S. (1990). Family-based interventions for helping drug-abusing adolescents. *Journal of Adolescent Research, 5,* 82–95.

Liddle, H. A., Dakof, G. A., Parker, K., Diamond, G., Garcia, R., Barrett, K., & Jurwitz, S. (1993, June). *Effectiveness of family therapy versus multi-family therapy and group therapy: Results of the Adolescents and Families Project—A randomized clinical trial.* Paper presented at the annual meeting of the Society for Psychotherapy Research, Pittsburgh, PA.

Liddle, H. A., & Dakof, G. A. (1995). Efficacy of family therapy for drug abuse: Promising but not definitive. *Journal of Marital and Family Therapy, 21,* 511–544.

Liddle, H. A., Diamond, G., Dakof, G. A., (1992). Adolescent substance abuse: Multidimensional family therapy in action. In E. Kaufman & P. Kaufmann, (Eds.), *Family therapy of drug and alcohol abuse* (2nd ed., pp. 120–171). Boston: Allyn & Bacon.

McCrady, B. S. (1986). The family in the change process. In W. R. Miller & N. Heather (Eds.), *Treating addictive behaviors* (pp. 305–318). New York: Plenum.

McCrady, B. S. (1989). Outcomes of family-involved alcoholism treatment. In M. Galanter (Ed.), *Recent developments in alcoholism* (Vol. 7, pp. 165–182). New York: Plenum.

McLellan, A., Arndt, I., Metzger, D., Woody, G., & O'Brien, C. (1993). The effects of psychosocial services in substance abuse treatment. *Journal of the American Medical Association, 269,* 1953–1959.

Miller, W. R., & Rollnick, S. (1991). *Motivational interviewing.* New York: Guilford.

Morris, S., Alexander, J. F., & Waldron, H. (1988). Functional Family Therapy: Issues in clinical practice. In I. R. H. Falloon (Ed.), *Handbook of behavioral family therapy* (pp. 107–127). New York: Guilford.

O'Farrell, T. J. (1995). Marital and family therapy. In R. K. Hester & W. R. Miller (Eds.), *Handbook of alcoholism treatment approaches: Effective alternatives* (2nd ed., pp. 195–220). Boston: Allyn & Bacon.

Scopetta, M. A., King, O. E., Szapocznik, J., & Tillman, W. (1979). *Ecological structural family therapy with Cuban immigrant families* (Report to the National Institute on Drug Abuse: Grant #H81DA 01696). Miami, FL: Department of Psychiatry, University of Miami.

Stanton, M. D., & Shadish, W. R. (1997). Outcome attrition and family/couples treatment for drug abuse: A meta-analysis and review of the controlled, comparative studies. *Psychological Bulletin, 122,* 170–191.

Stanton, M. D., Todd, T. C., & Associates. (1982). *The family therapy of drug abuse and addiction.* New York: Guilford.

Steinglass, P., Bennett, L., Wolin, S., & Reiss, D. (1987). *The alcoholic family.* New York: Basic Books.

Szapocznik, J., & Kurtines, W. M. (1989). *Breakthroughs in family therapy with drug-abusing and problem youth.* New York: Springer.

Szapocznik, J., Kurtines, W. M., Foote, F. H., Perez-Vidal, A., & Hervis, O. (1983). Conjoint versus one-person family therapy: Some evidence for the effectiveness of conducting family therapy through one person. *Journal of Consulting and Clinical Psychology, 51,* 889–899.

Szapocznik, J., Kurtines, W. M., Foote, F. H., Perez-Vidal, A., & Hervis, O. (1986). Conjoint versus one-person family therapy: Further evidence for the effectiveness of conducting family therapy through one person with drug-abusing adolescents. *Journal of Consulting and Clinical Psychology, 54,* 395–397.

Szapocznik, J., Perez-Vidal, A., Brickman, A. L., Foote, F. H., Santisteban, D., & Hervis, O. (1988). Engaging adolescent drug abusers and their families in treatment: A strategic structural systems approach. *Journal of Consulting and Clinical Psychology, 56,* 552–557.

Szapocznik, J., Perez-Vidal, A., Hervis, O. E., Brickman, A. L. & Kurtines, W. M. (1990). Innovations in family therapy: Strategies for overcoming resistance to treatment. In R. A. Wells & V. J. Giannetti (Eds.), *Handbook of brief psychotherapies* (pp. 93–114). New York: Plenum.

Waldron, H. B. (1994a). *Drug abuse treatments for adolescents* (National Institute on Drug Abuse Grant Project Number RO1 DA09422). Albuquerque: Department of Psychology, University of New Mexico.

Waldron, H. B. (1994b) *Functional Family Therapy for substance-abusing adolescents: A treatment manual.* Unpublished therapy manual, University of New Mexico.

Waldron, H. B. (1997). Adolescent substance abuse and family therapy outcome: A review of randomized trials. In T. H. Ollendick & R. J. Prinz (Eds.), *Advances in clinical child psychology* (Vol. 19, pp. 199–234). New York: Plenum.

Waldron, H. B., & Slesnick, N. (1997, November). *The effectiveness of Functional Family Therapy for adolescent substance abuse: Preliminary findings.* Paper presented at the annual meeting of the Association for Advancement of Behavior Therapy, Social Learning and the Family. Miami Beach, FL.

Ziegler-Driscoll, G. (1977). Family research study at Eagleville Hospital and Rehabilitation Center. *Family Process, 16,* 175–190.

21

Mutual-Help Groups
Research and Clinical Implications

J. SCOTT TONIGAN AND RADKA T. TOSCOVA

OVERVIEW

In a text for clinicians, one may ask, why a chapter on mutual-help groups? By definition, these groups of individuals share a common problem and are *not led by a professional*. In a word, prevalence. It is estimated, for example, that 1 in 10 Americans have attended an AA meeting (McCrady & Miller, 1993), and that a majority of clients seeking professional treatment for alcohol problems in the United States have had prior involvement in a 12-step program (Tonigan, Connors, & Miller, 1996). In addition, about 40% of successful AA members report seeking professional counseling after achieving abstinence, and most of these people say that such counseling was important for their recovery (Alcoholics Anonymous, 1997). We believe that the effectiveness of psychotherapy is enhanced when clinicians are sensitive to client beliefs about the nature and process of recovery. With so many people choosing to participate in mutual-help programs, clinicians are well advised to become familiar with the basic tenets and practices associated with membership in these programs.

The purpose of this chapter is to address some basic questions clinicians may have about mutual-help programs, focusing on change mechanisms and outcomes associated with these programs. As background, the first section describes the defining characteristics of some of the more popular mutual-help programs. The second section reviews the research literature on the effectiveness of mutual-help programs.

J. SCOTT TONIGAN • Center on Alcoholism, Substance Abuse, and Addictions, Family and Child Guidance Center, University of New Mexico, Albuquerque, New Mexico 87106. RADKA T. TOSCOVA • Albuquerque Family and Child Guidance Center, Albuquerque, New Mexico 87108.

Treating Addictive Behaviors, 2nd ed., edited by Miller and Heather. Plenum Press, New York, 1998.

Attention is directed to distinctions between attendance and engagement in mutual-help programs. The third section of the chapter examines specific processes of change in mutual-help programs. The final section identifies important considerations in making referrals to mutual-help programs, paying some attention to factors of social context and the special needs of clients.

TYPES OF MUTUAL-HELP PROGRAMS

As previously mentioned, a mutual-help organization is a group of individuals with a common problem, who seek relief from the problem using a common plan, and who are not led by a professional. Mutual-help programs are now available for an array of problems, including chronic psychiatric problems (Kennedy, 1990), manic depression (Kurtz, 1988), diabetes (Simmons, 1992), and bereavement (Caserta & Lund, 1993), to name only a few. Numerous mutual-help organizations are available for individuals with substance abuse problems, and this section highlights some of the basic tenets and practices of the more popular programs in the United States. All of the mutual-help programs described in this chapter are abstinence-based. Programs differ, however, in their prescriptions about how long members are expected to participate in mutual-help programs, and about the consequences of disaffiliation.

12-STEP PROGRAMS

Alcoholics Anonymous is the largest mutual-help program, currently estimated as having 96,000 groups (Alcoholics Anonymous, 1997) with an annual membership of about 3.5 million (Room, 1993). The core literature of AA (Alcoholics Anonymous, 1976 and 1981) describes the nature of alcoholism and offers a curative program for recovery embodied in the 12 steps. In AA's view, alcoholism is a threefold malady consisting of mental, physical, and spiritual aspects. The 12 steps are intended as a blueprint to recover from alcoholism, and central in AA philosophy is the development of a faith in a power greater than oneself. It is suggested that the 12 steps be done sequentially, generally with the aid of a more experienced AA member called a sponsor. It is estimated that a majority of AA members have sponsors (76%) and that sponsors are often enlisted within the first 90 days of affiliation (Alcoholics Anonymous, 1997).

The *program* of AA is encapsulated in the 12 steps while the *fellowship* of AA refers to the practice of AA principles. General guidelines for the practice of the AA program are enumerated in the 12 traditions, and AA group processes and activities as a rule tend to adhere closely to these traditions. Twelve-step meetings can be described along two dimensions. First, meetings are offered in "open" and "closed" formats. Any interested person can attend an open meeting, but closed meetings are reserved for individuals who acknowledge having problems with alcohol. A second dimension is the content or structure of a meeting. Open discussion meetings generally use approved AA literature to introduce a topic, with group members having an opportunity to share; speaker meetings have 1 or 2 members share in detail their experiences of alcoholism and recovery with a larger group; and study meetings have members take turns reading from the core literature of AA. Characteristic of all AA meetings, cross-talk is discouraged, individuals can decline sharing, meetings typically are 1 hour, and meetings begin with readings of the AA preamble, "How It Works," and the 12 traditions, and close with members joining hands and reciting the Lord's Prayer.

RATIONAL MUTUAL-HELP PROGRAMS

A number of alternatives to 12-step programs have emerged in the past 25 years. In general, origins for these mutual-help programs can be traced to perceived deficiencies in 12-step ideology and practices or as reactions against certain aspects of 12-step programs. Women for Sobriety (WFS) is a mutual-help program attuned to meet the special needs of women, needs felt to be overlooked in perceived male-dominated 12-step programs. Rational Recovery (RR) is based upon rational emotive therapy (Ellis, 1962), underscores how irrational beliefs drive addictive behaviors, and proposes cognitive strategies for achieving sobriety. Secular Organizations for Sobriety (SOS) does not emphasize reliance upon a *higher power*, stressing instead the need to take personal responsibility for achieving and maintaining sobriety (Christopher, 1988).

Women for Sobriety (WFS)

Founded in 1976 by Jean Kirkpatrick, WFS is a mutual-help organization designed to meet the specific needs of women with alcohol problems. Membership is restricted to females, and more than 200 WFS groups are in operation in the United States and overseas. Based on the "New Life" program, the WFS program consists of 13 affirmations or statements, largely intended to improve self-worth and value as well as to reduce perceived shame of group members. Four books form the core literature of the WFS program, the most important one being *Turnabout: New Help for the Woman Alcoholic*.

WFS meetings can range in size from 2 to 20 participants although the recommended group size is 6 to 10 women. Meetings are led by a certified moderator who must have 1 year of continuous sobriety and who is well versed in the WFS philosophy and program. Certification is not a process leading to any licensure, and moderators are not compensated for their effort. The format of WFS meetings can be divided into three sections. The introductory section is led by the moderator and includes reading of the 13 statements of the new life program followed by a review of the WFS purpose. The discussion section of the meeting is based on a topic from the WFS literature. Cross-talk is encouraged. Closing of the meeting is accomplished by holding hands and reciting the WFS motto, "We are capable and competent, caring and compassionate, always willing to help another, bonded together in overcoming our addictions."

Rational Recovery (RR)

Rational Recovery (RR) is most accurately termed a self-help movement because of its rejection of the need for regular attendance at group meetings. Instructional in tone, RR endorses the addictive voice recognition technique (AVRT) in which individuals learn that abstinence is a planned activity. Learning of cognitive strategies to recognize drinking cues is done in an instructional format with groups as large as 40 individuals. The core philosophy of RR is contained in two texts, The "small book" (Trimpey, 1988) and *The Final Fix: AVRT.* The RR movement originated as a strong reaction against spiritual aspects of 12-step programs, and offers a secular approach to understanding addiction. Currently, the RR movement is institutionalized in the form of national RR centers offering courses for a fee and locally based in small groups that follow the tenets of the RR program without fees. At this time, the actual number of locally based RR groups and the total size of the RR membership is unknown.

Secular Organizations for Sobriety (SOS)

This mutual-help program was founded in 1986 by James Christopher and currently is estimated to have a membership of 20,000 (Connors & Derman, 1996). The core literature describing the Secular Organizations for Sobriety (SOS) program for recovery is contained in three texts, *How to Stay Sober* (Christopher, 1988), *Unhooked: Staying Sober and Drug-Free* (Christopher, 1989), and *SOS Sobriety* (Christopher, 1992). According to Connors and Derman (1996), SOS has three objectives: (1) offer peer support for sobriety, (2) be nonreligious in orientation, and (3) provide an opportunity for individuals to share their experiences and feelings in a supportive group setting. Individual responsibility for recovery is stressed and formal sponsor relationships are not utilized.

Considerable variation can be found among SOS meetings. In general, the format of SOS meetings is a reading of the organization's purpose, followed by group announcements and celebration of sobriety anniversaries. SOS guidelines are then reviewed. The remainder of the meeting (about 1 hour) is devoted to open discussion by group members on topics pertaining to individual struggles for achieving and/or maintaining sobriety. The SOS national newsletter is a popular means for the organization to communicate planned conventions and emergent SOS philosophy.

DO MUTUAL-HELP PROGRAMS REALLY HELP?

A fundamental question posed about mutual-help programs for addictive behaviors is, Are they effective? Nearly all research in this area has been conducted on AA affiliation and participation, and we look forward to future integration of findings relating to other 12-step–based and other mutual-help programs. How confident can we be in the findings of the effectiveness of AA? The few clinical trials that included randomization to AA may be of limited value because of threats to internal validity (e.g., Brandsma, Maultsby, & Welsh, 1980; Ditman, Crawford, Forgy, Moskowitz, & MacAndrew, 1967; Walsh *et al.,* 1991) and, equally important, because randomization to AA is insensitive to the self-selective processes of AA affiliation and engagement (McCrady & Miller, 1993; Montgomery, Miller, & Tonigan, 1993). Tonigan, Toscova, and Miller (1996) developed a global rating of study quality and rated 74 studies reporting findings on AA. This rating evaluated the extent to which studies corroborated self-report, used reliable assessment tools, and employed random selection and assignment. Their verdict was that, in general, the quality of AA studies was poor (mean rating of 1 on a 0 to 5 scale).

With this limitation in mind, how effective is AA? At the most global level, frequency of attendance at AA meetings reflects client action taking, and like other forms of action is positively related to abstinence (Emrick, Tonigan, Montgomery, & Little, 1993). When findings were divided according to whether studies were of poor or fair quality, better designed studies yielded, on average, stronger associations between AA attendance and *psychosocial outcomes* relative to poorly executed studies. Better designed studies, however, provided less support for the benefits of AA attendance after treatment than did poorly designed studies in regard to *abstinence* (Tonigan, Toscova, & Miller, 1996).

For individuals who use what AA has to offer, how often should they attend meetings? This is a complex question involving individual differences in problem severity, length of abstinence and affiliation with AA, the supportiveness of social networks for abstinence, and AA group characteristics. The recommendation is voiced in AA that newcomers should attend AA meetings daily for the first 90 days. Members of AA with a substantial length of abstinence, however, report attending meetings considerably less often, about two times per week (Alcoholics Anonymous, 1997). Practically, clients will determine the frequency of attendance. For those clients expressing an interest in or an affiliation with AA, we encourage clinicians to help clients examine the factors leading to self-defined attendance rates.

Frequency of AA meeting attendance has traditionally been equated with extent of commitment, engagement, or involvement in AA. An emergent view is that frequency of attendance and commitment to AA are not synonymous. Several excellent measures with known psychometric properties are available which, to varying degrees, summarize information about AA members' specific AA practices (Gorski, 1990; Morgenstern, Kahler, Frey, & Labouvie, 1996; Ouimette, Moos, & Finney, in press; Tonigan, Toscova, & Miller, 1996). In general, engagement measures inquire about experiences in at least one of three domains: (1) practicing of the 12 steps, (2) participation in the fellowship of AA, and (3) spirituality. These measures often yield summary scores reflecting extent of AA involvement, and some instruments have normative data to compare individual scores.

Research suggests that AA attendance and commitment are distinct constructs, offering clinicians different perspectives on mutual-help exposure. For example, among AA members who had achieved sobriety (range 3 weeks to 26 years, mean = 5.93 years), attendance and a three-item measure of involvement shared only 30% variance (Snow, Prochaska, & Rossi, 1994). Likewise, in Project MATCH, which included both outpatient and aftercare samples ($N = 1,726$), only 43% to 50% shared variance was found between AA attendance and involvement for clients with 9 or fewer months of sobriety (Tonigan, Miller, & Connors, in press). Of interest in the Project MATCH study was the finding that AA attendance and involvement were positively related up to the point at which clients attended AA meetings about 60% of the available days (more than 2 of 3 days). On average, those clients attending AA on more than 60% of the available days showed no further gains in AA involvement. This finding awaits replication in future research. It appears that recommendations to attend AA daily for the first 90 days should not be made to enhance engagement in AA per se, but may be warranted to offer a social network supportive of abstinence.

Given that attendance and engagement in AA are distinct, which is the more important aspect of mutual-help exposure to evaluate? With some exception, findings suggest that both attendance and engagement are positively associated with posttreatment abstinence. Ouimette and colleagues (in press), for example, found no difference between AA attendance and involvement; both positively and significantly predicted 1-year posttreatment abstinence. This finding has been replicated in Project MATCH with both aftercare and outpatient clients (Tonigan, Connors, & Miller, in press). In contrast, Mongomery, Miller, and Tonigan (1995) reported that after discharge from an inpatient treatment facility, AA meeting attendance did not predict percentage of abstinent days, but a summary measure of engagement in AA was significantly and positively related to abstinence. A clear advantage of multiple item measures of engagement is that they inform about the presence or absence of specific behaviors to effect change. Simple measures of the frequency of attendance are silent in this regard. In this context, we recommend assessment of specific behaviors related to participation in mutual-help groups.

HOW MUTUAL-HELP PROGRAMS WORK

Thus far it has been suggested that mutual-help programs offer positive benefit for some individuals and that popular mutual-help programs differ in their basic assumptions about the function of the group. This section addresses the topic of *how and why* participation in mutual-help groups is associated with positive gains. Empirical work on this topic pertains almost exclusively to participation in AA. This is unfortunate. At the outset of this discussion it is also important to acknowledge how group social functioning may influence the translation of prescribed activities into actual behaviors. Several studies (e.g., Montgomery *et al.*, 1993; Tonigan, Ashcroft, & Miller, 1995) report that AA groups differed in their perceived cohesiveness, aggressiveness, and expressiveness. Interestingly, AA member perceptions of the frequency that the 12 steps were discussed in meetings was significantly and positively related with perceived cohesiveness and expressiveness of groups and negatively associated with perceived group aggressiveness. An important implication of these studies is that the intensity of endorsement of change mechanisms in AA, for example, the steps, may vary according to the social dynamics of particular groups.

With this background, Table 1 shows the relationship between specific AA-related activities and abstinence. The column labeled *r* (weighted), provides the correlations (possible range −1.0 to 1.0) between a specific activity and abstinence, with greater weight given to studies with larger sample sizes. Ten of the 12 correlations were positive, suggesting that most of the activities studied in the literature were beneficial for achieving and maintaining sobriety. Reaching out for help, having an AA sponsor, and doing the first step of AA were most strongly related to abstinence. Within the context of the transtheoretical model, the first step involves the *recognition* and admission of an alcohol problem, and the remaining activities reflect action (0 to 6 months abstinence) and maintenance (more than 6 months abstinence) behavioral processes.

Activities in Table 1 generally associated with spiritual processes were of little import in predicting abstinence, that is, working steps 2 and 3. How do these

TABLE 1
Relationship between AA Related Activities and Abstinence: Metanalytic
Summary of the Research on Alcoholics[1]

Activity	r (weighted)[a]	No. of studies	No. of subjects
Reaching out for help	.29	1	47
Has an AA sponsor	.26	4	539
Work step 1	.26	1	188
Leads a meeting	.23	2	1,093
Does 12-step work	.20	3	1,140
Tells story at meeting	.07	3	1,142
Sponsors AA member	.17	2	1,091
Work steps 6–12	.11	2	1,096
Work step 2	.16	1	188
Work step 3	.07	1	188
Take-retake step 4	−.08	1	330
Take-retake step 5	−.12	1	332

[1]Table 1 summarizes findings initially reported in "Alcoholics Anonymous: What Is Currently Known," by C. D. Emrick, J. S. Tonigan, H. Montgomery, and L. Little, 1993, in B. S. McCrady and W. R. Miller (Eds.), *Research on Alcoholics Anonymous: Opportunities and Alternatives* (pp. 41–76).
[a]Mean weighted correlation.

findings from a single study compare with the findings of other studies? Christo and Franey (1995) reported that the spiritual beliefs of addicts were positively related to the extent of subsequent attendance at Narcotics Anonymous meetings, but not to subsequent drug use. Likewise, and at intake, Project MATCH outpatient clients with higher God consciousness and formal religious practices scores reported significantly more prior AA attendance and involvement (Connors, Tonigan, & Miller, 1996), but such beliefs were unrelated to frequency or intensity of subsequent alcohol consumption. Contrary with these findings, God consciousness and formal religious practices of aftercare clients in Project MATCH were predictive of less frequent and intense drinking. It is clear that the relationship between spiritual beliefs and practices and abstinence is not straightforward. We suspect that spiritual activities may play a mediating role in recovery, facilitating the initiation and maintenance of prescribed behaviors.

Twelve-step programs explicitly offer a spiritual path to recovery, and 7 of the 12 steps make direct reference to God or a *higher power*. Nevertheless, commonalities in practice between 12-step programs and cognitive-behavioral approaches have been described (DiClemente, 1993; McCrady, 1994). Twelve-step programs emphasize behavior change and the practice of these programs reflects the importance of environmental and stimulus control in facilitating change (Snow *et al.*, 1994). For example, the *meeting* represents the cornerstone of stimulus control in the 12-step program. AA meetings are generally offered between 5 P.M. and 7 P.M., a time that American bars traditionally offer discounted liquor (happy hour). It is also common for 24-hour AA meetings to be held on holidays when excessive drinking is considered normal, for example, New Year's Eve. Finally, it is often recommended to newcomers that they attend 90 meetings in 90 days, a time during which relapse is most likely.

Sponsorship in 12-step programs offers another means for experiential learning. Newcomers learn to contend with high-risk situations from the experiences of a sponsor and also develop a social network supportive of abstinence. Equally important, the explicit role of a sponsor is to assist and direct a member through the 12 steps. The role of sponsor thus may explain the finding that increased AA affiliation is associated with increased commitment to abstinence (Morgenstern, Labouvie, McCrady, Kahler, & Frey, in press). Some clinicians recommend that therapist and sponsors meet to discuss client/sponsee AA progress and goals (Thompson & Thompson, 1993). We have reservations about this recommendation. The 8th tradition states that AA will forever remain nonprofessional, and sponsor–therapist collaboration may violate this tradition. Such collaboration also may violate the confidential nature of therapy. From the perspective of the client, therapist–sponsor discussions may blur important boundaries between professional therapy and mutual-help participation.

Cognitive support and restructuring occurs in the context of new information and indoctrination learned through the reading and repeating of the 12 steps and traditions, slogans, and discussions of AA literature. The repetitive nature of the information serves to reinforce learning and memory, which may be compromised in the early stages of abstinence. Repetition of information serves to desensitize and decrease the stigma of the label of alcoholic or addict. Additional benefits may include increased consciousness raising (Snow *et al.*, 1994), hope, optimism, and the pursuit of shared goals and ideals. New members learn to correct and restructure cognitive distortions and self-defeating beliefs through the use of slogans such as "first things first," "one day at a time," "live and let live," "avoid stinking thinking," and "let go and let God." Slogans are utilized to cope with cravings, negative mood states, and organizational and support problems.

AA/NA group members provide support and confrontation for each other necessary to facilitate the restructuring of self-defeating cognitions and to assimilate program beliefs. Much has been stated recently about the negative effects of confrontation within the context of formal 12-step treatment. There is no indication that confrontation is, in itself, negative or that it inevitably results in resistance, denial, or both. Confrontation in the form of giving feedback and highlighting negative consequences can be beneficial in the context of a positive and supportive relationship. Here, writing and sharing a moral inventory of persons harmed (steps 4 and 5) may be helpful to correct distorted cognitions, perceptions, and blame of others. Change is further consolidated by working steps 8 through 10, in which individuals learn to monitor and correct behaviors by living "the examined life" (Kus, 1992). This process cumulates in steps 11 and 12, in which members actively pursue a deeper relationship with a higher power and with humanity by altruistic and empathic deeds.

MAKING REFERRALS TO MUTUAL-HELP GROUPS

Under many circumstances, AA referral may be very beneficial. However, we do not recommend routine referral to mutual-help programs. Under many circumstances, however, such referral may be very beneficial. After some preliminary remarks, this section identifies some salient dimensions to consider when deciding whether to refer clients to mutual-help programs. Dimensions to evaluate are the social networks of clients, client and therapist motivation, dual diagnoses, membership characteristics of 12-step and non–12-step programs, and useful strategies for locating mutual-help group meetings.

It is vital that clinicians discuss with clients whether they have had prior experiences with mutual-help programs. In determining whether referral is indicated, and what type of program to suggest, it is important to assess the nature and extent of prior engagement in mutual-help programs and the perceived benefits and harm of earlier participation. Barriers the client perceives in participation in a mutual-help program and the supportiveness of abstinence in the client's social network also should be considered. Sampling of different types of programs may be warranted and the clinician should be prepared to provide information about the types and schedules of mutual-help programs in the community.

SOCIAL SUPPORT FOR ABSTINENCE

Social support for abstinence is an important predictor of success (Project MATCH Research Group, 1997), and clients lacking such support may benefit from affiliation with a mutual-help program. Divergent lines of research point to the importance of this dimension for clinical evaluation. Specifically, examining factors related to selection of type of treatment, George and Tucker (1996) reported that individuals selected AA as the primary method to deal with alcohol problems when social networks provided inconsistent messages about the desirability of changing addictive behavior. Presumably, the social support and consistent messages about the importance of abstinence provided in mutual-help programs are perceived to be desirable by individuals lacking such support and messages. From another research perspective, one primary hypothesis in Project MATCH predicted that clients with social networks more supportive of *drinking* would fare better when assigned to a 12-step facilitation therapy than clients with similar social networks assigned to a four-session motivational enhancement therapy. At 3-year follow-up this hypothesis was supported in the outpatient arm of the trial. Analyses of the change mechanisms producing the effect revealed that, as predicted, engagement in AA by clients with social networks *unsupportive* of abstinence led to better 3-year outcomes than when clients with equally unsupportive networks did not become engaged in AA. This finding supports the belief that participation in AA provides a social environment that may offset an unsupportive social network.

CLIENT MOTIVATION

Compliance with referral to 12-step programs is positively related with client readiness for change. Ouimette and colleagus (in press), for instance, found that VA clients were more likely to attend AA meetings 1 year after treatment when they reported higher levels of problem determination and lower levels of precontemplation (SOCRATES; Miller & Tonigan, 1996) at the beginning of treatment. A similar pattern of problem recognition predicting AA attendance has been observed in both outpatient and aftercare samples in Project MATCH at both early and 1-year follow-ups. These findings support the assertion of DiClemente (1993) and others suggesting that 12-step programs may be more acceptable to clients high in readiness for change but less acceptable to clients in precontemplation and contemplation stages of change. This reasoning, in part, is based on the assumption that self-labeling and demands of admission of powerlessness would be less acceptable to persons less cognizant of their drinking problems. These findings, however, do not speak to the suggestion that persons lower in readiness for change may affiliate more readily with non–12-step programs that do not have such prescriptions.

DUALLY DIAGNOSED CLIENTS

What about clients with psychological problems besides substance abuse disorders? The most common psychiatric disorders among the substance-abusing population and mutual-help groups are depressive and anxiety disorders including PTSD, and less often bipolar disorder or varieties of psychosis. One concern of clinicians has been the negative attitude of many AA and NA members about the use of medications among its members. In particular, both new and long-standing members of 12-step programs are often informed that cessation of all alcohol and drugs is required to be clean and sober. Dually diagnosed persons may sometimes be advised that all of their problems are addressed in the core 12-step literature, and that having continued problems indicates that they are not working the steps or the "program" properly.

Clinicians may use several approaches to counter the negative messages about medications and sobriety. First, therapists may educate clients on the benefits of medications such as antidepressants for detoxification and for long-term maintenance. Benefits can be framed in terms of enhancement of abstinence, improvement in life problems, and better mutual-help program functioning. Antidepressants, for example, may improve cognitive functioning and the ability to identify and express appropriate affect. Improvements in these areas can facilitate social and other life functioning. Role-play and rehearsal can be initiated to practice responding to pressures to discontinue medication use and clients can be coached on appropriate responses. To normalize medication use, clients can be made aware that one of the founding fathers of AA suffered from long-standing depression and used antidepressants for many years (Alcoholics Anonymous, 1976). A third strategy, one that we do not recommend under most circumstances, is to simply advise a client not to disclose medication use. Advisement of silence without effective coping strategies may place clients in a vulnerable position and is not recommended.

THERAPIST MOTIVATION

Clinicians are divided about the desirability of referral to mutual-help groups. We do not wish to enter the debate. Rather, we would like to address three concerns commonly voiced about professional referral to mutual-help groups. These concerns also apply to client assessment and discussions about prior and current mutual-help participation. First, clinicians may have misgivings about mutual-help referral because of a potentially poor fit between therapeutic approach and mutual-help beliefs and practices. In three well-defined and distinct psychosocial treatments, only one of which was 12-step in focus, clients in all three modalities reported similar gains from mutual-help attendance (Tonigan, Connors, & Miller, in press). Thus, even in circumstances of documented mismatches between therapeutic and mutual-help philosophies, clients reported positive associations between abstinence and attendance in mutual-help programs.

Related to this is a second concern, involving the therapeutic relationship between a therapist who does not have substance abuse problems and a client who adopts the 12-step belief that only a recovering alcoholic can be of aid to a person seeking relief from an alcohol problem. The core literature of AA does not endorse this position, and should this belief enter the therapeutic process we encourage discussing the matter with the client, referring him or her to the approved AA literature. Third, a therapist trained in general mental health treatment may be ill equipped for treating substance abuse clients. Sometimes training and certification programs for these clinicians do not adequately focus on the nature and purpose of substance abuse treatment and of mutual-help programs. This may result in clinicians who are unfamiliar with, and perhaps even cynical about, the positive benefits associated with mutual-help programs. Reading core literature of these programs and attendance at meetings is strongly recommended for these clinicians.

MEMBERSHIP CHARACTERISTICS OF DIFFERENT PROGRAMS

Few studies have examined the defining characteristics of members in 12-step programs and non–12-step movements. Clinical referral to either set of mutual-help programs should therefore be sensitive to prior experiences, needs, and preferences of clients. Moreover, perhaps because of the limited number of non–12-step meetings, it is common for members of both RR (Galanter, Egelko, & Edwards, 1993) and SOS (Connors & Dermen, 1996) to continue AA attendance *while* participating in non–12-step groups. Likewise, migration across types of 12-step programs is not uncommon, with regular attenders of AA participating in meetings of Cocaine Anonymous (CA) and Narcotics Anonymous (NA) (e.g., Snow *et al.,* 1994).

Emrick and colleagues (1993) reviewed 107 studies and summarized the demographic and substance use characteristics of AA affiliates. In comparison to figures provided by Emrick and colleagues, it appears that members of RR and SOS are somewhat older, have more formal education, and report higher incomes than AA affiliates (Connors & Dermen, 1996; Galanter *et al.,* 1993).

STRATEGIES FOR LOCATING MUTUAL-HELP GROUPS

The availability of different types of mutual-help programs is substantial. In large metropolitan areas all of the programs described in this chapter (and others) should be available to the interested person, but it may be difficult to locate non–12-step programs in smaller communities. At times, real investigative effort is required to find alternatives to 12-step programs.

At the community and state levels, we recommend the use of local telephone directories and city and state agencies to identify possible mutual-help groups and their meeting schedules and locations. Often, clients may be one of the best sources of information, and such information may acquired when a therapist inquires about prior or current mutual-help participation of clients. Local, state, and regional counseling professional associations are also good sources for information on mutual-help meetings.

All of the non–12-step programs reviewed in this chapter maintain web sites on the Internet. These web sites generally provide a brief description of the goals and principles of the mutual-help program, and always include information on the group's core literature and how to find out about meetings nearest to the individual. We encourage clinicians to access these web sites for a tutorial on the mission and practices of mutual-help groups.

CONCLUSIONS

A substantial percentage of clients presenting for substance abuse treatment will have had prior contact with mutual-help programs. Other clients may initiate participation in mutual-help programs during and after treatment. AA attendance and involvement are associated with reductions in drinking and improved psychosocial functioning, and specific AA activities are related to abstinence. In the preparation of this chapter we reviewed the work of many researchers and clinicians. We are grateful for their effort. It has become apparent, however, that most of the empirical research is atheoretical, and most of the theoretical work on the causal mechanisms in mutual-help groups lacks empirical support (for exceptions, see Morgenstern *et al.*, in press; Snow *et al.*, 1994). Integrative approaches are needed to clarify the complex processes of change in mutual-help groups. In addition, little is known about non–12-step participation and outcome and future research is needed to evaluate the relative effectiveness of these alternative programs.

Many kinds of mutual-help programs are available, and strategies were provided to locate these programs. Candidates for mutual-help referral include clients with less social support for abstinence, although clients with supportive social networks may also benefit from affiliation with a mutual-help group. Client readiness for change is an important predictor of AA affiliation and may also predict non–12-step group affiliation. It is unclear whether clients who are ambivalent about change will be more receptive to non–12-step programs.

We encourage clinicians to become familiar with the practices and literature of mutual-help groups. Because definitive matching of clients with different kinds of mutual-help is beyond our current knowledge, it is most likely best for clients interested in mutual-help participation to sample a number of different kinds of programs. Clinicians can serve an important role in this regard by providing schedules and meeting locations for these programs.

REFERENCES

Alcoholics Anonymous. (1976). *Alcoholics Anonymous* (3rd ed.). New York: Alcoholics Anonymous World Services.

Alcoholics Anonymous. (1981). *Twelve steps and twelve traditions.* New York: Alcoholics Anonymous World Services.

Alcoholics Anonymous. (1997). *Alcoholics Anonymous 1996 membership survey.* New York: Alcoholics Anonymous World Services.

Brandsma, J. M., Maultsby, M. C. J., & Welsh, R. J. (1980). *Outpatient treatment of alcoholism: A review and comparative study.* Baltimore: University Park Press.

Caserta, M. S., & Lund, D. A. (1993). Intrapersonal resources and the effectiveness of self-help groups for bereaved older adults. *Gerontologist, 33*(5), 619–629.

Christo, G., & Franey, C. (1995). Drug users' spiritual beliefs, locus of control and the disease concept in relation to Narcotics Anonymous attendance and six-month outcomes. *Drug and Alcohol Dependence, 38,* 51–56.

Christopher, J. (1988). *How to stay sober.* Buffalo, NY: Prometheus.

Christopher, J. (1989). *Unhooked: Staying sober and drug-free.* Buffalo, NY: Prometheus.

Christopher, J. (1992). *SOS Sobriety.* Buffalo, NY: Prometheus.

Connors, G. J., & Dermen, K. H. (1996). Characteristics of participants in Secular Organizations for Sobriety (SOS). *American Journal of Drug and Alcohol Abuse, 22*(2), 281–295.

Connors, G., Tonigan, J. S., & Miller, W. R. (1996). The Religious Background and Behavior instrument: Psychometric and normed findings. *Psychology of Addictive Behaviors. 10,* 90–96.

DiClemente, C. C. (1993). Alcoholics Anonymous and the structure of change. In B. S. McCrady & W. R. Miller (Eds.), *Research on Alcoholics Anonymous: Opportunities and alternatives* (pp. 79–112). New Brunswick, NJ: Rutgers Center of Alcohol Studies.

Ditman, K. S., Crawford, G. G., Forgy, E. W., Moskowitz, H., & MacAndrew, C. (1967). A controlled experiment on the use of court probation or drunk arrests. *American Journal of Psychiatry, 124,* 160–163.

Ellis, A. (1962). *Reason and emotion in psychotherapy.* Northvale, NJ: Stuart.

Emrick, C. D., Tonigan, J. S., Montgomery, H., & Little, L. (1993). Alcoholics Anonymous: What is currently known? In B. S. McCrady & W. R. Miller (Eds.), *Research on Alcoholics Anonymous: Opportunities and alternatives* (pp. 41–76). New Brunswick, NJ: Rutgers Center of Alcohol Studies.

Fowler, J. W. (1993). Alcoholics Anonymous and faith development. In B. S. McCrady & W. R. Miller (Eds.), *Research on Alcoholics Anonymous: Opportunities and alternatives* (pp. 113–135). New Brunswick, NJ: Rutgers Center of Alcohol Studies.

Galanter, M., Egelko, S., & Edwards, H. (1993). Rational Recovery: Alternative to AA for addiction. *American Journal of Drug and Alcohol Abuse, 19*(4), 499–510.

George, A. A., & Tucker, J. A. (1996). Help-seeking for alcohol-related problems: Social contexts surrounding entry into alcoholism treatment and Alcoholics Anonymous. *Journal of Studies on Alcohol, 57,* 449–457.

Gorski, T. T. (1990). *Questionnaire of twelve step completion.* Independence, MO: Herald House, Independence Press.

Kennedy, M. (1990). *Psychiatric hospitalizations of GROWers.* Paper presented at the 2nd biennial conference on Community Research and Action, East Lansing, MI.

Kohlberg, L. (1984). *Essays on moral development: Vol. II. The psychology of moral development.* San Francisco: Harper and Row.

Kurtz, L. F. (1988). Mutual aid for affective disorders: The manic depressive and Depressive Association. *American Journal of Orthopsychiatry, 58*(1), 152–155.

Kus, R. J. (1992). Spirituality in everyday life: Experiences of gay men of Alcoholics Anonymous. In *Lesbians and gay men: Chemical dependency treatment issues* (pp. 49–66). London: Haworth.

McCrady, B. S. (1994). Alcoholics Anonymous and behavior therapy: Can habits be treated as diseases? Can diseases be treated as habits? *Journal of Consulting and Clinical Psychology, 6,* 1159–1166.

McCrady, B. S., & Miller, W. R. (1993). The importance of research on Alcoholics Anonymous. In B. S. McCrady & W. R. Miller (Eds.), *Research on Alcoholics Anonymous: Opportunities and alternatives* (pp. 3–12). New Brunswick, NJ: Rutgers Center of Alcohol Studies.

McCrady, B. S., Epstein, E. E., & Hirsch, L. S. (1996). Issues in the implementation of a randomized clinical trial that includes Alcoholics Anonymous: Studying AA-related behaviors during treatment. *Journal of Studies on Alcohol, 57,* 604–612.

McLellan, A. T., Luborsky, L., Cacciola, J., Griffith, J., Evans, F., Barr, H. L., & O'Brien, C. P. (1985). New data from the Addiction Severity Index: Reliability and validity in three centers. *Journal of Nervous and Mental Disease, 173*(7), 412–423.

Miller, W. R., & Marlatt, G. A. (1984). *Comprehensive drinker profile: Interview booklet.* Odessa, FL: Psychological Assessment Resources.

Miller, W. R., & Tonigan, J. S. (1996). Assessing drinkers' motivation for change: The Stages of Change Readiness and Treatment Eagerness Scale (SOCRATES). *Psychology of Addictive Behaviors, 10,* 81–89.

Montgomery, H. A., Miller, W. R., & Tonigan, J. S. (1993). Differences among AA groups: Implications or research. *Journal of Studies on Alcohol, 54*, 502–504.

Montgomery, H. A., Miller, W. R., & Tonigan, J. S. (1995). Does Alcoholics Anonymous involvement predict treatment outcome? *Journal of Substance Abuse Treatment, 12*(4), 241–24.

Monti, P. M., Abrams, D. B., Kadden, R. M., & Kooney, N. L. (1989). *Treating alcohol dependence*. New York: Guilford.

Moos, R. H. (1986). *Group Environment Scale manual* (2d ed.). Palo Alto, CA: Consulting Psychologist Press.

Morgenstern, J., Kahler, C., Frey, R., & Labouvie, E. (1996). Modeling therapeutic responses to 12 step treatment: Optimal responders, non-responders and partial responders. *Journal of Substance Abuse, 8*, 45–59.

Morgenstern, J., Labouvie, E., McCrady, B. S., Kahler, C. W., & Frey, R. M. (in press). Affiliation with Alcoholics Anonymous following treatment: A study of its therapeutic effects and mechanisms of action, *Journal of Consulting and Clinical Psychology*.

Ouimette, P. C., Moos, R. H., & Finney, J. W. (in press). Influence of outpatient treatment and 12-step group involvement on one-year substance abuse treatment outcomes, *Journal of Studies on Alcohol*.

Piaget, J. (1970). *Piaget's theory. Carmichael's manual of child psychology* (P. Mussen, ed., 3rd ed., Vol. 1). New York: Wiley.

Prochaska, J. O., & DiClemente, C. C. (1986). The transtheoretical approach: Towards a systematic eclectic framework. In J. C. Norcross (Ed.), *Handbook of eclectic psychotherapy* (pp. 163–200). New York: Brunner/Mazel.

Project MATCH Research Group. (1993). Project MATCH: Rationale and methods for a multisite clinical trial matching patients to alcoholism treatment. *Alcoholism: Clinical and Experimental Research, 17*, 1130–1145.

Project MATCH Research Group. (1997). Matching alcoholism treatments to client heterogeneity: Project MATCH Posttreatment drinking outcomes. *Journal of Studies on Alcohol, 58*(1), 7–29.

Project MATCH Research Group. (in press-a). Matching alcoholism treatments to client heterogeneity: Project MATCH three-year drinking outcomes. *Alcoholism: Clinical and experimental research*.

Project MATCH Research Group. (in press-b). Project MATCH secondary a priori hypotheses, *Addiction, 92*, 1671–1698.

Room, R. (1993). Alcoholics Anonymous as a social movement. In B. S. McCrady & W. R. Miller (Eds.), *Research on Alcoholics Anonymous: Opportunities and alternatives* (pp. 167–188). New Brunswick, NJ: Rutgers Center of Alcohol Studies.

Simmons, D. (1992). Diabetes self-help facilitated by local diabetes research: The Coventry Asian diabetes support group. *Diabetic Medicine, 9*, 866–869.

Snow, M. G., Prochaska, J. O., & Rossi, J. S. (1994). Processes of change in Alcoholics Anonymous: Maintenance factors in long-term sobriety, *Journal of Studies on Alcohol, 55*, 362–371.

Thompson, D. L., & Thompson, J. A. (1993). Working the 12 steps of Alcoholics Anonymous with a client: A counseling opportunity. *Alcoholism Treatment Quarterly, 10*(1/2), 49–61.

Tonigan, J. S., Ashcroft, F., & Miller, W. R. (1995). AA group dynamics and 12 step activity. *Journal of Studies on Alcohol, 56*, 616–621.

Tonigan, J. S., Connors, G. J., & Miller, W. R. (1996). The Alcoholics Anonymous Involvement scale (AAI): Reliability and norms. *Psychology of Addictive Behaviors, 10*, 75–80.

Tonigan, J. S., Toscova, R., & Miller, W. R. (1996). Meta-analysis of the Alcoholics Anonymous literature: Sample and study characteristics moderate findings. *Journal of Studies on Alcohol, 57*, 65–72.

Tonigan, J. S., Miller, W. R., & Connors, G. J. (in press). *Prior Alcoholics Anonymous involvement and treatment outcome: Matching findings and causal chain analyses* (NIAAA Project MATCH Monograph series).

Tonigan, J. S., Connors, G. J., & Miller, W. R. (in press).

Trimpey, J. (1988). *Rational recovery from alcoholism: The small book*. Lotus, CA: Lotus Press.

Walsh, D. C., Hingson, R. W., Merrigan, D. M., Levenson, S. M., Cupples, L. A., Heeren, T., Coffman, G. A., Becker, C. A., Barker, T. A., Hamilton, S. K., McGuire, T. G., & Kelly, C. A. (1991). A randomized trial of treatment options for alcohol-abusing workers. *New England Journal of Medicine, 325*, 775–782.

V

Sustaining Change

This section of our first edition focused heavily on the avoidance of "relapse," and included a chapter on "aftercare." In the ensuing years, much has changed. It is now widely recognized that outcomes are much more complex than can be captured by a dichotomous classification such as "relapsed" versus "successful." This perspective requires a somewhat broader conception of the challenges involved in maintainance of change. For this reason we have shifted the focus of this section away from the negative concept of relapse, toward the positive challenge of maintaining and continuing gains. A first step in this direction is to understand what factors do predict successful outcomes, and this is the focus of Chapter 22 by Verner Westerberg. Longitudinal research often emphasizes different determinants of success than might be reconstructed by looking back on failure.

There has been a dramatic shift away from inpatient and residential care, even in North America where it was so heavily emphasized. Because the term "aftercare" was usually applied to a period of outpatient care following residential treatment, the meaning of this term has become blurred. A prior review of aftercare research has now become Dennis Donovan's Chapter 23 on strategies for helping clients to maintain change, regardless of the setting in which it was accomplished. Finally, Kenneth Weingardt and Alan Marlatt offer practical advice on the quandary of what to do when clients continue using during treatment. Some programs have terminated treatment in this case, which constitutes discharging clients for the same reason they were admitted. If you choose to continue working with clients who do not abstain, how best can you help them? That is the subject of Chapter 24, which closes this section on the challenges of maintenance.

22

What Predicts Success?

WHAT CONSTITUTES SUCCESS?

An indisputably successful substance abuse therapy would result in the elimi-
nation of all substance use and substance-related problems. Perhaps the simplest
definition of success is total abstinence from the target drug for all time; a more
difficult-to-achieve variation would be total abstinence from all drugs being
used. If clients were to achieve either of these goals it would go a long way toward eliminating all substance-related problems. An added bonus would be that
using these criteria, calculation of success rates is straightforward: success if abstinent, failure if not. Unfortunately, the number of people who are successful by
either of these criteria is extremely low. Based on the consumption of a single
posttreatment alcoholic drink Orford and Edwards (1977) reported the now-fa-
miliar rate of 10% success at the end of 1 year. Twenty years later, Miller, Westerberg, Harris, and Tonigan (Relapse Replication and Extension Project [RREP],
1996) also reported that 10% of clients remained continuously abstinent at 12
months posttreatment. In the intervening years this pattern had repeated itself in
study after study. Four years after treatment Polich, Armor, and Braiker (1981) reported that only 9% of their clients had attained sustained abstinence, and a sev-
eral-year follow-up of those treated for alcohol problems indicated 15% of
clients sustained 3 years of abstinence (Helzer & Pryzbeck, 1988). Even in a
tightly controlled research trial, rates of continuous abstinence over 12 months
varied between 19% and 35% depending on the treatment modality (Project
MATCH Research Group, 1997).

However, *continuous* abstinence is only one of many posttreatment substance
abuse outcomes, and success rates will differ quite dramatically depending on

VERNER S. WESTERBERG • Center on Alcoholism, Substance Abuse, and Addictions, University
of New Mexico, Albuquerque, New Mexico 87106.

Treating Addictive Behaviors, 2nd ed., edited by Miller and Heather. Plenum Press, New York, 1998.

how outcome is defined. As a case in point, although the RREP study found that only a small percentage of clients had been continuously abstinent, many more (about 28%) were abstinent at any given 2-month measuring point. In a 10-year study of alcoholics, although only 4% remained continuously abstinent, about half of the individuals displayed a pattern of moderate drinking and abstinence (Taylor *et al.*, 1986). Thus, if some abstinence without a remission to heavy drinking is used as a criterion for success, many more people are successes. Furthermore, because people seem to cycle in and out of success, a person who might be classified as a treatment failure at one point might be a treatment success at another. This is not just statistical hocus pocus; it suggests that long-term success may not occur all at once, but perhaps as a series of approximations. If this is true it also gives a good handhold for treatment. Ultimate success may be achieved by building on lesser successes all along the path. However, there are numerous obstacles to achieving even short-term success. Some of these obstacles are really only stumbling blocks, but others, such as relapse, are more serious and are real threats to success.

For those who have stopped substance use for a time, a single drink does not necessarily mean a relapse (Miller *et al.*, 1996) nor does the first use of opioid (Gossop, Green, Phillips, & Bradley, 1987) mean a return to full-blown dependence. Therefore, slips are only stumbling blocks to success. However, reinstitution of diagnostic-level dependence occurs quite quickly after a return to drinking (Besançon, 1993) illustrating that although a slip does not mean a relapse, the first few drinks are events to be taken seriously by both clinicians and clients (and researchers). Furthermore, in the RREP study, a single drink was usually associated with a return, if only for a limited time, to heavy drinking. Even within this less optimistic scenario, however, there is considerable room for optimism. Twelve months after the baseline interview, about 10% of clients had had a drink but did not return to heavy drinking. Measures taken more proximal to treatment initiation looked better yet; if measured at 200 days, about 25% had had a drink, but did not return to heavy drinking. If the window for defining success is opened a bit to include those who have a first drink, may have had a heavy drinking day, but for whom that did not lead to 4 or more days of drinking, then about 50% are successful. These data are similar to those determined in Project MATCH where 54% to 60% of clients never drank for 3 consecutive days. If failure is determined as a return to pretreatment drinking levels, about 50% succeed (Armor, Polich, & Stanbul, 1978). Thus it appears that various definitions of success are possible from complete and continuous abstinence through slips and full-blown relapses, and that each of these leads to different views of success. More important, it shows that there is considerable opportunity for intervention at all stages of outcome, that even when one takes a step or even two down the failure path, not all is lost (at least for a significant number of clients).

However, in these days of multiple drug use, one needs to question whether continuous or even intermittent abstinence from a single drug is an adequate definition of success; is it perhaps an artificial criterion? Few studies that focus on multiple drug outcomes after treatment have been done, but it is probably a fair statement that successful outcomes from all psychoactive drugs would be a yet more rare occurrence than successful outcomes from just one drug. To complicate matters for treatment and measurement, outcomes differ for different drugs, with abstinence rates at 3 months after standard treatment ranging from 40% for injection drugs to 90% for hallucinogens (Paul, Barrett, Crosby, & Stall, 1996). Definitions of success (and failure) also become more complicated when several drugs are considered. For example, suppose a client is being treated for an alcohol use disorder, remains continuously abstinent from alcohol, but begins to use heroin. Is this a treatment success or a failure? Most substance abuse research has trod lightly on this area, usually focusing on predictors of a single class of drugs and not considering all classes together. Most researchers, clinicians, and clients, however, would likely subscribe to a more inclusive definition of what constitutes success, incorporating not only multiple substances, but physical and social problems associated with their use. Although substance abuse causes problems that are more extensive than the consumption of the substance, the problems associated with substance abuse are not highly related to one another (Miller, 1996). Clients with substance use disorders come in all varieties: heavy drinkers with apparently few other problems, lighter drinkers who have many problems, long-term chronic drinkers with surprisingly few physical problems, injecting drug users who steer clear of all the attendant infections, abscesses, and overdoses. The fact that substance abuse consists of a somewhat variable set of modestly related problems, and that success may be a series of approximations rather than an absolute standard, indicates that harm reduction may be a reasonable treatment approach toward the goal of long-term success at least in a particular focus area (see Chapter 24, this volume). Setting proximal goals of using substances in settings that are less harmful to oneself and others may be a good method of bringing about success on a number of fronts.

The picture so far is not as simple as one might wish for, but it is a rich and much more accurate reflection of human behavior than to approach success after treatment as unidimensional. If posttreatment outcomes are so multidimensional, how are they to be visualized? One way to help visualize and make sense of these data is to try to define groups of people who have different outcomes after they have finished treatment. Using a descriptive statistical technique called cluster analysis, Westerberg, Miller, Harris, and Tonigan (1998) defined meaningful groups of clients based on their outcomes. As a first step they focused solely on alcohol but measured it by both quantity and frequency. This relatively simple method still provided several reliable clusters of individuals comprising an abstinent group; a group that drank frequently, but not very much at any given time; a group that didn't drink very frequently, but drank a lot when they did drink; and a group that drank a lot and quite frequently. Not surprisingly, things became considerably more complicated with the addition of total illicit drug use and days of cigarette use. It is not necessary to go through all of these clusters, but these authors reported six distinct and reliable clusters covering the range from essentially abstinent to the heavy use of all substances. Thus, looking at all possible outcomes after they have occurred, rather than assuming client status a priori, clearly indicates that outcomes come in many shapes and sizes and the assumption that one can compress all of these into a simple dichotomy may be simply simplistic.

Assume for a time that we have decided on a single definition of success and are happy with the outcome, as is the client, the client's family, and the client's employer. At what point can a success be counted a success? Formal guidelines set up by the American Medical Association in 1970 recommended 3 years of abstinence from the primary drug, and no abuse of other substances. If randomized treatment outcome studies are used as the measure of success, these typically have a follow-up duration of 12, and maybe as long as 15 or 18 months, but rarely longer. Thus, success is typically defined within that range. Controlled longitudinal studies usually cover a longer span of time, as do studies that measure recovery without the aid of treatment. Nonhuman animal studies can be surprisingly informative about treatment success, but usually the temporal definition of failure is very short. For human studies, 6 to 12 months is generally accepted as a reasonable criterion of success and is commonly used in treatment outcome studies. In the "natural recovery" studies, 12 months is more the norm. For all studies cited in this chapter, duration of recovery (as it is defined by that study) must have continued for a minimum of 6 months, but most studies cited have continued for at least 12. Irrespective of the length of time success can be thought of as maintenance, what keeps initial change going?

WHAT DO SUCCESS AND RELAPSE HAVE IN COMMON?

In the substance abuse field we talk very little of success and quite a bit about relapse (failure). This is a particulary bleak view of substance abuse treatment outcomes; it has the appearance of waiting for the inevitable ax to fall. Part of the reason for this focus on failure is that for ease of measurement, failure is often treated as a single point: you failed or you didn't. For example, if the goal of therapy is for clients not to drink any alcohol ever again, then when they do drink the point of failure is easily identified. This gets around a lot of arguing about whether, for example, one drink followed by 6 months of continuous abstinence is a failure or not—it clearly is. As discussed earlier, however, just as all successes are not equal, neither are all failures. It seems as though everyone would be better served if substance abuse treatment outcomes were considered as continuous multidimensional events with everyone at some point being in a period of relative success eventually working to increase the percentage of time in success and decreasing the percentage of time in "not success."

Another problem, and one that is less philosophical, is that the actions, behaviors, and attitudes that predict relapse may not predict success. The scientific literature is quite clear that the better one's coping skills, the less likely is relapse, therefore good coping skills will be related to success. This may be true. But then what can be made of the repeated (and no doubt true) findings that relapse precipitants include unpleasant mood states, external events, euphoric states, and lessened vigilance or testing control (Cannon, Leeka, Patterson, & Baker, 1990; Isenhart, 1993; Litman, 1986)? Does that mean that if a trigger for relapse is a euphoric mood state the way to prevent the relapse is to become less euphoric, or perhaps even depressed? Apparently not, because depression is also a trigger for relapse. Thus relapse and success may not be sides of the same coin. This apparent dilemma may result from something not as complex as it first appears, and that is that prediction is not necessarily the same thing as causation. The fact that negative mood is associated with relapse does not mean that it causes relapse, it may just be a marker for something else more fundamental. Connors, Maisto, and Zywiak (1996) have lent credence to this argument by pointing out that therapies that concentrate on the management of negative mood states are considerably less successful than those that concentrate on social skills and coping, indicating that perhaps mood states are simply reflections of more fundamental processes.

WHAT DOES PREDICT SUCCESS?

So, what is success? It is, like relapse, subject to multiple definitions. Success can be defined as everything that relapse is not, a very broad definition of success but not a very likely one considering the aforementioned rates of relapse. Thus success, like relapse, is just one point on a continuum of outcomes that might be thought of as going from no change in any behavior as a result of therapeutic intervention to the living of a full, productive life. The rest of this chapter will be devoted to all those things that happen to people both in therapy and outside of it that seem to make a difference, that give us some clues as to what moves people along that continuum of approximations to success, by hitting all of the other successes along the way.

SUCCESS PREDICTS SUCCESS

Abstinence predicts success: The longer the abstinence the better the chance of maintaining that abstinence. In a 46-year follow-up of a cohort of male drinkers Vaillant (1996) reported that the longer the men were abstinent the more likely that they would achieve stable remission. The depressing side of Vaillant's findings was that 2 years of abstinence was not long enough for maintenance, 6 years was required, findings that had also been reported for both men and women (Vaillant, Clark, & Cyrus, 1983). An important finding was that rather than progressing, alcohol abuse seemed to fluctuate in severity if outcomes were viewed in long blocks of time (5 years) rather than shorter (months), echoing the earlier conclusion that a person may be considered a success or a failure depending on criteria for success and when they are measured. One does not have to be abstinent to be successful; serious approximations to success, such as controlling substance use, predict success (Armor *et al.*, 1978). But again success may be in the eye of the evaluator because although a significant percentage of those who wish to achieve controlled drinking do so, a stable pattern of trouble-free drinking is less likely than continued or renewed problem drinking (Miller, Leckman, Delaney, & Tinkcom, 1992). Last, the better the start someone gets toward abstinence while in treatment, the more likely that individual will have sustained (6-month) abstinence, as Budney, Higgins, Wong, and Bickel (1995) showed with cocaine addicts.

TRYING PREDICTS SUCCESS

This is a consistent finding—that trying does matter—going to treatment, going to AA, engaging in behaviors other than substance use, anything that is positive and moving toward something else and away from drinking. We found in the RREP study (Miller *et al.*, 1996) that a good predictor of success at 6 months was a high score on the "taking steps" (action) scale of the Stages of Change Readiness and Treatment Eagerness Scale (SOCRATES; Miller & Tonigan, 1996), which measures *doing something* about drinking. Many treatment outcome studies also indicate that trying predicts success. Project MATCH administered three different treatments, and over 15 months all treatments were effective in helping clients reduce alcohol consumption, problems related to drinking, and their use of other drugs (Project MATCH Research Group, 1997). In a 22-year follow-up of heroin users, those who remained in methadone programs showed a decline in mortality, a decreased use of all drugs (including alcohol, excluding tobacco), and improvement in many aspects of social behavior (Goldstein & Herrera, 1995). Trying and being compliant with medication predicts good outcomes. Clients given the medication acamprosate for drinking problems fared better at follow-up than did the nonmedicated group, and they also showed better treatment retention (Sass, Soyka, Mann, & Zieglgansberger, 1996). Longer treatment has been associated with better outcomes, and this finding indicates again that staying with treatment, doing something, increases the chances of good outcomes. Sometimes a little effort is necessary, however; just going to therapy is not good enough. For example, simply attending AA after treatment did not predict positive outcomes, but the degree to which clients became *involved* in AA after treatment did predict success (Montgomery, Miller, & Tonigan, 1995).

SEVERITY OF DRUG INVOLVEMENT

It is tempting to believe that the more severe the person's drug problem the less likely they will do well over the long term. Surprisingly, the data are not totally consistent, but generally better levels of pretreatment functioning (drinking, social, occupational, psychological) are predictive of better outcomes (Armor *et al.*, 1978; Sannibale, 1989). Over 12 months of posttreatment assessment Connors and colleagues (1996) found that increased alcohol involvement was consistently related to a wide range of poorer drinking outcomes including consumption and problems related to drinking. However, W. R. Miller and colleagues (1996) did not find that increased alcohol involvement was associated with outcome in either direction. A major difference between these two studies may have been that Connors and colleagues (1996) used a composite variable that comprised a problems scale in addition to a physical symptoms scale, whereas Miller and colleagues (1996) used a single instrument that focused on physical problems only. Thus there may have been a measuring artifact; more global severity rather than just the severity of consumption problems may be the more important factor. This latter postulation is backed up to some degree by Sannibale (1989), who found that the worse the problem drinking (blackouts, alcohol consumption, legal problems) at pretreatment the more likely the clients were to be problem drinkers at follow-up and, furthermore, the best statistical predictors of general client functioning at follow-up were measures of alcohol-related problems such as accidents, jail, morning drinking, and general deterioration.

However, drug use severity is by its nature complicated. In the Project MATCH study, higher alcohol involvement was found to be associated with more drinks per drinking day at follow-up, but not with the number of abstinent days, and only in the group that received inpatient treatment (but not the outpatient treatment group). Thus there is some complex interplay among at least severity, type of outcome measure chosen, treatment modality, and other variables. This complexity is further substantiated by the fact that more aftercare patients (those who had received inpatient treatment) were able to maintain complete abstinence than were the outpatients, in spite of the fact that they had more alcohol-dependence symptoms. If substance use severity is measured by the use of other drugs, especially prior to treatment, then severity certainly leads to poor outcomes as measured by premature dropout (Stark & Campbell, 1988). Furthermore, having more social problems because of alcohol use at treatment intake made good outcomes less likely at 12 months, but more social problems at intake were not related to poor outcomes for other drugs (Paul *et al.*, 1996). Cigarette smokers who have recently quit show similar effects (Killen, Fortmann, Newman, & Varady, 1991; Killen, Fortmann, Kraemer, Varady, & Newman, 1992), where those who had lower blood nicotine levels (a measure of use) were more likely to be abstinent at 2 months, whereas higher nicotine levels predicted failure at 12 and at 24 months.

PSYCHIATRIC COMORBIDITY

This is a broad area and is not easily contained, so for the purposes of this discussion, a very common definition of comorbidity will be used: a psychiatric disorder (most commonly depression, anxiety, or antisocial personality disorder) that co-occurs with a substance use disorder. Data in this area are inconsistent, but very generally speaking psychiatric comorbidities are predictive of poorer outcomes. One of the early studies in this area (Hatsukami & Pickens, 1982) indicated that a diagnosis of depression was predictive of poor outcomes in alcoholics. Loosen, Dew, and Prange (1990) also found that depression was a predictor of failure during a 2-year follow-up in abstinent alcoholic men, but that it operated through negative effects on length of abstinence at intake. Unfortunately, even these findings are not invariant because major depression also has been associated with lower intensity of drinking (Kranzler, Del Boca, & Rounsaville, 1996). However, the role of psychiatric comorbidities is complex. For example, severity of psychopathology (as measured by the Addiction Severity Index; ASI) at intake into a methadone program was predictive of *better* outcomes in regard to overall substance use at follow-up (conducted at 6, 12, 18, and 24 months postadmission), but was not predictive of treatment retention (Saxon, Wells, Fleming, Jackson, & Calsyn, 1996), which is in general agreement with at least one other report (Joe, Simpson, & Sells, 1994). However, antisocial personality disorder has been reported as related to poorer global alcohol-related outcomes (Kranzler *et al.*, 1996). On the surface, it seems wrong that an area in which clarity should occur is an area that is so unclear. For example, one of the strongest findings in Project MATCH was that psychiatric severity partly determines how well clients do in different therapies. This, however, does indicate that one reason for the inconsistencies may be different therapeutic regimens. Other reasons may be that psychiatric status can vary widely and the degree of psychiatric acuity helps determine the treatment into which these clients are placed. Thus, there may be great differences between two studies when one is conducted in an aftercare program, and the other in an inpatient program, because the clients are different.

MOOD STATES

Although mood states are related to psychiatric comorbidities, the mood states mentioned here are generally temporary and less severe than the states just discussed. Negative mood states traditionally have been seen as threats to success both in the short and long terms. Kadden (1996), commenting on findings from the RREP study, concluded that negative mood states as envisioned by Marlatt make "good clinical sense" in that clients and therapists see states such as depression, anger, anxiety, loneliness, and frustration not only as antecedents to previous failures but as risks to future successes. In a group of clients with alcohol dependence, unpleasant emotions and conflict with others were both strong predictors of relapse. Unfortunately, these were measured at only 3 months after treatment and may not be predictors of longer-term success (Hodgins, el-Guebaly, & Armstrong, 1992). Very often clients are asked to think back in time to events that may have led to successes or failures, which is a useful method, but may be subject to a number of problems, notably distortions of memory and attitude bias about the events. Overall, retrospective data are not as strong as are prospective data, but as Hodgins and el-Guebaly (1993) showed, although negative mood was inversely related to success, there was no bias in inquiring about these data retrospectively.

In experimental studies designed specifically to evaluate these variables, negative mood states have been identified as threats to success (e.g., Chaney, O'Leary, & Marlatt, 1978; Heather, Stallard, & Tebbutt, 1991). Analysis of the results of measuring these states through tools such as the IDS have consistently identified negative mood states as a common factor (Cannon et al., 1990; Isenhart, 1991). Connors and colleagues (1996) found that depression and anxiety occurring at the time of intake to treatment were related directly and indirectly to poorer success (defined by alcohol consumption and alcohol problem variables) at 12 months postintake. Miller and colleagues (1996) used the same instrument for measuring depression as did Connors and colleagues, and also measured anger, but found no relationship between these states and success or failure 2 or 10 months later.

COPING AND STRESS

Coping is one area where the results consistently point in the direction of success: The more and better the coping responses, the better the chances for success no matter how it is defined. Although negative stress is associated with failure, coping can moderate the impact of this negative stress (Billings & Moos, 1983; Marlatt & Gordon, 1980; Miller et al., 1996). There are several types of coping that seem to be related to both long- and short-term success (Donovan, 1996). Behavioral coping is involved in avoiding high-risk situations, and is thus related to short-term success. As an individual remains abstinent, coping changes to a cognitive type: thinking about the negative aspects of substance use in the past and the positive aspects of continued success. Confirming this complexity of different types of coping is the finding that self-blaming coping at entrance into treatment is related to a decreased likelihood of stopping alcohol use, whereas baseline support-seeking coping decreased the likelihood of reducing marijuana use (Paul et al., 1996).

Two studies that were part of the RREP indicated quite clearly the strong relationship between coping skills and recovery. As discussed earlier, Miller and colleagues (1996) measured people entering treatment for alcohol problems on several domains of functioning including pretreatment characteristics, mood states, craving, motivation, and risky drinking situations. Of all of these domains the strongest predictor of 12-month outcome was the use of positive coping behaviors. The use of avoidant coping was related to failure. Using a recursive path model Connors and colleagues (1996) also measured clients at baseline on several dimensions including consumption measures, treatment process, background characteristics, coping skills and responses, stressors, and general alcohol involvement. Conceptualizing outcome in four ways, as percent days abstinent, drinks per drinking day, drinking consequences, or craving experiences, only alcohol involvement severity and coping skills and responses showed direct effects on all four outcomes. In this regard both of these studies found that whereas coping was a good predictor of outcome, stressors did not seem to be related to outcomes, indicating that although stressors may be present, having and using good coping skills may mitigate stress.

SOCIAL SUPPORT

Social support can work both ways—as a positive factor for abstinence or as a negative factor for continued or renewed use. Furthermore, as with many of the variables already discussed, social support can have a direct effect and an indirect effect. As an example of a direct effect, greater social and environmental support for quitting cigarette smoking were predictive of both initial quitting and relapse at 12 and 24 months for both genders (Nides et al., 1995). As an example of an indirect effect on success, persons with greater general social support report higher levels of well-being, and those with higher well-being have better outcomes after alcohol treatment (Beattie et al., 1993; Longabaugh & Beattie, 1985). A prevalent theme in this literature has been that social support functions through buffering stressful life events, although this hypothesis has been seriously questioned (Mitchell, 1984), and it now appears that social support has an effect independent of stressful life events in addition to buffering (Cohen & Willis, 1985; Wesson, Havassy, & Smith, 1986). Furthermore, as with coping, social support is a complex construct that needs to be differentiated at least by source, kind, and specificity (Rice & Longabaugh, 1996). Generally the alcohol treatment literature consistently documents a relationship between greater social support and good posttreatment outcomes (Bromet & Moos, 1977; Cronkite & Moos, 1980) and of the inverse: poor support resulting in poorer long-term outcomes (e.g., Breteler, Van Den Hurk, Schippers, & Meerkerk, 1996).

However, one's social support may be those who use drugs, which most likely would not be supportive of successful outcomes. Indeed, Project MATCH found that those who had more social support for drinking were also more likely to show a higher intensity of drinking during posttreatment follow-up, and the less social support for drinking, the better were drinking outcomes after treatment in terms of both intensity and frequency of drinking. Even when the support is not support for drug use, family interactions may promote relapse (Coleman, 1980; Lichtenstein, 1982). When abstinence-specific social support was used experimentally, 10-year follow-up rates indicated that those who received high partner contact (effective helping relationship) were more successful in maintaining abstinence than those in the low partner contact condition (Janis & Hoffman, 1982). People who were previous tobacco smokers were more likely to become continuous abstainers if their spouses demonstrated fewer undermining behaviors. Again indicating the complexity involved in social support is the finding by the same group that smokers' recycling and attempting to quit were best predicted by a greater frequency of spouse supportive behaviors (Roski, Schmid, & Lando, 1996).

Closely related to social support is the concept of social adjustment. An early report by Platt and Labate (1976) reported that opioid addicts at the lowest risk for relapse were those who were married, older, better educated and employed, better psychologically adjusted, and less criminally involved: in other words, displaying a number of characteristics of social support. These findings were generally supported at 12-year follow-up in the DARP study (Simpson & Marsh, 1986), where it was found that the groups rated lowest in level of social adjustment displayed the poorest outcomes.

SELF-EFFICACY

Bandura (1982) postulated that self-efficacy might play a role in relapse, and there is a significant body of literature that bears this out. Again the role of self-efficacy might be direct or indirect, for example, self-efficacy might exert its influence through executing coping behaviors. Self-efficacy has been enormously influential in the substance abuse area, in large measure through the work of Marlatt and colleagues (Marlatt & Gordon, 1980) who postulated that those with high self-efficacy are less likely to relapse and more likely to use coping strategies than those with low self-efficacy. Using the Situational Confidence Questionnaire to measure self efficacy, Miller, Ross, Emerson, and Todt (1989) found in comparing those who were sober with those who were abstinent for at least 1 year, the long-term sober clients had significantly greater self-efficacy. DiClemente, Prochaska, and Gibertini (1985) found in a 2-year study of cigarette cessation and maintenance that higher self-efficacy scores were associated with quitting and maintenance of abstinence. This relationship was complex because self-efficacy was found to be a relevant variable only for contemplators and recent quitters, so depending on the stage of change, self-efficacy may be more or less important; this is a potentially important clinical finding. However, other measures, including substance abuse involvement, may be more important than motivation in predicting success. A prediction algorithm that combined several measures of cigarette smoking such as cigarettes smoked per day and the number of "quits" of at least a year, predicted smokers who stopped at 1 to 2 years better than did the stages of change. Concurring with this finding that self-efficacy is only important depending on the stage of change, Rist and Watzl (1983) reported that self-efficacy ratings were predictive of abstinence at a short-term outcome point (3 months) but not at a long-term outcome point (18 months). Furthermore, although self-efficacy does increase over the course of treatment, self-efficacy ratings at intake have been shown to be inversely related to relapse at both 6 and 12 months, but self-efficacy ratings at discharge were not predictive of success (Rychitarik, Prue, & Rapp, 1992). Conversely, McKay, Maisto, and O'Farrell (1993) found that low end-of-treatment self-efficacy was predictive of poorer drinking outcomes at one year but, echoing the complexity of these interactions, only for those men not in aftercare. Again, end-of-treatment self-efficacy is related to alcohol abstinence at 3 months (Goldbeck, Myatt, & Aitchison, 1997), but is not related to drug and alcohol use at 6 months follow-up (Burling, Reilly, Moltzen, & Ziff, 1989). Apparently confusing results such as these regarding level of motivation indicate that behavior can be predicted by multiple factors probably because behavior is determined from multiple sources.

EXPECTATIONS

A person's expectations cannot be totally separated from other factors discussed in this chapter because they *are* related. Bandura (1977), for example, postulated that a person's expectations of success and failure determine their coping behavior. However, expectations of the consequences of drug use is an area with a fair amount of scientific literature with some concordance of results, even over various data collection methodologies (Wood, Sher, & Strathman, 1996). MacAndrew and Edgerton (1969) proposed that people hold long-lasting beliefs about alcohol's effects, a concept that has developed into alcohol expectancies (George *et al.*, 1995). Nonlongitudinal data have indicated that positive expectancies about alcohol's effects are related to drinking (see George *et al.*, 1995), and several self-report questionnaires have been developed to measure the concept of expectations, most notably the Alcohol Expectancy Questionnaire (AEQ; Brown, Goldman, Inn, & Anderson, 1980). In longitudinal treatment outcome studies, positive outcome expectancies have been shown to be predictors of failure after 1 year in alcoholics (Brown, 1985), although Miller and colleagues (1996) in the RREP project did not find a variant of the AEQ predictive of relapse at any time point tested, even when explicitly tested in a proxy of Marlatt and Gordon's (1980) model of relapse.

CONCLUSIONS

Success is not easily defined in the treatment of addictive behaviors. What is encouraging is the convergence of research on factors associated with more successful outcomes, broadly defined. Clients with more favorable outcomes tend to be those with active rather than avoidant coping skills, with social support for change, with expectancies (including self-efficacy) that favor change, and with greater motivation for change as manifested in *trying,* in actively taking steps to overcome the problem.

The evidence is mixed on those factors that often come to mind as predictors of doom. Greater severity of alcohol and drug problems is sometimes associated with poorer outcomes, but in other settings has been found to be a positive prognostic sign, consistent with the notion of hitting bottom. The presence of additional comorbid diagnoses and psychological problems is found to predict poorer response in some treatment studies but not others, and the difference here may be in the extent to which treatment addresses these additional problems (see Chapter 13, this volume). Similarly, a high level of life stressors does not necessarily predispose to relapse; what seems to matter more is the presence of positive coping skills for dealing with the negative experiences that life brings to everyone.

Taken together, these pieces of evidence suggest that treatment for addictive behaviors could fruitfully focus on strengthening clients for success, rather than placing primary emphasis on avoiding failure. This mirrors, in fact, the finding that positive rather than avoidant coping skills are associated with more successful outcomes. In practical terms, this might include (1) examining and building social support for sobriety, (2) encouraging the trying out of various approaches for change, (3) reinforcing any and all active steps toward change, rather than focusing on slips and relapses, (4) strengthening self-efficacy by emphasizing positive aspects of previous attempts at change and linking them to prior successes, and (5) taking seriously the client's other life problems and addressing them in treatment by enhancing positive coping styles that do not involve addictive behaviors.

It is no coincidence that these attributes resemble those of successful cognitive-behavioral and other empirically supported treatment approaches described in other chapters of this volume. The findings of Project MATCH Research Group (1997) do warrant acceptance of a broad range of treatment philosophies and strategies in the search for ways to help clients recover from addictive behaviors. The literature on what predicts success rather than failure may provide a guiding model for pulling these diverse strategies together in programs for helping people change.

REFERENCES

Annis, H. M. (1984). *Inventory of Drinking Situations.* Toronto: Addiction Research Foundation.

Armor, D., Polich, J., & Stanbul, H. (1978). *Alcoholism and treatment.* New York: Wiley.

Bandura, A. (1977). Self-efficacy: Towards a unifying theory of behavioral change. *Psychological Review, 84,* 191–215.

Bandura, A. (1982). Self-efficacy mechanism in human agency. *American Psychologist, 37,* 122.

Beattie, M. C., Longabaugh, R., Elliott, G., Stout, R. L., Fava. J., & Noel, N. E. (1993). Effect of the social environment on alcohol involvement and subjective well-being prior to alcoholism treatment. *Journal of Studies on Alcohol, 54,* 283–296.

Besançon, F. (1993). Time to alcohol dependence after abstinence and first drink. *Addiction, 88,* 1647–1650.

Billings, A. G., & Moos, R. H. (1983). Psychosocial processes of recovery among alcoholics and their families: Implications for clinicians and program evaluators. *Addictive Behaviors, 8,* 205–218.

Breteler, M. H. M., Van Den Hurk, A. A., Schippers, G. M., & Meerkerk, G. J. (1996). Enrollment in a drug-free detention program: The prediction of successful behavior change of drug-using inmates. *Addictive Behaviors, 21*(5), 665–669.

Bromet, E., & Moos, R. H. (1977). Environmental resources and the posttreatment functioning of alcoholic patients. *Journal of Health and Social Behavior, 18,* 326–338.

Brown, S. A. (1985). Reinforcement expectancies and alcoholism treatment outcome after a one-year follow-up. *Journal of Studies on Alcohol, 46,* 304–308.

Brown, S. A., Goldman, M. S., Inn, A., & Anderson, L. R. (1980). Expectancies of reinforcement from alcohol: Their domain and relation to drinking patterns. *Journal of Consulting and Clinical Psychology, 48,* 419–426.

Budney, A. J., Higgins, S. T., Wong, C. J., & Bickel, W. K. (1995, Nov.). *Early abstinence predicts outcome in behavioral treatment for cocaine dependence.* Poster presented at the 29th annual convention of the Association for the Advancement of Behavior Therapy, Washington, D.C.

Burling, T. A., Reilly, P. M., Moltzen, J. O., & Ziff, D. C. (1989). Self-efficacy and relapse among inpatient drug and alcohol abusers: A predictor of outcome. *Journal of Studies on Alcohol, 50*(4), 354–360.

Cannon, D. S., Leeka, J. K., Patterson, E. T., & Baker, T. B. (1990). Principal components analysis of the Inventory of Drinking Situations: Empirical categories of drinking by alcoholics. *Addictive Behaviors, 15,* 265–269.

Chaney, E. F., O'Leary, M. R., & Marlatt, G. A. (1978). Skill training with alcoholics. *Journal of Consulting and Clinical Psychology, 46,* 1092–1104.

Cohen, S., & Willis, T. A. (1985). Stress, social support, and the buffering hypothesis. *Psychological Bulletin, 98*(2), 310–357.

Coleman, S. B. (1980). Incomplete mourning and addict/family transactions: A theory for under-standing heroin abuse. In J. Grabowski, M. Stitzer, & J. Henningfield (Eds.), *Behavioral interven-tion techniques in drug abuse treatment* (National Institute on Drug Abuse Research Monograph No. 46, DHHS Publ. No. (ADM) 84-1282, pp. 83–99). Washington, DC: U.S. Government Printing Office.

Connors, G. J., Maisto, S. A., & Zywiak, W. H. (1996). Understanding relapse in the broader context of post-treatment functioning. *Addiction, 91* (Suppl.), S173–S189.

Cronkite, R. C., & Moos, R. H. (1980). Determinants of the post treatment functioning of alcohol pa-tients: A conceptual framework. *Journal of Consulting and Clinical Psychology, 48,* 305–316.

DiClemente, C. C., Prochaska, J. O., & Gibertini, M. (1985). Self-efficacy and the stages of self-change of smoking. *Cognitive Therapy and Research, 9*(2), 181–200.

Donovan, D. M. (1996). Assessment issues and domains in the prediction of relapse. *Addiction, 91* (Suppl.), S29–S36.

George, W. H., Frone, M. R., Cooper, M. L., Russell, M., Skinner, J. B., & Windle, M. (1995). A revised alcohol expectancy questionnaire: Factor structure confirmation and invariance in a general pop-ulation sample. *Journal of Studies on Alcohol, 56,* 177–185.

Goldbeck, R., Myatt, P., & Aitchison, T. (1997). End-of-treatment self-efficacy: A predictor of absti-nence. *Addiction, 92*(3), 313–324.

Goldstein, A., & Herrera, J. (1995). Heroin addicts and methadone treatment in Albuquerque: A 22-year follow-up. *Drug and Alcohol Dependence, 40,* 139–150.

Gossop, M., Green, L., Phillips, G., & Bradley, B. (1987). What happens to opiate addicts immediately after treatment: A prospective follow up study. *British Medical Journal, 294*(30), 1377–1380.

Hatsukami, D., & Pickens, R. W. (1982). Post-treatment depression in an alcohol and drug abuse popu-lation. *American Journal of Psychiatry, 139,* 1563–1566.

Heather, N., Stallard, A., & Tebbutt, J. (1991). Importance of substance cues in relapse among heroin users: Comparison of two methods of investigation. *Addictive Behaviors, 16,* 41–49.

Helzer, J. E., & Pryzbeck, T. R. (1988). The co-occurrence of alcoholism with other psychiatric disorders in the general population and its impact on treatment. *Journal of Studies on Alcohol, 49*(3), 219–224.

Hodgins, D. C., & el-Guebaly, N. (1993). *Prospective and retrospective reports of mood states prior to relapse to substance use.* Paper presented at the 6th International Conference on Treatment of Ad-dictive Behaviors, Santa Fe, New Mexico.

Hodgins, D. C., el-Guebaly, N., & Armstrong, S. (1992, Nov.). *Do past heavy drinking situations predict future relapses in alcohol abusers seeking abstinence?* Poster presented at the 26th annual con-vention of the Association for Advancement of Behavior Therapy, Boston.

Isenhart, C. E. (1991). Factor structure of the Inventory of Drinking Situations. *Journal of Substance Abuse, 3,* 59–71.

Isenhart, C. E. (1993). Psychometric evaluation of a short form of the Inventory of Drinking Situations. *Journal of Studies on Alcohol, 54,* 345–349.

Janis, I., & Hoffman, D. (1982). Effective partnerships in a clinic for smokers. In I. Janis (Ed.), *Counsel-ing on personal decisions: Theory and research on short-term helping relationships* (pp. 75–93). New Haven, CT: Yale University Press.

Joe, G. W., Simpson, D. D., & Sells, S. B. (1994). Treatment process and relapse to opioid use during methadone maintenance. *American Journal of Drug and Alcohol Abuse, 20,* 173–197.

Kadden, R. M. (1996). Is Marlatt's relapse taxonomy reliable or valid? *Addiction, 91* (Suppl.), 139–145.

Killen, J. D., Fortman, S. P., Newman, B., & Varady, A. (1991). Prospective study of factors influencing the development of craving associated with smoking cessation. *Psychopharmacology, 105,* 191–196.

Killen, J. D., Fortmann, S. P., Kraemer, H. C., Varady, A., & Newman, B. (1992). Who will relapse? Symptoms of nicotine dependence predict long-term relapse after smoking cessation. *Journal of Consulting and Clinical Psychology, 60,* 797–801.

Kranzler, H. R., Del Boca, F. K., & Rounsaville, B. J. (1996). Comorbid psychiatric diagnosis predicts three-year outcomes in alcoholics: A posttreatment natural history study. *Journal of Studies on Al-cohol, 57,* 619–626.

Lichtenstein, E. (1982). The smoking problem: A behavioral perspective. *Journal of Consulting and Clinical Psychology, 50,* 804–819.

Litman, G. K. (1986). Alcoholism survival: The prevention of relapse. In W. R. Miller & N. Heather (Eds.), *Treating addictive behaviors: Processes of change* (pp. 391–405). New York: Plenum.

Longabaugh, R., & Beattie, M. C. (1985). Optimizing the cost effectiveness of treatment for alcohol abusers. In B. S. McCrady, N. E. Noel, & T. D. Nirenberg (Eds.), *Future directions in alcohol abuse treatment research* (NIAAA Research Monograph No. 15, DHHS Publication No. ADM 85-1322, pp. 104–136). Washington, DC: U.S. Government Printing Office.

Loosen, P. T., Dew, B. W., & Prange, A. J. (1990). Long-term predictors of outcome in abstinent alcoholic men. *American Journal of Psychiatry, 147,* 1662–1666.

MacAndrew, C., & Edgerton, R. B. (1969). *Drunken comportment: A social explanation.* Chicago: Aldine.

Marlatt, G. A., & Gordon, J. R. (1980). Determinants of relapse: Implications for the maintenance of behavior change. In P. Davidson & S. Davidson (Eds.), *Behavioral medicine: Changing health lifestyles* (pp. 410–452). New York: Brunner/Mazel.

McKay, J. R., Maisto, S. A., O'Farrell, T. J. (1993). End-of-treatment self-efficacy, aftercare, and drinking outcomes of alcoholic men. *Alcoholism: Clinical and Experimental Research, 17*(5), 1078–1083.

Miller, P. J., Ross, S. M., Emmerson, R. Y., & Todt, E. H. (1989). Self-efficacy in alcoholics: Clinical validation of the situational confidence questionnaire. *Addictive Behaviors, 14,* 217–224.

Miller, W. R. (1996). What is relapse? Fifty ways to leave the wagon. *Addiction, 91* (Suppl.) S15–S28.

Miller, W. R., & Tonigan, J. S. (1996). Assessing drinkers' motivation for change: The Stages of Change Readiness and Treatment Eagerness Scale (SOCRATES). *Psychology of Addictive Behaviors, 10,* 81–89.

Miller, W. R., Leckman, A. L., Delaney, H. D., & Tinkcom, M. (1992). Long-term follow-up of behavioral self-control training. *Journal of Studies on Alcohol, 53*(3), 249–261.

Miller, W. R., Westerberg, V. S., Harris, R. J., & Tonigan, J. S. (1996). What predicts relapse? Prospective testing of antecedent models. *Addiction, 91,* S155–S171.

Mitchell, R. E. (1984). *Stress, social support and functioning: Beyond the stress buffering effect.* Paper presented at the annual meeting of the American Psychological Association, Toronto, Ontario, Canada.

Montgomery, H. A., Miller, W. R., & Tonigan, J. S. (1995). Does Alcoholics Anonymous involvement predict treatment outcome? *Journal of Substance Abuse Treatment, 12*(4), 241–246.

Nides, M. A., Rakos, R. F., Gonzales, D., Murray, R. P., Tashkin, D. P., & Bjornson-Benson, W.M. (1995). Predictors of initial smoking cessation and relapse through the first 2 years of the lung health study. *Journal of Consulting and Clinical Psychology, 63*(1), 60–69.

Orford, J., & Edwards, G. (1977). *Alcoholism: A comparison of treatment and advice, with a study of influence of marriage* (Maudsley Monographs No. 26). New York: Oxford University Press.

Paul, J. P., Barrett, D. C., Crosby, G. M., & Stall, R. D. (1996). Longitudinal changes in alcohol and drug use among men seen at a gay-specific substance abuse treatment agency. *Journal of Studies on Alcohol, 57,* 475–485.

Platt, J. J., & Labate, C. (1976). *Heroin addiction: Theory, research and treatment.* New York: Wiley.

Polich, J. M, Armor, D. J., & Braiker, H. B. (1981). *The course of alcoholism: Four years after treatment.* New York: Wiley.

Project MATCH Research Group. (1997). Matching alcoholism treatments to client heterogeneity: Project MATCH posttreatment drinking outcomes. *Journal of Studies on Alcohol, 58,* 7–29.

Rice, C., & Longabaugh, R. (1996). Measuring general social support in alcoholic patients: Short forms for perceived social support. *Psychology of Addictive Behaviors, 10*(2), 104–114.

Rist, F., & Watzl, H. (1983). Self assessment of relapse risk and assertiveness in relation to treatment outcome of female alcoholics. *Addictive Behaviors, 8,* 121–127.

Roski, J., Schmid, L. A., & Lando, H. A. (1996). Long-term associations of helpful and harmful spousal behaviors with smoking cessation. *Addictive Behaviors, 21*(2), 173–185.

Rychtarik, R. G., Prue, D. M., & Rapp, S. R. (1992). Self-efficacy, aftercare and relapse in a treatment program for alcoholics. *British Journal of Addiction, 85,* 25–29.

Sannibale, C. (1989). A prospective study of treatment outcome with a group of male problem drinkers. *Journal of Studies on Alcohol, 50*(3), 236–244.

Sass, H., Soyka, M., Mann, K., Zieglgansberger, W. (1996). Relapse prevention by acamprosate. *Archives of General Psychiatry, 53,* 673–680.

Saxon, A. J., Wells, E. A., Fleming, C., Jackson, T. R., & Calsyn, D. A. (1996). Pre-treatment characteristics, program philosophy and level of ancillary services as predictors of methadone maintenance treatment outcome. *Addiction, 81*(8), 1197–1209.

Simpson, D. D., & Marsh, K. L. (1986). *Relapse and recovery among opioid addicts 12 years* (NIDA Research Monograph Series No. 72, pp. 86–103). Rockville, MD: Department of Health and Human Services.

Stark, M. J., & Campbell, B. K. (1988). Personality, drug use and early attrition from substance abuse treatment. *American Journal of Drug and Alcohol Abuse, 14,* 475–485

Taylor, C., Brown, D., Duckitt, A., Edwards, G., Oppenheimer, E., & Sheehan, M. (1986). Multivariate description of alcoholism careers: A 10-year follow-up. In F. M. Tims & C. G. Leukefeld (Eds.), *Relapse and recovery in drug abuse* (pp.72–85). Rockville, MD: National Institute on Drug Abuse.

Vaillant, G. E. (1996). A long-term follow-up of male alcohol abuse. *Archives of General Psychiatry, 53,* 243–249.

Vaillant, G. E., Clark, W., & Cyrus, C. (1983). Prospective study of alcoholism treatment: Eight-year follow up. *American Journal of Medicine, 75,* 455–463.

Wesson, D. R., Havassy, B. E., & Smith, D. E. (1986). *Theories of relapse and recovery and their implications for drug abuse treatment* (NIDA Research Monograph Series No. 72, pp. 5–19). Rockville, MD: Department of Health and Human Services.

Westerberg, V. S., Miller, W. R., Harris, R., & Tonigan, J. S. (1998). The topography of relapse in clinical samples. *Addictive Behaviors.*

Wood, M. D., Sher, K. J., & Strathman, A. (1996). Alcohol outcome expectancies and alcohol use and problems. *Journal of Studies on Alcohol, 57,* 283–288.

23

Continuing Care

Promoting the Maintenance of Change

DENNIS M. DONOVAN

INTRODUCTION

A number of fundamental changes, driven largely by efforts to contain health care costs, have taken place in the recent past in the conceptualization and delivery of substance abuse treatment (McCaul & Furst, 1994; McCrady & Langenbucher, 1996). These changes are reflected in a decreased reliance on and reduced length of acute care stays in inpatient treatment settings, and a corresponding increased reliance on outpatient care (Alterman, O'Brien, & McLellan, 1991; McCrady & Langenbucher, 1996; McKay & Maisto, 1993; Moos, King, & Patterson,1996). This has led to the development of "stepped care" approaches to treatment, which initially use the least costly, yet effective, outpatient interventions appropriate to the severity and complexity of the individual's condition, with treatment being "stepped up" to more intensive inpatient approaches if the initial interventions are not effective. Patients are then "stepped down" from more structured inpatient settings to less structured outpatient treatment (Donovan & Marlatt, 1993; Marlatt, 1988; Miller, 1989).

There also has been an increased focus on substance use disorders as similar to other chronic health problems, such as diabetes, hypertension, or asthma, which require continuing long-term treatment of varying degrees of intensity across time (O'Brien & McLellan, 1996). This suggests that continued monitoring and maintenance treatment, either psychosocial or pharmacological, or both, is required to maintain treatment gains (O'Brien & McLellan, 1996). Such long-term support and continuing care contribute significantly to the long-term effectiveness of substance

DENNIS M. DONOVAN • Alcohol and Drug Abuse Institute and Department of Psychiatry and Behavioral Sciences, University of Washington, Seattle, Washington 98105.

Treating Addictive Behaviors, 2nd ed., edited by Miller and Heather. Plenum Press, New York, 1998.

abuse treatment, regardless of the approach used for initiating behavior change (Allen, Lowman, Mattson, & Litten, 1992). This view is also consistent with Prochaska and DiClemente (1986, and Chapter 1, this volume), whose model of behavior change suggests that maintenance is a separate stage of change characterized by continued action by the individual to consolidate, reinforce, and more firmly establish the new behavior change that occurred earlier in the action stage.

Services provided by treatment agencies to help maintain the therapeutic gains achieved through more intensive interventions were previously termed "aftercare." They are now described as "continuing care" to reflect more accurately that such services represent a continuation of therapy or an extension of treatment rather than something that takes place after "treatment" has been completed (McLatchie & Lomp, 1988; Scott, 1987). Continuing care services focus primarily on helping the client maintain his or her goal of abstinence or reduced, moderated substance use (Alterman et al., 1991; Donovan & Ito, 1988; Marlatt & Gordon, 1985). However, a potentially more realistic and intermediate goal is to help promote and maintain the therapeutic gains made in more intensive treatment, minimize the likelihood of relapse, and reduce the harm to the individual and others if substance use does recur (Marlatt & Tapert, 1993). Continuing care involvement does not necessarily prevent an initial lapse from occurring, but one of its most important functions is early identification and intervention in the relapse process, helping to keep an initial lapse from developing into a full-blown relapse (Ito & Donovan, 1986; McLatchie & Lomp, 1988).

The role and importance of continuing care has increased as inpatient treatment has been reduced in scope and duration (Walker, Donovan, Kivlahan, & O'Leary, 1983). Treatment programs should explicitly plan to provide continuing care services that are low in intensity but longer in duration and that may be used intermittently across time for supportive purposes. Such services should be integrated systematically into the continuum of care and a client's treatment plan rather than being seen as an optional add-on (Mattick & Jarvis, 1994a; McCrady & Langenbucher, 1996). Continuing care services might include "booster sessions" to maintain clients' motivation and skills developed during more intensive treatment, or simple support and monitoring of progress as the individual attempts to reintegrate into his or her social environment (Mattick & Jarvis, 1994a).

There continue to be questions raised about continuing care services and their efficacy, due in part to the equivocal conclusions found in the literature (e.g., Alterman et al., 1991). The purpose of this chapter is to review literature on continuing care and the maintenance of behavior change that has been published since our previous review (Ito & Donovan, 1986), with a hope of being able to address some of the questions about continuing care and its role in the recovery process.

WHAT HAVE WE LEARNED?

CLIENTS PERCEIVE BOTH COSTS AND BENEFITS OF CONTINUING CARE INVOLVEMENT

There appears to be considerable interest in and demand for continuing care services among alcoholics who are given an option to volunteer for such services (McLatchie & Lomp, 1988). However, this does not always lead to high rates of attendance. When asked about their expectation of continuing care (Whorley, 1996b), patients report that they perceive a number of potential short- and long-term benefits from their involvement in continuing care. These include intimate resources (e.g., affection, respect, service exchanged among relatives and friends) which are perceived to occur in the long term rather than in the short term. Certain impersonal resources (e.g., information on coping skills) are expected to be provided in the short term. At the same time, participants anticipate a number of potential costs from continuing care involvement (e.g., losses or rewards forgone as a result of aftercare attendance) in the short term in both intimate and impersonal resources. In addition, participants expect that they may experience one or more general categories of barriers that will possibly prevent their continuing care participation. These include personal barriers (e.g., thinking errors such as denial, physical or psychiatric disabilities that were expected to hinder continuing care attendance), interpersonal barriers (e.g., codependent relationships or relationships with other addicts who were expected to oppose continuing care), and socioeconomic and organizational barriers (e.g., agency waiting lists, inadequate shelter or homelessness, inadequate transportation system, alcohol- and drug-saturated neighborhoods or social settings with communal pressure to use or drink). Conducting a cost-benefits analysis, in which the individual expects short-term costs and potential barriers while anticipating delayed meaningful personal and intimate benefits, suggests that it is difficult clinically to motivate patients for continuing care involvement (Whorley, 1996b). This may help to explain in part the relatively high rates of noncompliance with continuing care plans. Clinicians should explore their patients' expectations of short- and long-term benefits and costs and barriers as a routine component of continuing care planning and seek opportunities to emphasize short-term gains (especially intimate resources) in order to offset immediate costs (through loss and denial of resources) in upcoming continuing care treatment.

IT IS POSSIBLE TO PREDICT CONTINUING CARE ATTENDANCE

Many substance abusers may feel that the relative costs of continuing care are sufficiently high and the barriers sufficiently difficult to overcome that they will choose not to begin or to drop out of continuing care. A number of potential predictors of continuing care involvement have been investigated. These have included both client characteristics and programmatic and logistical issues. Based on a study of male veterans, travel barriers appear to reduce continuing care participation significantly, especially for elderly individuals living in rural areas (Fortney, Booth, Blow, & Bunn, 1995). Those living farther from the treatment program are less likely to attend their continuing care appointments. Older alcoholics appear to be more negatively affected by such travel barriers than are younger alcoholics. However, increasing age has a positive effect on attendance for those in close proximity to the treatment program. The adverse effects of distance are more pronounced for patients living in rural areas than for those living in metropolitan areas. Both younger and older subjects appear less likely than middle-aged individuals to keep their aftercare appointments. Married patients are more likely to attend aftercare than unmarried patients. Ethnic status (African American), severity of illness (greater severity), and urban size (those living in large metropolitan areas) negatively affect the likelihood of aftercare attendance.

A number of investigators have evaluated the relative impact of continuing care on treatment outcome for clients who have been classified based on some empirical, theoretical, or diagnostic subgroups. The possibility of matching client characteristics and the therapeutic orientation and content of continuing care has been examined (e.g., Kadden, Cooney, Getter, & Litt, 1989). Clients received 26 weeks of either coping skills and relapse prevention or an interpersonal/interactional group therapy following an inpatient stay. Substantial and significant improvements, regardless of the type of continuing care received, were found with reduced heavy drinking days and psychological problems over the 6 months of continuing care involvement. However, significant treatment-by-client characteristic interaction effects were found. Clients who were higher in psychiatric severity and sociopathy had better outcomes in the coping skills and relapse prevention group than in an interpersonal/interactional group therapy, which had better outcomes for those lower in sociopathy and psychopathology as well as those who had higher levels of cognitive impairment. However, the results involving the coping skills condition were not replicated in Project MATCH, in which continuing care was administered as individual rather than group therapy (Project MATCH Research Group, 1997).

Another subtype involves indices of risk vulnerability and problem severity. These subtypes, described as Types A and B (Babor et al., 1992) or Types I and II (Cloninger, Sigvardsson, & Bohman, 1996), share a number of common features. Type A or Type I alcoholics are characterized by later onset of alcohol problems, fewer childhood risk factors, less severe dependence, fewer alcohol-related problems, and less psychopathology. Type B or Type II alcoholics are characterized by multiple childhood risk factors, familial alcoholism, early onset of alcohol problems, greater severity of dependence, polydrug use, higher incidence of antisocial behavior and sociopathy, and more life stress. Type A alcoholics were found to do better in an interactional aftercare group and more poorly in a coping skills training group, while Type B alcoholics did better in more structured coping skills treatment and worse in interactional group therapy (Litt, Babor, DelBoca, Kadden, & Cooney, 1992). However, this finding of differential outcomes across treatments for Type A or B alcoholics also was not supported by the results of Project MATCH (1997). Similarly, Type I and Type II alcoholics did not differ in the probability of relapse during continuing care treatment; however, the temporal pattern of relapse did differ, with most Type II relapses occurring less than a month following entry into continuing care, while most of Type I relapses occurred from 1 to 3 months following entry into aftercare (Shanks, Bell, Nessman, Arredondo, & Johnson, 1995).

Individuals having a substance use disorder and at least one other Axis I comorbid psychiatric diagnosis typically have low rates of compliance with continuing care. Two diagnostic measures appear to be significant predictors of continuing care compliance in this group, defined as visiting the continuing care site at least three times (Wolpe, Gorton, Serota, & Sanford, 1993). Cocaine users with a diagnosis of cocaine dependence rather than abuse, a discharge diagnosis involving any type of depression disorder versus those not having such a discharge diagnosis, and, among depressed subjects, those with major depression versus those with other depressive disorders, are less compliant with continuing care.

Similarly, patients who have relatively circumscribed alcohol- or drug-related problems and no other concomitant psychiatric disorders appear to benefit most from community-based residential care, whereas those with substance abuse problems and concomitant psychiatric problems benefit more from hospital-based residential care (Moos *et al.*, 1996).

While a given type of continuing care service provided may show little or no differential effectiveness over other approaches when dealing with undifferentiated samples of substance abusers, a number of client characteristics may interact with the type of continuing care to suggest the possibility of client–treatment matching. However, the findings from Project MATCH (1997), which found relatively little evidence to support treatment matching in its continuing care treatments, raise questions about the viability of client–treatment matching (Project MATCH Research Group, 1997).

IT IS POSSIBLE TO INCREASE COMPLIANCE VIA SPECIFIC INTERVENTIONS

While the rationale for a treatment recommendation to continuing care appears sensible to the clinician, the likelihood is high that substance abuse patients view continuing care as less of a priority than do staff, and it is difficult to get substance abuse clients to comply with referrals for continuing care (Gilbert, 1988; Whorley, 1996b). This has led to a recommendation that continuing care providers take a more proactive stance toward client attendance and compliance in order to increase participation rates (Foote & Erfurt, 1988; Fortney *et al.*, 1995). Although there has been relatively little research exploring effective means of increasing continuing care participation (Ito & Donovan, 1986; Lash & Dillard, 1996), a number of relatively low-cost interventions have been tried.

Orientation Groups

A possible factor contributing to early attrition from continuing care is that clients may not know what to expect from their attending. A number of approaches to deal with this issue have been evaluated. One approach involves transition planning groups for problem drinkers during inpatient treatment. Such groups help sensitize clients to the need for ongoing continuing care, explore their expectations about the benefits and costs associated with future participation in continuing care, familiarize them with the services of the continuing care outpatient clinic, provide them with support as they make the transition to outpatient care, facilitate identification of potential personal, social, or environmental barriers to continuing care involvement, and develop solutions to these barriers (Hanson, Foreman, Tomlin, & Bright, 1994; Whorley, 1996a). Orientation sessions also might include current outpatients discussing the importance of continuing care, accompanying inpatients to an outpatient continuing care group, and working with inpatients to complete a contract for participation in continuing care (Lash & Dillard, 1996). These transitional planning groups appear to lead to greater acceptance of continuing care referrals, better initial contact with programs providing the continuing care, better attendance, and more favorable outcomes than a general orientation to aftercare services (e.g., Whorley, 1996a).

Predischarge Continuing Care Involvement

A second approach to increasing attendance and compliance is to have patients attend at least one continuing care therapy meeting while they are still inpatients (Lash & Dillard, 1996; Verinis & Taylor, 1994). This procedure also may be combined with brief orientation sessions. Placing inpatients in outpatient continuing care groups and mixing the inpatients with existing outpatients whenever possible familiarizes them with the continuing care clinic milieu, breaks down some of the inhibitions about attending a new clinic, exposes them to some successful role models, communicates the clinic atmosphere of mutual support and acceptance, and provides an opportunity for informal socialization. Results, with some exceptions (e.g., Lash & Dillard, 1996), indicate that participation in continuing care groups while still an inpatient increases the likelihood of continued participation (Donovan, Cooney, Rychtarik, & Rice, 1995; Verinis & Taylor, 1994). The continuity of having the same counselor from inpatient to outpatient continuing care, however, does not appear to add meaningfully to continuing care compliance over and above initiating continuing care before discharge from inpatient treatment (Verinis & Taylor, 1994).

Behavioral Contracting

The effectiveness of behavioral contracting procedures has also been evaluated (Ossip-Klein & Rychtarik, 1993; Singh & Howden-Chapman, 1987). Alcoholics sign a contract to attend a specified number of continuing care meetings; this is combined with active follow-up if the client fails to meet the conditions of the contract. Spouse involvement in the contracting process has also been evaluated. During the last portion of inpatient treatment, the counselor presents the patient with an appointment calendar for continuing care meetings and assists in negotiating an attendance contract between the patient and spouse. This contract involves the patient's agreeing to post the appointment calendar in a prominent location at home, attend all scheduled continuing care sessions, and call to reschedule if an appointment must be missed. In exchange for adhering to these behaviors, the spouse agrees to provide a mutually negotiated incentive within one week of the appointment. The contract is then referred to and reviewed at each subsequent continuing care session. These easy to implement behavioral contracting procedures, involving either the patient alone or the patient and spouse, appear to increase continuing care attendance substantially. The contracting procedures appear to be most useful in increasing attendance at the first continuing care session. The increased attendance when contracting only with the patient is not related consistently to drinking status at follow-up, but behavioral contracting with spouse involvement has led to increased continuing care attendance, which appears to be associated with greater rates of abstinence, clinical improvement, and employment at 1-year follow-up when compared with standard care (Ahles, Schlundt, Prue, & Rychtarik, 1983).

VOLUNTARY COMPLIANCE WITH AFTERCARE PREDICTS OUTCOME

While it seems intuitive clinically to attempt to increase participation in and compliance with continuing care, a basic and fundamental question is whether continuing care contributes to improved outcome. The results of previous studies would suggest an affirmative answer to this question (Ito & Donovan, 1986). A number of more recent studies bear on this question.

Correlational Studies

Readmission following inpatient substance abuse treatment is a key measure of service utilization, an indicator of poor posttreatment functioning, and a factor contributing to increased treatment costs (Peterson, Swindle, Phibbs, Recine, & Moos, 1994). Patients treated for substance abuse problems are at high risk for relapse during the first year following discharge, with resultingly high readmission rates. Programs that discharge more patients who then attend at least two outpatient aftercare sessions within the first month following their inpatient stay have fewer patients readmitted. However, the percentages of patients attending two or more continuing care sessions in the first postdischarge month is typically quite low (e.g., 20%). Increased efforts need to be made by programs to get more patients to attend continuing care sessions, which may help to reduce readmission rates.

As is typically found in general psychotherapy literature, an increased level of continuing care attendance is associated with better outcomes. For example, treatment outcome was evaluated in the study of the effectiveness of behavioral contracting with spouse involvement (Ahles et al., 1983). Regardless of the type of intervention used, subjects with six or more aftercare sessions were significantly more likely to be abstinent at both 6 months (100% and 30.4% of attendees and nonattendees, respectively) and 1 year (58.3% and 12.5% of attendees and nonattendees, respectively). Similarly, the number of weekly sessions attended during the first 8 weeks of continuing care is related inversely to the amount of alcohol consumed and the number of drinking days over a 6-month postintervention period even after the effects of client characteristics, such as demographics, chronicity, and coping, had been taken into account (Ito & Donovan, 1990). Also, patients who were abstinent over the entire 6-month postintervention period attended more continuing care sessions during the initial 8-week period of therapy than did nonabstainers.

Randomized Trials

There has been relatively little research in which the provision of continuing care has been experimentally manipulated (McLatchie & Lomp, 1988). However, the results of two randomized clinical trials dealing with continuing care following initial treatment in either an inpatient or outpatient setting do not support the findings from correlational studies (Connors, Tarbox, & Faillace, 1992; McLatchie & Lomp, 1988). When continuing care is presented as a mandatory or standard component of treatment, rather than voluntary, there is a relatively high level of attendance. Despite the differences in therapy attendance across treatment conditions or the nature of the therapy delivery (e.g., standard group therapy versus individual counseling through telephone contacts), no differences were found with respect to relapse rates. Also, the absence of aftercare services during the critical 3-month period following discharge from inpatient treatment did not increase relapse vulnerability. From this pattern of results it has been recommended that the focus of continuing care should be shifted from relapse prevention to the processing of relapses if and when they occur and helping the individual cope with and recover from relapsing (McLatchie & Lomp, 1988).

Despite an ongoing belief by clinicians in its efficacy, the results of controlled randomized trials suggest that continuing care may play a less prominent role in the recovery process than has been thought previously. Experimental tests of continuing care, as limited as they are, do not support the efficacy of special "after-care" programs. Added "relapse prevention" measures do not appear to prevent relapse; if they have a salutary effect it is to decrease the duration and severity of lapses. The more positive results from correlational studies must be interpreted with caution since there almost certainly is some self-selection bias among patients who attend continuing care (Peterson *et al.,* 1994), with those entering and complying with continuing care being more highly motivated than those who do not. It may be that attendance at continuing care influences compliance, as defined by attendance and completion, rather than attendance leading to improving outcomes (Foote & Erfurt, 1988; Gilbert, 1988; Hitchcock, Stainback, & Roque, 1995; Peterson *et al.,* 1994).

THE TYPE OF CONTINUING CARE AND THE MODE OF ITS DELIVERY MAY NOT MAKE MUCH DIFFERENCE

Type of Therapy

A number of studies have evaluated the therapeutic orientation of continuing care interventions as well as the method through which these are delivered. It appears that most types of continuing care are equivalent with respect to their influence on treatment outcome. For example, while eight 90-minute cognitive-behavioral relapse prevention groups led to somewhat higher rates of completion of a 6-month commitment to continuing care, no differences were found in drinking-related outcomes at a 6-month postdischarge follow-up between this relapse prevention group and an interactional/interpersonal process therapy group (Ito, Donovan, & Hall, 1988). Even when patients received up to 6 months of either cognitive-behavioral or interpersonal continuing care therapy groups, there still were no differences in outcome (Kadden *et al.,* 1989). Similarly, while substantial decreases were found in drinking-related behaviors and consequences from pretreatment to posttreatment, no clinically significant differences were found between individually delivered cognitive-behavioral coping skills–relapse prevention training, motivational enhancement therapy, and 12-step facilitation therapy with respect to drinking-related and psychosocial outcomes (Project MATCH Research Group, 1997).

Mode of Therapy Delivery

As noted previously, continuing care services have been presented in a variety of delivery modes, including telephone counseling, group therapy, and individual therapy. A question has been raised about the relative effectiveness of individual counseling versus group therapy in delivering continuing care services. Few studies have evaluated this issue. A comparison has been conducted of cognitive-behavioral relapse prevention continuing care, delivered as either individual or group therapy during the first 3 months following completion of either inpatient or intensive out-patient alcohol treatment. Both approaches demonstrated a high rate of attendance and client satisfaction, as well as substantial reductions in substance use over a 12-month follow-up. However, no differences were found between the group or individual therapy conditions on any of the alcohol or drug use outcome measures (Graham, Annis, Brett, & Venesoen, 1996).

Cocaine-dependent patients who participated in an intensive outpatient or day hospital program received one of two types of continuing care twice weekly over a 5-month period: "treatment as usual" consisting of group sessions with an interactional, 12-step focus, or an individual relapse prevention session plus one group session per week (McKay *et al.*, 1997). No overall differences were found between the two interventions with respect to the percent days of cocaine use over a 6-month period. Patients in the relapse prevention condition were more likely to report some use of cocaine than were those in the standard group condition. However, among patients who had some cocaine use in the first 3 months of continuing care, those in the relapse prevention condition had fewer days of cocaine use than did those in the standard continuing care group. These results are consistent with previous suggestions that continuing care may provide harm reduction rather than relapse prevention. Significant interaction effects suggestive of a client attribute-by-treatment match were also found. Patients who were able to achieve remission of cocaine use during the intensive outpatient phase of treatment had relatively good outcomes in both treatments; however, those who failed to achieve remission had much worse outcomes in the standard condition than in the relapse prevention condition.

These findings suggest that the therapeutic approach employed or the method of delivering continuing care services (e.g., individual versus group therapy) may have minimal impact on continuing care attendance or treatment outcome. However, important interactions may exist between the form of therapy delivery and therapeutic orientation and client characteristics, suggesting the possibility of treatment matching (McKay *et al.*, 1997).

WHAT SHOULD WE DO TO HELP CLIENTS AFTER AN INITIAL TREATMENT EPISODE?

INVOLVE THE SOCIAL SUPPORT SYSTEM

There is evidence that involving available family and significant others in the treatment and continuing care process can improve outcome. The involvement of family or friends in the assessment and treatment planning process results in fewer readmissions in the year following discharge from inpatient care (Peterson *et al.*, 1994). The previously described behavioral contracting procedure involving patient and spouse has been shown to increase continuing care attendance and improve treatment outcome (Ahles *et al.*, 1983; Ossip-Klein, Vanlandingham, Prue, & Rychtarik, 1984; Ossip-Klein & Rychtarik, 1993). Attendance at the first seven sessions was nearly twice as high for contracting subjects compared to usual care, with the greatest impact on attendance at the first session. Subjects in the behavioral contracting condition were significantly more likely to have been abstinent, to be considered treatment successes, and to be employed at 1-year follow-up than the standard care group.

Couples who receive behavioral marital therapy as an adjunct to individual outpatient alcoholism treatment have better outcomes with respect to their relationship (e.g., better dyadic adjustment and less time separated), and the husbands in the behavioral marital therapy have better substance-related outcomes (fewer days of drug use, longer periods of abstinence, fewer drug-related arrests and rehospitalizations) than participants in standard individual outpatient treatment (Fals-Stewart, Birchler, & O'Farrell, 1996). The incremental benefit of adding 15 additional sessions of conjoint therapy focusing specifically on relapse prevention as continuing care during the year following an initial 5 months of weekly behavioral marital therapy has been evaluated (O'Farrell, Chequette, Cutter, Brown, & Mc-Courti, 1993). All participants evidenced significant improvements as a result of their participation in the initial behavioral marital therapy. Those who received the subsequent conjoint relapse prevention sessions had more days abstinent, fewer days of drinking, and more improved relationships with spouses than those who received no further continuing care treatment beyond the initial behavioral marital therapy (O'Farrell *et al.,* 1993).

USE RECOVERY HOUSES AND TRANSITIONAL LIVING SETTINGS

Community residential facilities such as halfway or recovery houses play an increasingly important role in the continuum of care for the treatment of substance abuse as episodes of acute inpatient care are shortened and patients are more likely to be placed directly into outpatient or day hospital care (Ross, Booth, Russell, Laughlin, & Brown, 1995). Many substance abusers need transitional residential and other support services to help them maintain sobriety and establish a more functional lifestyle (Moos, Pettit, & Gruber, 1995). The milieu associated with halfway houses offers recovering substance abusers a supportive environment from which to negotiate the tasks associated with the recovery process, such as learning effective affiliation skills to decrease social isolation, developing effective relapse prevention strategies, overcoming educational and vocational deficits, and engaging in leisure time activities not associated with substance use (Fischer, 1996; Hitchcock *et al.,* 1995). Many substance abusers hold positive expectations about and intend to go to a halfway house as a part of their treatment plan; furthermore, they relatively consistently follow through by actually entering the halfway house (Fischer, 1996). As an example, approximately one third of a group of veterans who enrolled in an ongoing continuing care program chose to live concurrently in a nearby halfway house while the remaining two thirds made community-based living arrangements (Hitchcock *et al.,* 1995). Although these two groups were similar on most demographic measures and indices of substance dependence, the halfway house group had significantly better compliance with continuing care attendance and were more likely to have achieved a number of major treatment milestones than those in the community-based group.

Individuals living in recovery-oriented community-based transitional residential care programs are much more likely to engage in outpatient continuing care, obtain much more intensive care, and are less likely to be readmitted for acute hospital care in comparison to patients who received either hospital-based residential care or who lived in the community but not in a therapeutic program (Moos *et al.,* 1995; Moos *et al.,* 1996). Longer stays in these residential care programs, particularly for those having a concurrent psychiatric disorder, are associated with better outcomes. The results highlight the value of providing adequate amounts of residential care and outpatient continuing care for patients in substance abuse treatment, especially those who are considered at increased risk due to their poor social support system and increased psychiatric comorbidity (Ross *et al.,* 1995). By increasing patients' involvement in outpatient continuing care, treatment in community residential facilities may lessen the need for subsequent readmission to acute inpatient care.

SET UP A MONITORING SYSTEM TO CATCH LAPSES EARLY

As noted previously, the value of continuing care involvement rests less in its ability to keep lapses from occurring than its ability to intervene in the relapse process early and prevent an initial lapse from becoming a relapse. Based on this, a number of relatively simple methods may be employed to facilitate this task. These include sending reminders to clients prior to their next scheduled appointment and following up on the clients who fail to attend a continuing care appointment, and/or developing a more systematic call system to allow ongoing monitoring.

Ongoing continuing care sessions with individuals over the phone have led to outcomes comparable to those found with in-person group therapy (Connors *et al.,* 1992). Such phone counseling appears to be well liked by alcoholic clients, who report wanting them to continue and view them as part of good treatment (Fitzgerald & Mulford, 1985). It is also possible for therapists who make periodic calls to clients during the continuing care phase of treatment to collect outcome data at the same time, thus fulfilling both clinical and program evaluative goals and needs (Breslin, Sobell, Sobell, Buchan, & Kwan, 1996).

An extended case monitoring approach has been suggested recently (Stout, Rubin, Zwick, & Zywiak, 1997). This approach is meant to maximize long-term benefits of treatment with a low-cost supplement to current clinical practice. It involves periodic telephone contacts with clients, with more frequent calls being made earlier in the continuing care period when relapse risk is high. The phone counseling services are provided by bachelor's level therapists who adhere to and are trained and supervised in the basic principles of motivational interviewing, such as nonjudgmental attitude, reflective listening, interpersonal warmth, and empathy (Miller & Rollnick, 1991). This approach, which is longer and less intensive than case management, has as its goals the prevention of crises and the facilitation of treatment reentry before a full-blown crisis or relapse occurs. The effectiveness of this approach is currently being evaluated.

ENCOURAGE SAMPLING OF SELF-HELP SUPPORT GROUPS

Self-help groups represent a readily available resource to provide or augment continuing care services. Alcoholics Anonymous (AA), the most prominent of such groups, is free and quite accessible in most communities. Involvement in AA, including both meeting attendance and the incorporation of the 12-step philosophy and specific recovery steps, appears to be associated with reduced drinking (e.g., Johnsen & Herringer, 1993; Timko, Finney, Moos, & Moos, 1995) and better psychosocial functioning (e.g., Watson *et al.*, 1997). Further, the greater the involvement, the better the outcome (e.g., Montgomery, Miller, & Tonigan, 1995). The reductions in drinking-related measures associated with AA involvement are more consistent and often exceed those attributable to the effects of social support from friends and family (Humphreys, Moos, & Finney, 1996). Also, AA attendance provides considerable cost savings over professional treatment (Humphreys & Moos, 1996). It also appears that combining AA and professional treatment may lead to better outcomes over and above that attributable to either approach independently (McCrady & Delaney, 1995; Timko *et al.*, 1995; see Chapter 21, this volume).

No single approach is suited to meet the needs of all substance abusers. Some alcoholics choose not to attend AA because of its emphasis on spirituality (Connors & Dermen, 1996). Men and women appear to respond differently to AA, with involvement appearing less beneficial for women (Tonigan & Hiller-Strumhofel, 1994). Similarly, substance abusers with comorbid psychiatric disorders feel that they receive little understanding, acceptance, or support at 12-step meetings (Hastings-Vertino, 1996). This has led to the development of a number of alternative self-help groups. These include Rational Recovery (RR), Secular Organizations for Sobriety (SOS), Support Together for Mental and Emotional Serenity and Sobriety (STEMSS) for alcoholics with comorbid psychiatric problems, Women for Sobriety (WFS), and Self-Management and Recovery Training (SMART). These groups share in common philosophical and theoretical differences from AA and a goal to help the individual in his or her attempts at recovery and maintenance; however, each has distinctive features meant to address the specific needs and expectations of its participants. Little controlled research has been conducted on these alternatives. It will be important to develop studies concerning the characteristics of individuals who choose to affiliate with one or more of these approaches and the relative benefits achieved. Given the heterogeneity of styles within a given self-help support organization, as well as that which exists across organizations, and given the heterogeneity of client characteristics of those who choose to participate in different groups, it is possible to explore client–treatment matching (Galaif & Sussman, 1995; Morgenstern, Kahler, Frey, & Labouvie, 1996; Tonigan, Toscova, & Miller, 1996).

It is important for clinicians to familiarize themselves with AA and its alternatives, learning about the characteristics of those substance abusers who seem to benefit from different approaches, and to learn ways to facilitate referrals to and involvement in these groups (Johnson & Chappel, 1994; McCrady & Delaney, 1995). A special 12-step facilitation therapy was developed for and evaluated in Project MATCH (Nowinski, Baker, & Carroll, 1992). This individual therapy was successful in increasing AA attendance and had outcomes comparable to or slightly better than the other therapies evaluated (Project MATCH Research Group, 1997).

CONSIDER MEDICATIONS THAT MAY BE HELPFUL IN MAINTENANCE

A variety of pharmacological therapies have begun to emerge as potentially effective interventions to help clients achieve abstinence, maintain therapeutic gains, and minimize relapse or its consequences (see Chapters 15 and 16, this volume). Consideration should be given to their incorporation into the continuing care phase of treatment. Disulfiram, or Antabuse, has been available for some time. The findings concerning its efficacy have been mixed. Much of the apparent response to Antabuse may be an expectancy and motivational effect, in that those individuals whose compliance is high, regardless of whether they are taking active disulfiram or placebo, tend to have more positive outcomes than those who are less compliant (Fuller *et al.*, 1986). A recent review of controlled trials of Antabuse suggests that while it may not promote higher rates of abstinence among those taking it versus those who are not, its use is associated with reduced quantity of alcohol consumed and a reduced number of drinking days (Hughes & Cook, 1997). If Antabuse is prescribed its use should be monitored and should be a component part of a comprehensive treatment program in order to increase complaince (O'Farrell, Allen, & Litten, 1995).

Medications, such as naltrexone and acamprosate, have been used increasingly as adjuncts to alcoholism treatment. These two drugs, although having different sites and mechanisms of action, appear to decrease craving and the reinforcing properties of alcohol. Evaluations of naltrexone in alcohol-dependent patients who also received psychosocial treatments found rates of abstinence to be higher with naltrexone; naltrexone-treated subjects also exhibited significantly lower rates of serious relapse and fewer drinking days without any serious adverse events (O'Malley *et al.*, 1992; Volpicelli, Alterman, Hayashida, & O'Brien, 1992). A similar pattern of results has been observed for acamprosate (Sass, Soyka, Mann, & Zieglgansberger, 1996; Whitworth *et al.*, 1996).

In general, subjects on supervised disulfiram or those prescribed naltrexone or acamprosate appear to do better than placebo-treated subjects in terms of number of drinking days, total alcohol consumption, and avoidance of serious relapse. Given these encouraging results, the continued evaluation of medications in conjunction with different forms of continuing care treatment is an important area of research (Annis & Peachey, 1992; Anton, 1996; Jaffe *et al.*, 1996).

PROVIDE CASE MANAGEMENT SERVICES

It has been suggested that relapse prevention approaches pay too little attention to clients' social context and that very few attempts are made to help substance abusers modify their posttreatment environment (Barber, 1992). It has been argued that clinic-based care is not able to compete successfully with the substance abuser's community and may never prove sufficient to deal with the multiplicity of problems of such clients (Saunders & Allsop, 1991). These concerns have led some to suggest that continuing care practice has a critical need for "case management" services after discharge in order to help provide a bridge between client and treatment programs and other social services and facilitate the transition from structured treatment to unstructured community living (Gray, 1993; Whorley, 1996b).

Case management represents a form of managed service delivery which includes the clinical management of client services (Gray, 1993). The case manager is often not a direct treatment provider; rather, he or she serves to coordinate, advocate, and broker services for the client (Godley, Godley, Pratt, & Wallace, 1994; Gray, 1993). The case manager plays a critical role during the continuing care phase of treatment. This includes routinely assessing the client's progress and determining when the individual is ready to be discharged from continuing care; taking the lead in developing and implementing the continuing care plan; monitoring the care process to ensure that services listed in the care plan are delivered appropriately; helping encourage the client's attendance at medication monitoring appointments, group meetings, and other therapeutic activities; monitoring the client's individualized relapse precipitants; and advocating for the client and family to obtain appropriate services. The support activities provided by the case manager during aftercare include problem-solving assistance on an ongoing basis and at times of crisis; review and reinforcement of skills training that the client has received while emphasizing how to become involved in productive, substance-free social and leisure activities in the community; and help in learning to cope with stress and "negative emotional states" without resorting to alcohol or drug use and to cope with a slip or lapse without allowing it to become a full-blown relapse. While a goal of continuing care is relapse prevention, the case manager must also work with clients to minimize the harm associated with relapse and to rebound functionally after relapse occurs.

The inclusion of such case management activities in the continuing care process appears to contribute positively to the outcomes of substance abusers. As an example, alcoholics were assigned to a case management condition in which they received structured outpatient problem-solving therapy and received a call from their therapists 2 to 3 days before a continuing care appointment to remind them of the date and time of their appointment (Gilbert, 1988). Other subjects were assigned to a home visit condition. They received the standard structured outpatient therapy but therapy appointments were not scheduled at the hospital; instead the therapist agreed to meet the patient at a location that was convenient for the patient (e.g., his home, a coffee shop near his home or place of employment, or any other convenient location). These two conditions were compared to standard continuing care which included the same structured outpatient therapy but no attention paid to improving attendance at regularly scheduled aftercare meetings. As predicted, the two active follow-up methods had significantly higher compliance with scheduled outpatient appointments, with the home visit group having more visits than either of the other two groups. Patients in the home visit condition also were more likely to complete the 12-month aftercare contract and had longer stays in continuing care than either the case management or the traditional treatments. However, increasing continuing care attendance rates did not improve treatment outcome with respect to drinking-related variables, emotional functioning, socioeconomic status, or social functioning.

More positive results have been found with respect to the impact of case management on treatment outcome (Patterson, McCourt, & Shiels, 1991). Following completion of a 6-week inpatient alcoholism treatment, participants received either standard clinic-based outpatient continuing care or a special condition which involved continuing care provided by a community psychiatric nurse in the alcoholic's home. Those who received the community-based program had considerably higher rates of continuous abstinence (54% versus 20%), were more likely to be classified as having successful outcomes (72% versus 37%), had greater attendance at hospital open meetings (60% versus 20%), and had fewer hospital admissions (19% versus 37%) during the year postdischarge compared with the

control condition. These positive results for participants receiving the community psychiatric nurse continuing care have been found to persist as long as 5 years after treatment (Patterson, MacPherson, & Brady, 1997).

Despite the apparent increased positive outcomes associated with the home visit continuing care, advocates have suggested that it is unlikely that such an approach will be widely adopted (Barber, 1992; Gilbert, 1988; Patterson *et al.*, 1991; Whorley, 1996a). Case management approaches in general, and home visit procedures in particular, are considered to be quite expensive to conduct in terms of therapist time and transportation costs. The staff intensity and resultant costs may make such approaches impractical since most treatment programs lack adequate resources to provide case management support. However, further research should be conducted to determine whether these more intensive and expensive approaches may provide sufficient cost offsets in the future by reducing relapse, readmission to acute care treatment, and other service utilization to justify their use.

CONCLUSIONS AND FUTURE DIRECTIONS

This review attempted to address a number of issues and questions that have been posed in the literature about continuing care and its contributions to outcome. Based on the findings reviewed, the following tentative conclusions can be drawn:

- It is possible to increase continuing care compliance through relatively concrete interventions such as orientations to continuing care, beginning attendance before discharge from the more intensive primary treatment, and behavioral contracting that also involves contingency management.
- It is not clear whether this increased compliance and attendance will positively impact treatment outcome. Studies in which aftercare attendance has been shown to be related to improved substance-related outcomes have most often been correlational in nature; studies using random assignment or quasi-experimental designs typically do not support, or provide only equivocal support for, the effectiveness of continuing care. The fact that experimental manipulations that improve retention in continuing care do not appear to improve outcomes, combined with the positive findings of continuing care participation in the correlational studies, suggests that the prognostic effect of voluntary compliance is not a "dose–response" effect, but perhaps a marker of motivation or some other third factor.
- It appears that subtypes of substance abusers may have differential outcomes across continuing care therapy differing in theoretical orientations, content, or method of delivery. This suggests that the continued examination of possible client-by-treatment matching is warranted. Recommendations have also been made to consider the possibility of matching patients to different self-help support groups.
- As had been noted in our previous review (Ito & Donovan, 1986), an increasing body of evidence indicates that continuing care may more appropriately serve to minimize the duration, severity, and harm associated with relapse rather than prevent relapse from occurring.

- There is a growing sense that clinic-based continuing care programs may be insufficient and that more intensive community-based programs, including case management, community reinforcement, and transitional living and residential services such as halfway houses, may lead to better outcomes, particularly with the growing segment of the substance abuse population that also has comorbid psychiatric problems. Despite the increased expense involved in providing this greater intensity, future studies should attempt to determine whether these approaches are associated with greater cost offsets than are less intense treatments.
- The greater the degree of social support that can be generated by including family and significant others in the treatment and continuing care processes, the greater the likelihood of improved outcome. This appears to be particularly true when specific contracts and contingencies are made between patient and spouse.
- Alcoholics Anonymous and its alternative self-help support groups represent widely available and accessible low-cost networks that may serve as or augment continuing care. Further research into the profiles of individuals who benefit from these groups as well as outcome evaluations of their effectiveness are warranted. Clinicians also need to increase their knowledge of and make more frequent referrals to these support groups.
- Recent developments in pharmacological treatments for alcohol and drug abuse provide additional avenues to help substance abusers achieve their treatment goals and maintain therapeutic gains. Further investigation into the effects of combining different psychotherapeutic approaches and different medications is needed.

Although this review has provided information concerning a number of important issues, even if unable to provide unequivocal answers to them, a number of questions remain (Alterman *et al.*, 1991; Foote & Erfurt, 1988). It has been suggested that future studies might examine

- techniques that are successful in engaging people in continuing care, in part to determine predictors of compliance but also to allow sufficient attendance to fully evaluate the effectiveness of continuing care;
- the effects of different types of therapies (e.g., unstructured support groups versus groups focused on the prediction and control of relapse);
- the impact of continuing care on relapse prevention and harm reduction over varying lengths of time;
- the cost-effectiveness, cost-benefit, and cost-offsets of various continuing care and relapse prevention strategies;
- the typical length of stay in continuing care or the proportion of alcoholics who complete the designated program of continuing care;
- whether patients who complete continuing care treatment have fewer problems and more resources upon entry to treatment than those who drop out;
- the optimal combination of shorter inpatient or intensive outpatient treatment duration and longer continuing care that maximizes treatment outcome and that is maximally cost-effective;
- the client attributes and types of continuing care therapies that may lead to clinically useful client–treatment matching.

The ultimate question that should continually serve as the guiding principle of clinical practice and future research is what approaches best serve to maintain the therapeutic gains achieved in a preceding treatment episode, to reduce the likelihood of relapse, and to minimize harm if relapse does occur.

REFERENCES

Ahles, T. A., Schlundt, D. G., Prue, D. M., & Rychtarik, R. G. (1983). Impact of aftercare arrangements on the maintenance of treatment success in abusive drinkers. *Addictive Behaviors, 8,* 53–58.

Allen, J. P., Lowman, C., Mattson, M. E., & Litten, R. Z. (1992). Promising themes in alcoholism treatment research. In R. R. Watson (Ed.), *Drug and alcohol abuse reviews* (Vol. 3, pp. 33– 64). Totowa, NJ: Humana.

Alterman, A. I., O'Brien, C. P., & McLellan, A. T. (1991). Differential therapeutics for substance abuse. In R. J. Francis & S. I. Miller (Eds.), *Clinical textbook of addictive disorders* (pp. 369–390). New York: Guilford.

Annis, H. M., & Peachy, J. E. (1992). The use of calcium carbimide in relapse prevention counseling: Results of a randomized controlled trial. *British Journal of Addictions, 87,* 63–72.

Anton, R. F. (1996). Neurobehavioral basis for the pharmacotherapy of alcoholism: Current and future directions. *Alcohol and Alcoholism, 31* (Suppl. 1), 43–53.

Babor, T. F., Hofman, M., DelBoca, F. K., Hesselbrock, V., Meyer, R. E., Dolinsky, Z., & Rounsaville, B. (1992). Types of alcoholics: I. Evidence for an empirically derived typology based on indicators of vulnerability and severity. *Archives of General Psychiatry, 49,* 599–608.

Barber, J. G. (1992). Relapse prevention and the need for brief social interventions. *Journal of Substance Abuse Treatment, 9,* 157–158.

Breslin,C., Sobell, L. C., Sobell, M. B., Buchan, G., & Kwan, E. (1996). Aftercare telephone contacts with problem drinkers can serve a clinical and research function. *Addiction, 91,* 1359–1364.

Cloninger, C. R., Sigvardsson, S., & Bohman, M. (1996). Type I and type II alcoholism: An update. *Alcohol Health & Research World, 20,* 18–23.

Connors, G. J., & Dermen, K. H. (1996). Characteristics of participants in Secular Organizations for Sobriety (SOS). *American Journal of Drug and Alcohol Abuse, 22,* 281–296.

Connors, G. J., Tarbox, A. R., & Faillace, L. A. (1992). Achieving and maintaining gains among problem drinkers: Process and outcome results. *Behavior Therapy, 23,* 449–474.

Donovan, D. M., & Ito, J. R. (1988). Cognitive behavioral relapse prevention strategies and aftercare in alcoholism rehabilitation. *Psychology of Addictive Behaviors, 2,* 74–81.

Donovan, D. M., & Marlatt, G. A. (1993). Behavioral treatment of alcoholism: A decade of evolution. In M. Galanter (Ed.), *Recent developments in alcoholism* (Vol. 11, pp. 397–411). New York: Plenum.

Donovan, D. M., Cooney, N. L., Rychtarik, R., & Rice, C. (1995, June). *Therapy attendance in Project MATCH.* Paper presented at the annual scientific meeting of the Research Society on Alcoholism, Steamboat Springs, CO.

Fals-Stewart, W., Birchler, G. R., & O'Farrell, T. J. (1996). Behavioral couples therapy for male substance-abusing patients: Effects on relationship adjustment and drug-using behavior. *Journal of Consulting and Clinical Psychology, 64,* 959–972.

Fischer, E. H. (1996). Alcoholic patients' decisions about halfway houses: What they say, what they do. *Journal of Substance Abuse Treatment, 13,* 159–164.

Fitzgerald, J. L., & Mulford, H. A. (1985). An experimental test of telephone aftercare contacts with alcoholics. *Journal of Studies on Alcohol, 46,* 418–424.

Foote, A., & Erfurt, J. C. (1988). Posttreatment follow-up, aftercare, and worksite reentry of the recovering alcoholic employee. In M. Galanter (Ed.), *Recent developments in alcoholism* (Vol. 6, pp. 193–204). New York: Plenum.

Fortney, J. C., Booth, B. M., Blow, F. C., & Bunn, J. Y. (1995). The effects of travel barriers and age on the utilization of alcoholism treatment aftercare. *American Journal of Drug and Alcohol Abuse, 21,* 391–406.

Fuller, R. K., Branchey, L., Brightwell, D. R., Derman, R. M., Emrick, C. D., Iber, F. L., James, K. E., Lacoursiere, R. B., Lee, K. K., Lowenstam, I., Maany, I., Neiderheiser, D., Nocks, J. J., & Shaw, S. (1986). Disulfiram treatment of alcoholism: A Veterans Administration cooperative study. *Journal of Nervous and Mental Disease, 256,* 1449–1455.

Galaif, E. R., & Sussman, S. (1995). For whom does Alcoholics Anonymous work? *International Journal of the Addictions, 30,* 161–184.

Gilbert, F. S. (1988). The effect of type of aftercare follow-up on treatment outcome among alcoholics. *Journal of Studies on Alcohol, 49,* 149–159.

Godley, S. H., Godley, M. D., Pratt, A., & Wallace, J. L. (1994). Case management services for adolescent substance abusers: A program description. *Journal of Substance Abuse Treatment, 11,* 309–317.

Graham, K., Annis, H. M., Brett, P. J., & Venesoen, P. (1996). A controlled field trial of group versus individual cognitive-behavioural training for relapse prevention. *Addiction, 91,* 1127–1139.

Gray, M. (1993). Relapse prevention. In S. L. A. Straussner (Ed.), *Clinical work with substance-abusing clients* (pp. 351–368). New York: Guilford.

Hanson, M., Foreman, L., Tomlin, W., & Bright, Y. (1994). Facilitating problem drinking clients' transition from inpatient to outpatient care. *Health and Social Work, 19,* 23–28.

Hastings-Vertino, K. A. (1996). STEMSS (Support Together for Mental and Emotional Serenity and Sobriety): An alternative to traditional forms of self-help for the dually diagnosed consumer. *Journal of Addictions Nursing, 8,* 20–28.

Hitchcock, H. C., Stainback, R. D., & Roque, G. M. (1995). Effects of halfway house placement on retention of patients in substance abuse aftercare. *American Journal of Drug and Alcohol Abuse, 21*(3), 379–390.

Hughes, J. C., & Cook, C. C. H. (1997). The efficacy of disulfiram: A review of outcome studies. *Addiction, 92,* 381–395.

Humphreys, K., & Moos, R. H. (1996). Reduced substance-abuse-related health care costs among voluntary participants in Alcoholics Anonymous. *Psychiatric Services, 47,* 709–713.

Humphreys, K., Moos, R. H., & Finney, J. W. (1996). Life domains, Alcoholics Anonymous, and role incumbency in the 3-year course of problem drinking. *Journal of Nervous and Mental Disease, 184,* 475–481.

Ito, J. R., & Donovan, D. M. (1986). Aftercare in alcoholism treatment: A review. In W. R. Miller & N. Heather (Eds.), *The addictive behaviors: Processes of change* (pp. 435–456). New York: Plenum.

Ito, J. R., & Donovan, D. M. (1990). Predicting drinking outcomes: Demography, chronicity, coping and aftercare. *Addictive Behaviors, 15,* 553–559.

Ito, J. R., Donovan, D. M., & Hall, J. J. (1988). Relapse prevention in alcohol after care: Effects on drinking outcome, change process, and aftercare attendance. *British Journal of Addictions, 83,* 171–181.

Jaffe, A. J., Rounsaville, B., Chang, G., Schottenfeld, R. S., Meyer, R. E., & O'Malley, S. S. (1996). Naltrexone, relapse prevention, and supportive therapy with alcoholics: An analysis of patient treatment matching. *Journal of Consulting and Clinical Psychology, 64,* 1044–1053.

Johnsen, E., & Herringer, L. G. (1993). Note on the utilization of common support activities and relapse following substance abuse treatment. *Journal of Psychology, 127,* 73–78.

Johnson, N. P., & Chappel, J. N. (1994). Using AA and other 12-step programs more effectively. *Journal of Substance Abuse Treatment, 11,* 137–142.

Kadden, R. M., Cooney, N. L., Getter, H., & Litt, M. D. (1989). Matching alcoholics to coping skills or interactional therapies: Posttreatment results. *Journal of Consulting and Clinical Psychology, 57,* 698–704.

Lash, S. J., & Dillard, W. (1996). Encouraging participation in aftercare group therapy among substance-dependent men. *Psychological Reports, 79,* 585–586.

Litt, M. D., Babor, T. F., DelBoca, F. K., Kadden, R. M., & Cooney, N. L. (1992). Types of alcoholics: II. Application of an empirically derived typology to treatment matching. *Archives of General Psychiatry, 49,* 609–614.

Marlatt, G. A. (1988). Matching clients to treatment: Treatment models and stages of change. In D. M. Donovan & G. A. Marlatt (Eds.), *Assessment of addictive behaviors* (pp. 474–483). New York: Guilford.

Marlatt, G. A., & Gordon, J. R. (Eds.). (1985). *Relapse prevention: Maintenance strategies in the treatment of addictive behaviors.* New York: Guilford.

Marlatt, G. A., & Tapert, S. F. (1993). Harm reduction: Reducing the risks of addictive behaviors. In J. S. Baer, G. A. Marlatt, & R. McMahon (Eds.), *Addictive behaviors across the lifespan* (pp. 243–273). Newbury Park, CA: Sage.

Mattack, R. P., & Jarvis, T. (1994a). Brief or minimal intervention for "alcoholics"? The evidence suggests otherwise. *Drug and Alcohol Review, 13,* 137–144.

Mattack, R. P., & Jarvis, T. (1994b). In-patient setting and long duration for the treatment of alcohol dependence? Out-patient care is as good. *Drug and Alcohol Review, 13,* 127–135.

McCaul, M. E., & Furst, J. (1994). Alcoholism treatment in the United States. *Alcohol Health & Research World, 18*, 253–260.

McCrady, B. S., & Delaney, S. I. (1995). Self-help groups. In R. K. Hester & W. R. Miller (Eds.), *Handbook of alcoholism treatment approaches: Effective alternatives* (2nd ed., pp. 160–175). Needham Heights, MA: Allyn & Bacon.

McCrady, B. S., & Langenbucher, J. W. (1996). Alcohol treatment and health care system reform. *Archives of General Psychiatry, 53*, 737–746.

McKay, J. R., & Maisto, S. A. (1993). An overview and critique of advances in the treatment of alcohol use disorders. *Drugs & Society, 8*, 1–29.

McKay, J. R., Alterman, A. I., Cacciola, J. S., Rutherford, M. J., O'Brien, C. P., & Koppenhaver, J. (1997). Group counseling vs. individualized relapse prevention aftercare following intensive outpatient for cocaine dependence: Initial results. *Journal of Consulting and Clinical Psychology, 65*, 778–788.

McLatchie, B. H., & Lomp, K. G. E. (1988). An experimental investigation of the influence of aftercare on alcoholic relapse. *British Journal of Addiction, 83*, 1045–1054.

Miller, W. R. (1989). Matching individuals with interventions. In R. K. Hester & W. R. Miller (Eds.), *Handbook of alcoholism treatment approaches: Effective alternatives* (pp. 261–271). New York: Pergamon.

Miller, W. R., & Rollnick, S. (Eds.). (1991). *Motivational interviewing: Preparing people to change addictive behavior.* New York: Guilford.

Montgomery, H. A., Miller, W. R., & Tonigan, J. S. (1995). Does Alcoholics Anonymous involvement predict treatment outcome? *Journal of Substance Abuse Treatment, 12*, 241–246.

Moos, R. H., Pettit, B., & Gruber, V. (1995). Longer episodes of community residential care reduce substance abuse patients' readmission rates. *Journal of Studies on Alcohol, 56*, 433–443.

Moos, R. H., King, M. J., & Patterson, M. A. (1996). Outcomes of residential treatment of substance abuse in hospital and community-based programs. *Psychiatric Services, 47*(1), 68–74.

Morgenstern, J., Kahler, C. W, Frey, R. M., & Labouvie, E. (1996). Modeling therapeutic response to 12-step treatment: Optimal responders, nonresponders, and partial responders. *Journal of Substance Abuse, 8*, 45–60.

Nowinski, J., Baker, S., & Carroll, K. (1992). *Twelve step facilitation therapy manual: A clinical research guide for therapists treating individuals with alcohol abuse and dependence* (Project MATCH Monograph Series, Vol. 1. DHHS Pub. No. (ADM) 92-1893). Washington, DC: National Institute on Alcohol Abuse and Alcoholism.

O'Brien, C. P., & McLellan, A. T. (1996). Myths about the treatment of addiction. *Lancet, 347*, 237–240.

O'Farrell, T. J., Chequette, K. A., Cutter, H. S. G., Brown, E. D., & McCourti, W. F. (1993). Behavioral marital therapy with and without additional couples relapse prevention sessions for alcoholics and their wives. *Journal of Studies on Alcohol, 54*, 652–666.

O'Farrell, T. J., Allen, J. P, & Litten, R. Z. (1995). Disulfiram (Antabuse) contracts in treatment of alcoholism. In L. S. Onken, J. D. Blaine, & J. J. Boren (Eds.), *Integrating behavioral therapies with medications in the treatment of drug dependence* (NIDA Research Monograph No. 150, pp. 65–91). Rockville, MD: National Institute on Drug Abuse.

O'Malley, S. S., Jaffe, A. J., Chang, G., Schottenfeld, R. S., Meyer, R. E., & Rounsaville, B. (1992). Naltrexone and coping skills therapy for alcohol dependence: A controlled study. *Archives of General Psychiatry, 49*, 881–887.

Ossip-Klein, D. J., & Rychtarik, R. G. (1993). Behavioral contracts between alcoholics and family members: Improving aftercare participation and maintaining sobriety after inpatient alcoholism treatment. In T. J. O'Farrell (Ed.), *Treating alcohol problems: Marital and family interventions* (pp. 281–304). New York: Guilford.

Ossip-Klein, D. J., Vanlandingham, W., Prue, D. M., & Rychtarik, R. G. (1984). Increasing attendance at alcohol aftercare using calendar prompts and home based contracting. *Addictive Behaviors, 9*, 85–89.

Patterson, D. G., McCourt, M. W., & Shiels, J. R. A. (1991). Community psychiatric nurse aftercare for alcoholics. *Irish Journal of Psychological Medicine, 8*, 4–14.

Patterson, D. G., MacPherson, J., & Brady, N. M. (1997). Community psychiatric nurse aftercare for alcoholics: A five-year follow-up. *Addiction, 92*, 459–468.

Peterson, K. A., Swindle, R. W., Phibbs, C. S., Recine, B., & Moos, R. H. (1994). Determinants of readmission following inpatient substance abuse treatment: A national study of VA programs. *Medical Care, 32*, 535–550.

Prochaska, J. O., & DiClemente, C. D. (1986). Toward a comprehensive model of change. In W. R. Miller & N. Heather (Eds.), *Treating addictive behaviors: Processes of change* (pp. 3–27). New York: Plenum.

Project MATCH Research Group. (1997). Matching alcoholism treatments to client heterogeneity: Project MATCH posttreatment drinking outcomes. *Journal of Studies on Alcohol, 58,* 7–29.

Ross, R., Booth, B. M., Russell, D. W., Laughlin, P. R., & Brown, K. (1995). Outcome of domiciliary care after inpatient alcoholism treatment in male veterans. *Journal of Substance Abuse Treatment, 12,* 319-32226.

Sass, H., Soyka, M., Mann, K., & Zieglgansberger, W. (1996). Relapse prevention by acamprosate: Results from a placebo-controlled study on alcohol dependence. *Archives of General Psychiatry, 53,* 673–680.

Saunders, B., & Allsop, S. (1991). Alcohol problems and relapse: Can the clinic combat the community? *Journal of Community and Applied Social Psychology, 1,* 213–221.

Scott, N. (1987). Eliminating aftercare. *Alcoholism & Addiction, July–August,* 5.

Shanks, D. A., Bell, R. W., Nessman, D., Arredondo, R., & Johnson, J. P. (1995). Alcoholic typology and the risk of relapse in an aftercare program. *Alcoholism Treatment Quarterly, 12,* 73–82.

Singh, J., & Howden-Chapman, P. (1987). Evaluation of effectiveness of aftercare in alcoholism. *New Zealand Medical Journal, 100,* 596–598.

Stout, R. L., Rubin, A., Zwick, W., & Zywiak, W. (1997). *Optimizing the cost-effectiveness of alcohol treatment: A rationale for extended case monitoring.* Unpublished manuscript, Center for Alcohol and Addiction Studies, Brown University, Providence, Rhode Island.

Timko, C., Moos, R. H., Finney, J. W., & Moos, B. S. (1994). Outcome of treatment for alcohol abuse and involvement in Alcoholics Anonymous among previously untreated problem drinkers. *Journal of Mental Health Administration, 21,* 145–160.

Timko, C., Finney, J. W., Moos, R. H., & Moos, B. S. (1995). Short-term treatment careers and outcomes of previously untreated alcoholics. *Journal of Studies on Alcohol, 56,* 597–610.

Tonigan, J. S., & Hiller-Strumhofel, S. (1994). Alcoholics Anonymous: Who benefits? *Alcohol Health & Research World, 18,* 308–310.

Tonigan, J. S., Toscova, R., & Miller, W. R. (1996). Meta-analysis of the literature on Alcoholics Anonymous: Sample and study characteristics moderate findings. *Journal of Studies on Alcohol, 57,* 65–72.

Verinis, J. S., & Taylor, J. (1994). Increasing alcoholic patients' aftercare attendance. *International Journal of the Addictions, 29,* 1487–1494.

Volpicelli, J. R., Alterman, A. I., Hayashida, M., & O'Brien, C. P. (1992). Naltrexone in the treatment of alcohol dependence. *Archives of General Psychiatry, 49,* 876–880.

Walker, R. D., Donovan, D. M., Kivlahan, D. R., & O'Leary, M. R. (1983). Length of stay, neuropsychological performance and aftercare: Influences on alcohol treatment outcome. *Journal of Consulting and Clinical Psychology, 51,* 900–911.

Watson, C. G., Hancock, M., Gearhart, L. P., Mendez, C. M., Malovrh, P., & Raden, M. (1997). A comparative outcome study of frequent, moderate, occasional, and nonattenders of Alcoholics Anonymous. *Journal of Clinical Psychology, 53,* 209–214.

Whitworth, A. B., Fischer, F., Lesch, O. M., Nimmerrichter, A., Oberauer, H., Platz, T., Potgieter, A., Walter, H., & Fleischhacker, W. W. (1996). Comparison of acamprosate and placebo in long-term treatment of alcohol dependence. *Lancet, 347,* 1438–1442.

Whorley, L. W. (1996a). Cognitive therapy techniques in continuing care planning with substance-dependent patients. *Addictive Behaviors, 21,* 223–231.

Whorley, L. W. (1996b). Exploring inpatient expectations of continuing care treatment: Focus groups with substance-dependent veterans. *Alcoholism Treatment Quarterly, 14,* 59–66.

Wolpe, P. R., Gorton, G., Serota, R., & Sanford, B. (1993). Predicting compliance of dual diagnosis inpatients with aftercare treatment. *Hospital and Community Psychiatry, 44,* 45–48.

24

Sustaining Change
Helping Those Who Are Still Using

KENNETH R. WEINGARDT AND G. ALAN MARLATT

Despite the development of effective new approaches to treating addictive behaviors, our commitment to using these approaches to help our clients remain abstinent, and our clients' determined efforts to maintain changes in their behavior, a significant proportion of clients who receive treatment return to use (McLellan *et al.*, 1996; Sobell, Cunningham, & Sobell, 1996). Whether their focal problem behavior is drinking, using drugs, gambling, overeating, or engaging in unsafe sexual activity, helping clients who are struggling with addictive behaviors inevitably involves dealing with some individuals who periodically revert to the old behavior patterns that have caused them so many problems in the past. In the pages that follow, we outline a conceptual framework that acknowledges this clinical reality, as well as a host of strategies and techniques intended to guide practicing clinicians in their efforts to reach out and help those who are still engaging in the behavior that they are trying to eliminate or control.

RETURNING TO USE IS PART OF THE THERAPEUTIC PROCESS

The first step toward helping those who are still using is the examination of one's own attitudes and beliefs as a clinician about what it means for someone who is in treatment to engage in the behavior that they are trying to eliminate or control. In the traditional view, an individual who, after a period of abstinence, indulges an urge or craving to reengage in addictive behavior is said to have "relapsed," and

KENNETH R. WEINGARDT AND G. ALAN MARLATT • Department of Psychology, University of Washington, Seattle, Washington 98195.

Treating Addictive Behaviors, 2nd ed., edited by Miller and Heather. Plenum Press, New York, 1998.

the problematic behavior is thus expected to increase in the direction of the pre-treatment baseline level. As Brownell, Marlatt, Lichtenstein, and Wilson (1986) put it, "A metaphor that describes traditional thought on relapse is of a person existing perilously close to the edge of a cliff. The slightest disruption can precipitate a fall from which there is no return. A person is always on the brink of relapse, ready to fall at any disturbance" (p. 766).

In order to help those who are still using, it is important to move beyond this overly simplistic concept of treatment outcome. The reality of clinical work in the addictive behaviors is that outcomes are much more complex. For example, Miller, Westerberg, Harris, and Tonigan (1996) conducted extensive analyses of prospective data on clients in alcohol treatment and found that almost every client in their sample drank at some time during the first year following treatment, and that most people drank heavily on at least one day. Does this suggest that treat-ment was a total failure for this sample? Decidedly not, for as Miller and col-leagues (1996) pointed out, despite their failure to remain completely abstinent, treated clients were found to drink much less often, for shorter periods of time, and to consume far less alcohol when they did drink. Furthermore, while some in-dividuals did return to a high-frequency, high-quantity pattern of consumption, many more clients could be classified at 1-year follow-up as mostly abstainers, regular moderate drinkers, or occasional heavy (binge) drinkers.

The term *relapse* has two common definitions. One is "a recurrence of symp-toms of a disease after a period of improvement" (Webster's, 1998). This definition refers to an outcome and is consistent with the traditional dichotomous view of re-lapse long embraced by those in the chemical dependency field—either the person is ill and has symptoms or is well and does not, either the person is abstinent or is using (Brownell *et. al.,* 1986). As discussed previously, this conceptualization of relapse has little bearing on clinical reality.

The word *relapse* has another definition that focuses on a process; namely "the act or an instance of backsliding, worsening, or subsiding" (Webster's, 1998). Marlatt and Gordon embraced this process-oriented definition in their develop-ment of the relapse prevention model (Marlatt & Gordon, 1980, 1985). By inter-preting the all-but-inevitable episodes of use that occur during treatment as slips, mistakes, or "lapses," Marlatt and Gordon's relapse prevention (RP) model implies that corrective action can be taken and that a return to pretreatment levels of use (i.e., "full-blown relapse") can be avoided. The definition of relapse as a process is also implicit in Prochaska and DiClemente's (1982, 1984) transtheoretical model of the stages of change (see Chapter 1, this volume). In the transtheoretical model, a client's return to use is interpreted as a stage of change during which he or she may acquire skills that could prove helpful in future change attempts.

Our challenge as clinicians is to follow the lead of these theoreticians and view the individual who uses during or soon after treatment not as a treatment failure, but rather as someone who is in the midst of a long and difficult learning process. There is considerable evidence to suggest that multiple attempts to change an addictive behavior occur before many people succeed (e.g., Schachter, 1982). As Miller (1996) puts it, "permanent perfection is not the ordinary course of human behavior change. . . . [T]he more typical course of recovery is a change in the flow of drinking, with generally decreased quantity and frequency, some waves, and eventual stabilization. It resembles the approximations of a developmental or learning curve" (p. S23). Our general approach to helping those who are still using is to accelerate the incremental learning that naturally occurs by helping individuals analyze their slips, acquire information about their weaknesses, and learn new ways to prevent lapses in the future (Brownell *et. al.*, 1986).

THE COGNITIVE-BEHAVIORAL MODEL OF RELAPSE

Since the techniques that we recommend for intervening with those who return to use following abstinence-oriented treatment are based on Marlatt and Gordon's (1985) cognitive-behavioral model of relapse prevention, a brief overview of this theoretical framework is in order. The foundation of what has become known as the relapse prevention (RP) approach is a causal chain of processes through which clients might move as they experience a return to pretreatment levels of use (i.e., a "full-blown relapse"). This linear model is depicted schematically in Figure 1, and is labeled "the process of relapse."

FROM ABSTINENCE TO USE: PROCESSES LEADING UP TO AN EPISODE OF USE

In the RP model, high-risk situations are thought to serve as precipitants of relapse. Three broad classes of high-risk situations have been identified as precursors to relapse: (1) negative emotional states (e.g., anger, frustration, anxiety, depression, boredom), (2) interpersonal conflict (e.g., situations involving conflict associated with any interpersonal relationship, particularly family or love relationships), and (3) social pressure (e.g., situations in which the person is responding to the influence

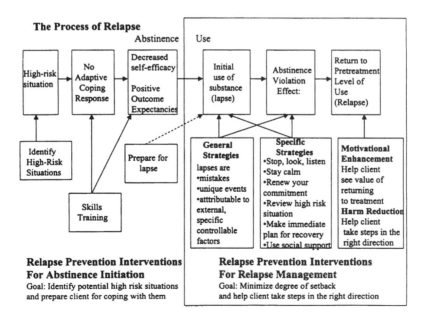

FIGURE 1. The process of relapse: Relapse prevention interventions for abstinence initiation and relapse management.

of another person or group of people who exert pressure on the person to engage in the proscribed behavior). In a sample of 311 initial relapse episodes in clients with a variety of problem behaviors (problem drinking, smoking, heroin addiction, compulsive gambling, and overeating) these three classes of high-risk situations were found to be associated with almost 75% of all relapses reported (Cummings, Gordon, & Marlatt, 1980; Marlatt & Gordon, 1980).

Although recent research has called into question the validity and reliability of the taxonomy of relapse precipitants originally outlined by Marlatt and Gordon (1980, 1985) (see Lowman, Allen, Stout, & Relapse Research Group, 1996), the RP model maintains that specific, dynamic intra- and interpersonal factors may predispose an individual client to return to use at a particular time (Marlatt, 1996b). The RP model further posits that high-risk situations, however identified or defined, will serve as precipitants of relapse only if the individual lacks an adaptive response for coping with that situation (see Figure 1). Individuals who encounter high-risk situations without an adaptive coping response are then thought to experience decreased confidence in their ability to cope with an impending high-risk situation (i.e., decreased *self-efficacy,* cf. Bandura, 1977). *Positive outcome expectancies* for the effects of engaging in the addictive behavior (e.g., "using will help me relax") are then thought to interact with this lowered self-efficacy to increase the probability of a lapse.

To summarize, the RP model suggests that the processes leading up to a lapse in a hypothetical case example might proceed as follows: a client who is anxious about an upcoming performance review (high-risk situation), but does not have any means of decreasing her subjective psychological distress other than using (no adaptive coping response) may lack confidence in her ability to deal with her anxiety (low self-efficacy) and think that using will be an effective way of coping with it (positive outcome expectancies). Given this scenario, it would certainly not be surprising for this client to use her substance of choice.

FROM LAPSE TO RELAPSE: PROCESSES THAT MIGHT LEAD FROM AN
INITIAL EPISODE OF USE TO A RETURN TO PRETREATMENT LEVELS OF USE

One of the most important features of the RP model is the acknowledgment that a discrete episode of use (i.e., an initial lapse) need not necessarily lead to an increase in use in the direction of pretreatment baseline levels (i.e., a "full-blown relapse"). Whether a lapse is followed by a total relapse is thought to depend primarily on the person's attributions about the cause of the lapse and how they cope with the cognitive and affective reactions that they have to it.

A lapse is thought to be more likely to lead to a full relapse if a client attributes the lapse to a cause that is internal, stable, and global, such as personal weakness or failure (e.g., "I'm a failure, I can't do this"). In such cases, clients are more likely to blame themselves for the lapse, feel guilty about it, and experience decreased self-efficacy. A lapse is also thought to be more likely to lead to a full relapse if the client has a strong self-image as a recovering addict who has made a long and effortful commitment to abstinence. In this case, a slip is thought to result in an uncomfortable state of internal inconsistency between that self-image (e.g., "I don't use anymore") and the occurrence of a behavior that directly contradicts that self-image (e.g., using). This state of inconsistency, termed *cognitive dissonance* (cf. Festinger, 1964) is typically experienced as guilt, shame, or general upset.

Taken together, the two cognitive-affective components (personal attribution and cognitive dissonance) comprise the *abstinence violation effect* (AVE; Marlatt & Gordon, 1985). Returning to our case example, the AVE dictates that our client's lapse is most likely to lead to continued use if (1) she interprets the slip as meaning that she is "a failure" or that she lacks willpower (personal attribution) and (2) after a long period of abstinence, she thinks of herself as a recovering addict for whom abstinence is the only solution, and thus experiences significant guilt and conflict over her slip (cognitive dissonance).

HELPING THOSE WHO RETURN TO USE: INTERVENTIONS FOR RELAPSE MANAGEMENT

RP interventions fall into two main categories: interventions that take place before a slip has occurred, and relapse management interventions that take place after a lapse and are designed to help prevent an initial use of a substance from escalating into a full-blown relapse (see Figure 1). A full discussion of RP interventions for the initiation and maintenance of abstinence is beyond the scope of this chapter. The interested reader is referred to Marlatt and Gordon (1985), Annis & Davis (1989) and to a recent manualized version of these interventions (Daley & Marlatt, 1997).

RELAPSE MANAGEMENT: GENERAL STRATEGIES

Once a client experiences a lapse, relapse management interventions can be employed in an effort to minimize the degree of harm associated with substance use (Marlatt & Tapert, 1993). In general terms, these interventions are intended to alter the individual's maladaptive attributions and attitudes about their recent lapse. Recall that in the RP model, cognitive errors and maladaptive assumptions associated with the AVE are thought to increase the probability that an initial slip will escalate into a return to pretreatment levels of use. Relapse management interventions specifically target and attempt to modify these problematic cognitions, thereby helping the individual who has experienced a lapse respond constructively to it.

Drawing on techniques that were developed to modify the cognitive errors and maladaptive assumptions associated with depression (e.g., Beck, Rush, Shaw, & Emery, 1979), Marlatt & Gordon (1985) formulated a number of general strategies designed to counter faulty assumptions and cognitive errors associated with initial lapses. These strategies attempt to help clients see their recent lapse as a mistake rather than a failure, that their lapse was a unique event that can be attributed to things other than their own weakness, and that all it takes to regain abstinence is to refrain from using next time.

A Lapse Is Similar to a Mistake or Error in the Learning Process

By helping the client appreciate that changing addictive behavior is a learning process, lapses can be reframed as valuable opportunities for corrective learning rather than indicators of total failure. Just as the novice bicycle rider can learn from a painful slip (e.g., by learning to apply the brakes more gently when coming to a stop, not to take the next curve so fast), so the ex-user learns from a slip what to do the next time (e.g., avoid the high-risk situation, use an adaptive coping mechanism). From this perspective, clients can be taught that slips are a normal and expected part of changing their addictive behavior, not a symptom of psychopathology or a failure of free will.

A Lapse Is a Specific, Unique Event in Time and Space

Clients often interpret a lapse as a sign or symptom of total relapse; the occurrence of a single isolated event is overgeneralized as a sign of total failure, thereby increasing the probability of recurrence over time and across situations. A general strategy that can be used to counter this cognitive error of overgeneralization is to help clients to view their lapse as a unique, independent event occurring at a specific time and place. One means of helping clients acquire this perspective is teaching them to focus on the here and now when a lapse occurs. By focusing on the specific circumstances surrounding the lapse, clients are discouraged from bringing in "excess baggage" from the past (e.g., "Last time I slipped I ended up using for two months"), or projecting the lapse into the future ("Now that I've used, there's no way to stop; I might just as well keep on using").

The Lapse Can Be Reattributed to External, Specific, and Controllable Factors

Recall that the magnitude of the AVE (and thus the likelihood that a lapse will escalate) is hypothesized to increase if the individual attributes the cause of the lapse to internal, stable, and global factors such as lack of willpower or the influence of powerful physical factors (physical dependency or disease). Such attributions result in increased feelings of guilt about the lapse and perceptions of loss of control. Relapse management focuses on helping clients to reattribute the cause of their lapse to external, specific, and controllable factors. Careful examination of the lapse episode with a client can be useful in helping them to identify such external, controllable factors as the difficulty level of the high-risk situation that they encountered, the adequacy of the coping response (if any) that they employed, and the transitory motivational deficits (e.g., excessive fatigue or stress) that might have played a role in their lapse.

Abstinence or Control Is Always Only a Moment Away

"Just as a cloud that momentarily passes before the sun on an otherwise clear sunny day does not mean that the weather has taken an inevitable turn for the worse, so a transitory lapse does not necessarily mean that the previous state of abstinence is lost forever. It can be regained at a moment's notice" (Marlatt & Gordon, 1985, p. 255). Many individuals who are struggling with addictive behaviors believe that once they violate the absolute rule of abstinence, even by a single discrete slip, they have lost something that they cannot regain. They may believe that a single use episode will trigger the disease process within them, and that their return to pretreatment levels of use is inevitable because the resulting biological symptoms (e.g., craving, subclinical withdrawal state) cannot be voluntarily controlled. The general strategy that is used to restructure these maladaptive cognitions is to impress upon the client that abstinence or control is always only a moment away: If the individual is not engaging in the problematic addictive behavior at this moment, a state of abstinence exists. The only requirement for abstinence is a commitment to refrain from use the next time around.

RELAPSE MANAGEMENT: SPECIFIC STRATEGIES

In this section, we describe a number of different strategies that may be used to help clients take advantage of the learning opportunity that a recent lapse presents, while addressing the very real danger that their use might escalate following the initial lapse. These strategies are listed in order of temporal priority, with the most important steps to take in the event of a lapse listed first. Marlatt and Gordon (1985) have recommended that clients be provided with a pocket-sized reminder card summarizing this information for use in moments of crisis.

Stop, Look, and Listen

Clients can be taught that a lapse is a warning signal indicating that they are in danger, similar to the way that a warning light on a car's dashboard indicates mechanical trouble. Just as the driver who sees the red light come on pulls over to the side of the road to assess the situation, so should the client who has just experienced a lapse stop the ongoing flow of events by getting out of the high-risk situation, and look and listen to what is happening. The client should be encouraged to retire to a quiet, safe place and review these strategies as they are summarized on their reminder card.

Stay Calm

Normal reactions to a lapse include feelings of guilt and self-blame. It is important for clients to understand that unless they allow themselves to give in to these feelings, this reaction is essentially harmless. Clients can be instructed to calmly allow the expected AVE reaction to arise and pass away, allowing it to occur without evaluating it or themselves negatively. It may be helpful at this critical time for clients to remind themselves that their slip was a single independent mistake that represents an opportunity for learning and is not a sign of total failure.

Renew Your Commitment

Due to the AVE, clients may feel hopeless after a lapse, in effect saying to themselves, "What's the use—I've blown it already." This normal reaction can be remedied by encouraging clients to (1) think back over the reasons they decided to change their behavior in the first place, (2) think of the long-range benefits that they stand to gain from the changes that they are trying to make, and ask themselves whether they are worth giving up just because they had a slip, (3) appreciate how far they have already come in changing their addictive behavior, and (4) remind themselves that they are attempting to change their habits as a way of caring for themselves, their health, and their life.

Review the Situation Leading Up to the Lapse

In order to learn from their mistake, it may be helpful for clients to identify and understand the high-risk situation that prompted this particular lapse. Encouraging clients to ask themselves the following questions will help them review the situation leading up to the lapse: What events led up to the slip? Were there any early warning signals that preceded the lapse? What was the setting? The time of day? Were others present? What mood was I in? Did I make any attempt to cope with the situation before the lapse occurred? If not, why not? Was my motivation weakened because of fatigue, the effects of other drugs, social pressure from others, or other transitory factors? What could I do next time to cope more effectively?

Make an Immediate Plan for Recovery

Immediately after a slip, time is of the essence. The more quickly clients can turn their renewed commitment into an immediate plan of action, the more likely it is that their lapse will not lead to further use. Components of an immediate action plan that might be suggested to clients include (1) getting rid of all drugs or other stimuli associated with the addictive behavior, (2) removing yourself from the high-risk situation physically, or if that is impossible, leaving psychologically—closing your eyes, meditating for a few moments, or taking a few breaths to clear your mind, and (3) planning a substitute activity that will also meet your needs at the moment. For example, it may be helpful to engage in robust physical exercise or other overt activity in order to drain off excess energy or negative feelings.

Use Your Support Network

After a lapse, it is often helpful to remind clients about the importance of asking family, friends, or others in treatment for their help and support. Social support can come in the form of offering encouragement, providing alternative activities, suggesting alternative ways of coping, or often just "being there" for someone who is struggling with an addictive behavior. If a client is without a support network, the clinician can suggest ways that he or she might go about developing one (e.g., calling other members of one's treatment group, finding an AA sponsor). In the meantime, it is suggested that clients be provided with the phone numbers of available community resources such as treatment and crisis centers that they can call in time of need.

MOTIVATIONAL ISSUES IN RELAPSE MANAGEMENT

While RP is often characterized as an approach based exclusively on skills training, this model also recognizes the importance of motivation as a prerequisite for initiating and maintaining behavior change. The specific strategies outlined earlier that are intended to renew commitment to change in the face of a recent slip are a good example of how the RP model acknowledges the importance of building motivation. Another technique that Marlatt proposes as a means of helping clients build their motivation to maintain changes in their behavior is described as a decisional balance exercise (Marlatt & Gordon, 1985; cf. Janis & Mann, 1977). Using this exercise, a therapist may help a client who has recently experienced a slip examine the positive and negative consequences of a return to pretreatment levels of use in both the long and short term. In this way, the decisional balance exercise builds motivation by reminding clients of the reasons they decided to stop using in the first place, and of the consequences they may suffer if they choose to continue using.

Many other techniques designed to help build clients' motivation to initiate and maintain changes in their behavior have been elaborated in the motivational interviewing (MI) approach to treating addictive behaviors (see Miller & Rollnick, 1991; see Chapter 9, this volume). These strategies and techniques may be successfully used in conjunction with the relapse management interventions described earlier. Stylistic elements of the MI approach, including empathic listening and an avoidance of judgmental, confrontational interactions between client and therapist are very much in line with the attitudes of acceptance and unconditional positive regard that are crucial in relapse management interventions. Furthermore, specific MI techniques designed to support self-efficacy, minimize resistance, explore cognitive discrepancies, and avoid argumentation can all nicely complement the relapse management strategies outlined above.

The MI approach may prove particularly useful in dealing with those clients for whom efforts at relapse management have been unsuccessful. For clients who have returned to pretreatment levels of use, the task at hand is to help them cycle through the stages of change once again, moving from "relapse" through precontemplation, contemplation, and returning to action. The MI approach was designed explicitly to help guide the client from precontemplation to action. With adequate client motivation to work toward abstinence once again in place, RP interventions can be used to accelerate the incremental learning that occurs during the action stage, thereby preventing relapse and thus another cycle through the stages of change.

Another motivational issue in relapse prevention and management concerns the quality of clients' overall abstinent lifestyles. What do individual clients do with free time when they have stopped using? Are they able to identify other positive reinforcers that they might enjoy and pursue them? The community reinforcement approach (CRA; Meyers & Smith, 1995; see Chapter 11, this volume) suggests that clients are motivated to change their addictive behavior to the extent that they are reinforced for doing so. For example, the client who finds herself able to play tennis again, get her driver's license back, and have a more satisfying relationship with her significant other is less likely to return to use. If a client has returned to use, the CRA suggests that it would be a good idea to help the client (re)identify positive reinforcers as a means of building motivation for continued abstinence. Along similar lines, Marlatt and Gordon (1985) point out that a comprehensive RP self-management program should attempt to improve the client's overall lifestyle balance. They outline a number of intervention strategies that may help clients develop more balanced daily lifestyles, including the adoption of "positive addictions" such as exercise and meditation.

EFFICACY OF INTERVENTIONS FOR RELAPSE MANAGEMENT

A consistent picture has yet to emerge regarding the prophylactic value of relapse prevention interventions for abstinence initiation (see Carroll, 1996), but considerable evidence suggests that aftercare interventions sharing common goals and conceptual underpinnings with the interventions outlined in this chapter may be particularly effective at reducing the intensity of relapse episodes when they do occur (see Ito & Donovan, 1986, and Chapter 23, this volume, for a review). For example, in their evaluation of the efficacy of two aftercare treatments for cocaine dependent clients (an RP condition and a "treatment as usual" control condition), McKay and colleagues (1997) found that clients in the RP condition who used cocaine during the first 3 months of the study relapsed significantly less often than clients in the control condition who used cocaine during this same period. In this study, relapse was operationally defined as meeting the criteria of experiencing 15% or more days of cocaine use. In sum, Donovan (Chapter 23, this volume) has suggested on the basis of his exhaustive literature review that continuing care has as one of its most important functions the early identification and intervention in the relapse process (i.e., relapse management interventions), helping to keep an initial use of a substance from developing into a full-blown relapse.

There is evidence to suggest that RP interventions undertaken during treatment can also have the important effect of minimizing the degree of setback experienced by clients who return to use. For example, in a clinical trial evaluating naltrexone (an opioid antagonist) and two manual-guided psychotherapies (RP or a supportive therapy without coping skills training), O'Malley and colleagues (1992) found that of those clients who initiated drinking, clients who received naltrexone and coping skills therapy were the least likely to return to pretreatment levels of use. Earlier studies found this same pattern of results in RP interventions for cigarette smokers (Davis & Glaros, 1986; Supnick & Colletti, 1984); relapse prevention interventions may reduce the intensity of relapse episodes if they do occur.

In a broad sense, interventions for relapse management can be thought of as attempts to minimize the harm associated with a return to substance use after a period of abstinence (Marlatt, 1996a; Marlatt & Tapert, 1993). When a client experiences a lapse, the empirical work outlined earlier suggests that RP interventions, particularly those targeted toward relapse management, can be an effective means of reducing or minimizing the harm that might occur as a result of that lapse. We now turn our attention to a host of other harm-reduction strategies that can be used with clients who are either unwilling or unable to maintain abstinence after treatment.

HARM REDUCTION

Some individuals who return to use after a period of abstinence are no longer interested in abstinence-oriented treatment. Other individuals who are still using have not recently been engaged in treatment and have yet to commit to any treatment goals. These individuals have decided to continue using, and our entire battery of motivational techniques cannot persuade them to consider doing otherwise. From the traditional perspective, these clients are often thought to be "relapsed," or "beyond help." From our perspective, however, even such protracted and extreme deviations from abstinence do not necessarily mean that treatment was a failure.

While there is general agreement that abstinence from all drug use is the ideal means of reducing the harm that can result from engaging in addictive behavior, "harm reduction" approaches also embrace alternative goals that can "step down" the harmful consequences of continued addictive behavior. We believe that familiarity with the principles and practices of harm reduction is important in helping clients maintain the gains that they have achieved during treatment (as is the primary focus of this chapter) and helping those who are still using and are currently unwilling or unable to enter conventional treatment programs. In the section that follows, we briefly outline the basic principles, assumptions, and values of the harm reduction model and the general classes of intervention that can be employed in an effort to reduce the harm associated with ongoing addictive behavior. The interested reader is referred to O'Hare, Newcombe, Matthews, Buning, and Drucker (1992), and Heather, Wodak, Nadelmann, and O'Hare (1994) for detailed discussions of the harm-reduction approach.

BASIC PRINCIPLES

The basic principles of harm reduction are straightforward. (1) Harm reduction views drug use and addiction as a public health problem rather than a criminal justice problem. Thus, harm reduction shifts the focus away from drug use itself and its moral or legal permissibility, to the consequences or effects of addictive behavior that can be evaluated primarily in terms of whether they are harmful or helpful to the drug user and to the larger society. (2) Harm reduction recognizes absolute abstinence as an ideal outcome but accepts alternatives to reduce harm. Abstinence is included as an ideal endpoint along a continuum ranging from excessively harmful to less harmful consequences along which individuals are encouraged to gradually take "one step at a time" to reduce the harmful consequences of their behavior. (3) Harm reduction has emerged primarily as a "bottom-up" approach based on addict advocacy, rather than "top-down" public policy. (4) Harm reduction promotes low-threshold access to services. Rather than setting abstinence as a high-threshold precondition for receiving treatment or assistance, low-threshold programs make it easier to "get on board" by reaching out and cooperating with the population in need when developing new programs and services, reducing stigma associated with getting help for these kind of problems, and providing integrated, comprehensive services that embrace and consolidate a variety of high-risk behaviors including, but not limited to, substance abuse. (5) Harm reduction is a compassionate, pragmatic approach that does not denigrate people who engage in high-risk addictive behaviors.

INTERVENTION STRATEGIES

There are three general classes of intervention that can be employed in an effort to reduce the harm associated with ongoing addictive behavior: (1) changing the route of administration of a substance, (2) providing a safer alternative substance or drug to replace the more harmful substance, and (3) reducing the frequency and/or intensity (quantity, dose level) of the target behavior. This third general class of intervention—reducing quantity and frequency of use—is an integral part of the relapse management approach described in this chapter. Applied to relapse management, RP represents a tertiary prevention approach to harm reduction designed to reduce the frequency and intensity of relapse episodes, to keep the client involved in the treatment process, and to motivate renewed efforts toward behavior change (Marlatt, 1996a). It is important to note that reducing the quantity and/or frequency of a harmful addictive behavior is also a viable harm-reduction intervention for individuals who are still using and have not yet received any abstinence-oriented treatment. From a pragmatic perspective, it is clear that helping a client restrict drug use to weekends, rather than using every day, can be a valuable step in the direction of reducing the drug-related harm that client might experience.

The other two classes of harm-reduction interventions just outlined (changing route of administration and substance substitution) are more controversial means of helping those who are still using. Traditionally minded members of the American treatment community may interpret such efforts as "enabling" the addict to continue using thereby helping them to avoid "hitting bottom," and consequently keeping them out of abstinence-oriented treatment. In contrast, it can be argued that these approaches not only reduce the risks associated with ongoing addictive behavior, but may also be the most effective means of helping clients who have returned to pretreatment levels of use take positive steps in the direction of decreasing or eliminating their use.

A basic objective of harm-reduction interventions is to keep clients healthy and alive until such time as they are ready to initiate or renew a commitment to abstinence. After years of heated debate, a fair degree of consensus has emerged that needle-exchange programs constitute an effective means of reducing the transmission of the HIV virus in the intravenous drug-using community (DesJarlais, Friedman, & Ward, 1993; Lurie & Reingold, 1993). If clients have returned to pretreatment levels of injection drug use and are currently uninterested in further treatment, providing them with a referral to a needle-exchange program may well help keep them from contracting HIV and other major infections until such time as they are motivated to do further work toward maintaining abstinence. Along similar lines, the harm-reduction approach suggests that providing heroin addicts who are unable to achieve or maintain abstinence with a referral to a methadone clinic may well reduce the harm resulting from their drug use. Methadone is less harmful in terms of decreased risk of AIDS for the drug user (methadone is taken orally rather than by injection) and decreased crime costs for the community (addicts on methadone are less likely to engage in crime to pay for the cost of illegal opiates).

In keeping with the harm-reduction principles just outlined, clients who have returned to use and currently lack motivation to engage in further abstinence-oriented treatment may be best served by low-threshold programs that do not require a commitment to abstinence or drug testing as a prerequisite for admission. The only requirement of the addict in low-threshold programs such as needle exchanges, street outreach services, and open-door medical clinics is to show up and, it is hoped, to begin taking steps in the direction of reducing harm. An important benefit of these low-threshold programs is that they facilitate continued contact between the population of individuals who are still using, and the social and treatment resources that are available to help them. Maintaining helpful and respectful contact with those who are still using can then be used to build bridges that may help lead these persons to return to or engage in abstinence-oriented treatment in the future (Marlatt & Tapert, 1993).

INTERNATIONAL EFFORTS

Researchers and clinicians involved in the treatment of substance abuse in the United States have only recently given serious consideration to the principles and practice of harm reduction, but the harm-reduction movement has been flourishing in the Netherlands, the United Kingdom, Canada, and Australia for the past decade. This international movement arose in response to the growing AIDS crisis in the 1980s (cf. DesJarlais & Friedman, 1993), although earlier origins of this approach to drug problems can be traced back to the nineteenth century (Berridge, 1993). The success of innovative public health approaches introduced in Europe (particularly in the Netherlands and the United Kingdom) and in Australia, such as syringe-exchange programs and the medical prescription of addictive substances have further spurred the development of the harm-reduction (known in the United Kingdom as the harm-minimization) model.

Although a comprehensive review of the international literature on the effectiveness of harm-reduction approaches is certainly beyond the scope of this chapter, available data suggest that these creative and pragmatic alternative strategies for helping those who are still using have met with considerable success. In the Netherlands, the evidence in support of needle exchange and related harm-reduction programs in reducing HIV infection is strong (Buning, Brussel, & Santen, 1992), low-threshold programs have greatly augmented the range of treatment services available to the Dutch population of drug users, and the Dutch claim to be in contact with the majority of the addict population (Engelsman, 1989). In the United Kingdom, the Merseyside Health Authority has offered addicts a wide range of services including needle exchange and outreach education, prescription of drugs such as heroin and cocaine, counseling, employment, and housing services. Health and crime statistics for the Mersey region support the effectiveness of these services. As of 1991 the region had the second lowest rate of HIV-positive intravenous drug users of all 14 English regions, and from 1990 to 1991 the Merseyside police were the only force in the United Kingdom to register a decrease in crime rates (Riley, 1994). Furthermore, the approach to reformulating drug education and prevention programs in terms of harm reduction has been recommended by the Canadian Centre on Substance Abuse (Riley, 1994), and has been formally introduced as part of Australia's national drug policy (Crofts & Herkt, 1995).

CONCLUSION

Helping those who are still using represents a unique set of challenges for the clinician. Primary among these challenges is adopting the perspective that a return to use, either during or after treatment, is not an indicator of treatment failure, but rather a valuable opportunity for corrective learning. Familiarity with the relapse management strategies outlined in this chapter will allow the clinician to capitalize on these opportunities as clients present them. Furthermore, use of these strategies, in conjunction with the motivational principles outlined elsewhere in this volume, will help clients maintain the positive changes that they have made in treatment, and thus avoid the AVE and a return to precontemplation. Finally, it is our hope that the alternative harm-reduction approaches outlined in this chapter will help underline the fact that we as clinicians can continue to be of help to our clients even if they continue to use.

REFERENCES

Annis, H. M. (1982). *Inventory of Drinking Situations.* Toronto, Ontario, Canada: Addiction Research Foundation.

Annis, H. M., & Davis, C. S. (1989). Relapse prevention. In R. K. Hester & W. R. Miller (Eds.), *Handbook of alcoholism treatment approaches: Effective alternatives* (pp. 170–182). New York: Pergamon.

Annis, H. M., & Martin, G. (1985) *Inventory of Drug-Taking Situations.* Toronto, Ontario, Canada: Addiction Research Foundation.

Bandura, A. (1977) Self-efficacy: Toward a unifying theory of behavioral change. *Psychological Review, 84,* 191–215.

Beck, A. T., Rush, A. J., Shaw, B. F., & Emery, G. (1979). *Cognitive therapy of depression.* New York: Guilford.

Berridge, V. (1993). Harm minimisation and public health: An historical perspective. In N. Heather, A. Wodak, E. Nadelmann, & P. O'Hare (Eds.), *Psychoactive drugs and harm reduction: From faith to science* (pp. 55–64). London: Whurr.

Brownell, K. D., Marlatt, G. A., Lichtenstein, E., & Wilson, G. T. (1986). Understanding and preventing relapse. *American Psychologist, 41*(7), 765–782.

Buning, E. C., Brussel, G. V., & Santen, G. V. (1992). The impact of harm reduction drug policy on AIDS prevention in Amsterdam. In P. A. O'Hare, R. Newcombe, A. Matthews, E. C. Buning, & E. Drucker (Eds.), *The reduction of drug-related harm* (pp. 30–38). London: Routledge.

Carroll, K. M. (1996). Relapse prevention as psychosocial treatment: A review of controlled clinical trials. *Experimental and Clinical Psychopharmacology, 4*(1), 46–54.

Crofts, N., & Herkt, D. (1995). A history of peer-based drug-user groups in Australia. *Journal of Drug Issues, 25,* 599–616.

Cummings, C., Gordon, J. R., & Marlatt, G. A. (1980). Relapse: Prevention and prediction. In W. R. Miller (Ed.), *The addictive disorders: Treatment of alcoholism, drug abuse, smoking and obesity* (pp. 291–322). New York: Pergamon.

Daley, D. C., & Marlatt, G. A. (1997). *Managing your drug or alcohol problem: Therapist guide.* San Antonio, TX: The Psychological Corporation.

Davis, J. R., & Glaros, A. G. (1986). Relapse prevention and smoking cessation. *Addictive Behaviors, 11,* 105–114.

DesJarlais, D. C., & Friedman, S. R. (1993). AIDS, injecting drug use and harm reduction. In N. Heather, A. Wodak, E. Nadelmann, & P. O'Hare (Eds.), *Psychoactive drugs and harm reduction: From faith to science* (pp. 297–309). London: Whurr.

DesJarlais, D. C., Friedman, S. R., & Ward, T. P. (1993). Harm reduction: A public health response to the AIDS epidemic among injecting drug users. *Annual Review of Public Health, 14,* 413–450.

Engelsman, E. L. (1989). Dutch policy on the management of drug-related problems. *British Journal of Addiction, 84,* 211–218.

Festinger, L. (1964). *Conflict, decision and dissonance.* Palo Alto, CA: Stanford University Press.

Heather, N., Wodak, A., Nadelmann, E., & O'Hare, P. (1994). *Psychoactive drugs and harm reduction: From faith to science.* London: Whurr.

Ito, J. R., & Donovan, D.M. (1986). Aftercare in alcoholism treatment: A review. In W. R. Miller & N. Heather (Eds.), *Treating addictive behaviors: Processes of change* (pp. 435–456). New York: Plenum.

Janis, I. L., & Mann, L. (1977). *Decision making.* New York: Free Press.

Lowman, C. Allen, J., Stout, R. L., & Relapse Research Group. (1996). Replication and extension of Marlatt's taxonomy of relapse precipitants: Overview of procedures and results. *Addiction, 91* (Suppl.), S51–S71.

Lurie, P., & Reingold, A. L. (Eds.). (1993). *The public health impact of needle exchange programs in the United States and abroad.* Berkeley, CA School of Public Health, UC Berkeley, and San Francisco: Institute of Health Policy Studies, UC San Francisco.

Marlatt, G. A. (1996a). Harm reduction: Come as you are. *Addictive Behaviors, 21*(6), 779–788.

Marlatt, G. A. (1996b) Lest taxonomy become taxidermy: A comment on the relapse replication and extension project. *Addiction, 91* (Suppl.), S147–S153.

Marlatt, G. A., & Gordon, J. R. (1980). Determinants of relapse: Implications for the maintenance of behavior change. In P. O. Davidson & S. M. Davidson (Eds.), *Behavioral medicine: changing health life-styles* (pp. 410–452). Elmsford, NY: Pergamon.

Marlatt, G. A., & Gordon, J. R. (Eds.). (1985). *Relapse prevention: Maintenance strategies in the treatment of addictive behaviors.* New York: Guilford.

Marlatt, G. A., & Tapert, S. F. (1993). Harm reduction: Reducing the risks of addictive behaviors. In J. S. Baer, G. A. Marlatt, & R. J. McMahon (Eds.), *Addictive behaviors across the lifespan* (pp. 243–273). Newbury Park, CA: Sage.

McKay, J. R., Alterman, A. I., Cacciola, J. S., Rutherford, M. J., O'Brien, C. P., & Koppenhaver, J. (1997). A comparison of group counseling vs. individualized relapse prevention aftercare following intensive outpatient for cocaine dependence: Initial results. *Journal of Consulting and Clinical Psychology.*

McLellan, A. T., Woody, G. E., Metzger, D. S., McKay, J., Durell, J., Alterman, A. I., & O'Brien, C. P. (1996). Evaluating the effectiveness of addiction treatments: Reasonable expectations, appropriate comparisons. *Milbank Quarterly, 74*(1), 51–85.

Meyers, R. J., & Smith, J. E. (1995). *Clinical guide to alcohol treatment: The community reinforcement approach.* New York: Guilford.

Miller, W. R. (1996) What is a relapse? Fifty ways to leave the wagon. *Addiction, 91* (Suppl.), S15–S27.

Miller, W. R., & Rollnick, S. (1991). *Motivational interviewing: Preparing people to change addictive behavior.* New York: Guilford.

Miller, W. R., Westerberg, V. S., Harris, R. J., & Tonigan, J. S. (1996). What predicts relapse? Prospective testing of antecedent models. *Addiction, 91* (Suppl.), S155–S172.

O'Hare, P. A., Newcombe, R., Matthews, A., Buning, E. C., & Drucker, E. (Eds.). (1992). *The reduction of drug-related harm.* London: Routledge.

O'Malley, S. S., Jaffe, A. J., Chang, G., Schottenfeld, R. S., Meyer, R. E., & Rounsaville, B. J. (1992). Naltrexone and coping skills therapy for alcohol dependence: A controlled study. *Archives of General Psychiatry, 49,* 881–887.

Prochaska, J. O., & DiClemente, C. C. (1982). Transtheoretical therapy: Toward a more integrated model of change. *Psychotherapy: Theory, Research and Practice, 19,* 276–288.

Prochaska, J. O., & DiClemente, C. C. (1984). *The transtheoretical approach: Crossing traditional boundaries of therapy.* Homewood, IL: Dow Jones/Irwin.

Riley, D. (1994). *The Harm Reduction Model: Pragmatic approaches to drug use from the area between intolerance and neglect.* Ottawa, Ontario: Canadian Centre on Substance Abuse.

Schacter, S. (1982). Recidivism and self-cure of smoking and obesity. *American Psychologist, 37,* 436–444.

Sobell, L. C., Cunningham, J. A., & Sobell, M. (1996). Recovery from alcohol problems with and without treatment: Prevalence in two population surveys. *American Journal of Public Health, 86*(7), 966–972.

Supnick, J. A., & Colletti, G. (1984). Relapse coping and problem solving training following treatment for smoking. *Addictive Behaviors, 9,* 401–404.

Webster's. (1998). Meriam-Webster online: wwwebster's dictionary, World Wide Web edition of Merriam-Webster's collegiate dictionary, 10th ed. http//www.m-w.com/dictionary.htm

Index